# CARDIAC
## ARRHYTHMIAS

# CARDIAC ARRHYTHMIAS

## AN INTEGRATED APPROACH FOR THE CLINICIAN

### Eric N. Prystowsky, M.D.

*Director of Clinical Electrophysiology Laboratory*
*St. Vincent Hospital, Indianapolis, Indiana*
*Consulting Professor of Medicine*
*Duke University Medical Center, Durham, North Carolina*

### George J. Klein, M.D.

*Director of Arrhythmia Service*
*University Hospital*
*Professor of Medicine*
*University of Western Ontario*
*London, Ontario, Canada*

### McGraw-Hill, Inc.
#### HEALTH PROFESSIONS DIVISION

*New York  St. Louis  San Francisco  Auckland  Bogotá*
*Caracas  Lisbon  London  Madrid  Mexico City  Milan*
*Montreal  New Delhi  Paris  San Juan  Singapore*
*Sydney  Tokyo  Toronto*

## CARDIAC ARRHYTHMIAS
An Integrated Approach for the Clinician

2 3 4 5 6 7 8 9 0   KGPKGP   9 8 7 6 5

ISBN 0-07-050984-0

*This book was set in Garamond by Monotype Composition Company, Inc.*
*The editors were J. Dereck Jeffers and Muza Navrozov;*
*the production supervisor was Clare B. Stanley;*
*the cover was designed by Marsha Cohen/Paralellogram;*
*the index was prepared by Elizabeth Babcock-Atkinson.*
*Arcata Graphics/Kingsport was printer and binder.*

Library of Congress Cataloging-in-Publication Data

Prystowsky, Eric N.
    Cardiac arrhythmias : an integrated approach for the clinician /
  Eric N. Prystowsky, George J. Klein.
        p.      cm.
    Includes bibliographical reference and index.
    ISBN 0-07-050984-0 :
    1. Arrhythmia.    I. Klein, George J., M.D.    II. Title.
    [DNLM:   1. Arrhythmia—diagnosis.   2. Arrhythmia—therapy.
  WG 330 P973c 1994]
  RC685.A65P79   1994
  616.1′28—dc20
  DNLM/DLC
  for Library of Congress                                    93-30278
                                                                CIP

# Contents

# Part IV    *Methods and Therapy*

# Color Plates

# *Preface*

There have been major advances in the care of patients with cardiac arrhythmias since we began our training in clinical electrophysiology over 15 years ago at Duke University. Substantial new data on the pathophysiology and natural history of cardiac arrhythmias have become available. Clinical electrophysiologic techniques have progressed from purely diagnostic to therapeutic with the advent of endocardial catheter ablation. Many new antiarrhythmic drugs and electrical devices have been approved for the treatment of patients with cardiac arrhythmias. There is an abundance of specialized information available, in journals and books, for the practicing clinical electrophysiologist. However, this literature is often very technical and difficult to understand for the non-electrophysiologist. Our intent was to write a comprehensive textbook on an integrated approach to cardiac arrhythmias for individuals without a background in clinical electrophysiology. This book should be useful for clinicians taking care of patients with arrhythmias—for example, medical students, housestaff, family practitioners, internists, cardiologists, and nurses on the coronary care or telemetry units. Because of the comprehensive nature of this book, we hope that it will also be of value to clinical electrophysiologists.

To achieve our purpose, we present a practical application of theoretical information and stress electrocardiographic correlates of clinical electrophysiologic observations. Thus, the reader learns to look through the electrocardiogram into the heart. We used an abundance of illustrations and schematics to amplify teaching points. To allow for easier reading, there is some deliberate overlap of information between various chapters. Key references of classic and up-to-date articles are provided for each chapter. Most importantly, this book represents our personal approach to patients with cardiac arrhythmias, partially reflected in the commentary sections. There is often more than one approach to treatment, and on occasion we differed on our choice for first-line

therapy. Regardless, we made every effort to provide the reader with a rational treatment scheme for each arrhythmia.

The book is divided into four parts. Part I presents clinical electrophysiologic correlates of basic electrocardiographic observations. There are in-depth discussions of cardiac conduction, bundle branch block, effects of premature atrial and ventricular ectopy on conduction and automaticity, electrocardiographic changes due to alterations of the autonomic nervous system, and mechanisms of tachycardia. Part II deals with specific arrhythmias. Included are a clinical classification of supraventricular tachycardia, ventricular tachycardia, and bradycardia. Diagnostic information from patient history, physical examination, and laboratory tests is given, as well as an approach to therapy. Separate chapters are devoted to the preexcitation syndromes (Wolff-Parkinson-White) and sustained monomorphic ventricular tachycardia because of their common occurrence and importance to understanding mechanisms of arrhythmias. Part III includes chapters on common clinical presentations. An approach is given for patients who present with these clinical situations, which include electrocardiographic abnormalities in asymptomatic persons, wide and narrow QRS tachycardia, syncope, dizziness, palpitations, cardiac arrest, and arrhythmias during acute myocardial infarction. Part IV consists of chapters on diagnostic techniques and therapeutic modalities. Methods and application of electrophysiologic testing, including endocardial catheter ablation and mapping, and several noninvasive tests—for example, electrocardiographic monitoring and signal-averaged electrocardiography—are included. There are also chapters on pharmacologic, operative, and electrical therapy.

We acknowledge the many people who helped us with this book: our wives and children, for their constant patience and encouragement; John J. Gallagher, M.D., for giving us an appreciation for clinical electrophysiology and for his continued friendship and guidance; Edward L. C. Pritchett, M.D., for imparting to us his unique perspective on cardiac arrhythmias; Mrs. Mary Kay Franklin and Mrs. Linda Humenick, for their outstanding secretarial assistance; Ms. Jane E. Watson, C.M.I., and Mr. George Moogk, for their expert artwork; Augustus O. Grant, M.D., and Katherine T. Murray, M.D., for their critical review of Chapters 5 and 19, respectively; and Mr. J. Dereck Jeffers, our editor at McGraw-Hill, for his numerous helpful suggestions and patience.

# CARDIAC
## ARRHYTHMIAS

# Part I

## Basic Electrocardiographic Observations and Clinical Electrophysiologic Correlates

# Chapter 1

# *Cardiac Conduction*

## *General Concepts*

The normal cardiac impulse originates in the sinus node, a crescent-shaped structure approximately 9 to 15 mm long that is located at the juncture of the superior vena cava and right atrium.[1] After the electrical impulse exits the sinus node, it proceeds to activate the right and left atria. Activation of the atria is responsible for the P wave recorded on the electrocardiogram (ECG). Activation of the normal human atria takes approximately 90 to 100 ms, the right atrium being activated within approximately 65 ms.[2] The latest area to be activated is the left atrial appendage, although atrial tissue near the left inferior pulmonary vein can also be activated very late. It should be noted that as the spread of atrial activation occurs, some sections of the right and left atria are activated at the same time.[2]

A controversy has existed for decades concerning the existence of specialized internodal pathways for conduction between the sinoatrial (SA) node and the atrioventricular (AV) node. The essence of this controversy is whether preferential atrial conduction between the SA and AV nodes occurs over specialized pathways or whether the activation wavefront proceeds through nonspecialized or ordinary atrial myocardium.[1,3] In our opinion, most data strongly suggest that no specialized pathways of conduction exist. The observed preferential conduction of atrial impulses along various anatomical routes can be explained adequately by various factors, such as the complex anatomy of the right atrium, which includes multiple "holes" such as the orifices of the inferior and superior venae cavae and coronary sinus ostium, as well as the orientation of atrial fibers in longitudinal

and perpendicular directions, with conduction being faster in the longitudinal direction.[4]

The PR interval in the ECG encompasses activation in the atria, AV node, His-Purkinje system, and ventricles (Fig. 1-1). Activation through the AV node is a complex process, and prevailing opinion suggests that the AV node can be subdivided into three functional zones: the AN, N, and NH zones.[5–7] The N zone appears to be the most common area where block occurs in the AV node. The impulses exit from the AV node into the ventricular specialized conduction system, which consists of the His bundle, the left and right bundle branches with their subdivisions, and the peripheral network of Purkinje fibers, which terminate into ventricular myocardium. The left bundle branch is often described as having two primary functional divisions, the anterior and posterior fascicles. However, as early as 1906, Tawara[8] identified a third fascicle of the left bundle branch that enters into the left interventricular septum, an observation confirmed by others (Fig. 1-2).[9] In a classic study by Durrer et al.[2] on excitation of the human heart, three endocardial areas were consistently shown to be excited synchronously 0 to 5 ms after the beginning of the left ventricular cavity potential, giving credence to the concept of a functional trifascicular left bundle branch system.

In the absence of bundle branch block, ventricular activation is quite rapid, usually less than 100 ms, and is represented on the electrocardiogram by the QRS complex. Examples of ventricular epicardial activation in normal hearts of patients undergoing surgery for ablation of the accessory pathway in the Wolff-Parkinson-White syndrome are demonstrated in Figs. 1-3 to 1-5. These maps were computer-generated during activation of one QRS complex,

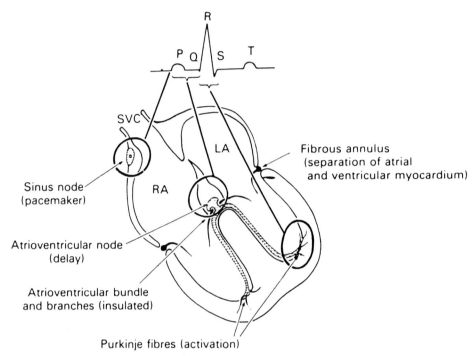

*Figure 1-1*   Schematic of the electrocardiogram and cardiac conduction system. *(Reproduced with permission from Davies MJ, Anderson RH, Becker AE: The Conduction System of the Heart. Butterworth, London, 1983.)*

using a 56-electrode array sock. Figure 1-3 shows normal ventricular activation; right bundle branch block and left bundle branch block are noted in Figs. 1-4 and 1-5, respectively.

### Electrophysiologic-Electrocardiographic Correlations

Electrophysiologic studies utilize several multipolar electrode catheters positioned at various locations in the heart (Fig. 1-6). These catheters make it possible to record electrical potentials from within the heart and to stimulate various cardiac chambers in the diagnosis and management of cardiac arrhythmias. Whereas the electrocardiographer analyzes the surface electrocardiogram, the clinical electrophysiologist peers through this tracing to analyze its component parts (Fig. 1-7). In essence, the more one knows about intracardiac events, the easier it is to analyze the surface electrocardiogram.

### PR Interval

Figure 1-8 demonstrates intracardiac electrophysiologic events.[10,11] The top tracing is surface ECG lead $V_1$; simultaneous intracardiac recordings are from one catheter in the high right atrium (HRA) and from another positioned across the tricuspid valve to record electrical signals coming from the AV junction near the His bundle electrogram (HBE). This was a quadripolar catheter, and the proximal two electrodes (HBE PROX) are closer to the atrial side of this juncture, recording a large atrial (A) depolarization along with a His bundle deflection (H) and a ventricular (V) electrogram that represents activation of the high ventricular septum. The distal bipolar electrode pair (HBE DIST) is situated more into the ventricle, and this enabled the recording of a right bundle branch (RB) potential.

The PA interval, a measure of atrial conduction, is taken from the onset of the surface P wave to local

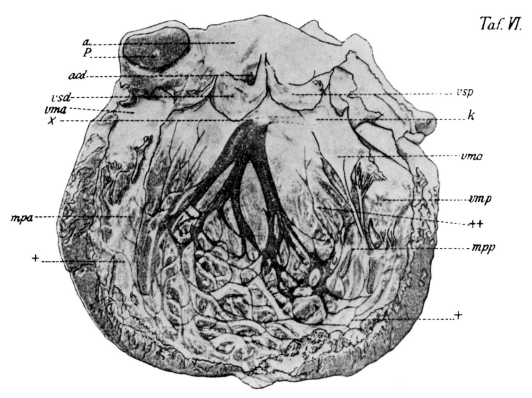

*Taf. VI.*

**Figure 1-2**   Photomicrograph demonstrating the distribution of the left bundle branch in the human heart taken from the original publication of Tawara. *(Reproduced with permission from Tawara S: Das Reizleitungssystem des Saugetierherzens. Fischer, Jena, Germany 1906.)*

atrial activation in the His bundle electrogram. In our opinion, this interval is of minimal value, since it only records atrial activation through a part of the right atrium. More important measurements are the atrio-His (AH) interval, which is an approximation of AV nodal conduction time, and the His-ventricle (HV) interval, which reflects conduction through the His-Purkinje system. Measurement of the AH interval is taken from the first rapid deflection in the atrial electrogram on the His bundle tracing to the onset of the His bundle deflection.[11] The first rapid deflection represents local atrial activation in the vicinity of the AV node, but the earliest identifiable His bundle activity is chosen because the measurement of interest is conduction time through the AV node—not conduction time to a specific local area in the His bundle. In other words, when the His

bundle activity is seen, conduction through the AV node is confirmed. In contrast, the HV interval is measured from the earliest identifiable His deflection to the earliest onset of ventricular activity recorded from either an intracardiac electrogram or any surface QRS complex. For this measurement the desired conduction time is from the earliest evidence of activity in the His bundle to any point confirming ventricular activity, regardless of the area from which this activity is generated. We consider an AH interval between 60 and 120 ms and an HV interval between 35 and 55 ms recorded during sinus rhythm as normal for our laboratories.

Abnormalities of AV conduction are discussed in more detail in Chap. 10, but some examples are offered here to illustrate the usefulness of intracardiac recordings in defining the location of conduction

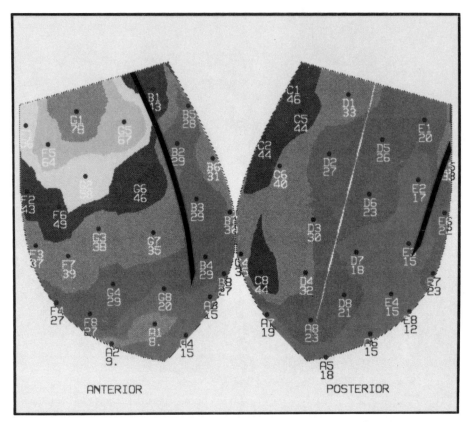

*Figure 1-3*  Normal epicardial ventricular activation. The format for Figs. 1-3, 1-4, and 1-5 is the same. At the time of surgery, a 56-electrode array sock was positioned on the epicardial surface of the heart; during one QRS complex, ventricular activation was obtained at all sites. Each site is noted by a letter and number that designate the electrode position and, underneath, the local activation time, using the initiation of the surface QRS complex as time 0. The left anterior descending (LAD) coronary artery is schematically represented in the anterior view and the posterior descending (PDA) coronary artery is represented similarly in the posterior view. These are approximate positions as noted during surgery. In this figure, note the rapid activation of the entire right and left ventricles. The last area activated is the base of the right ventricle, and activation time is complete within 78 ms. The right ventricle in the anterior view is to the left of the LAD and in the posterior view to the right of the PDA. This method of displaying the heart assumes that the posterior crux of the heart is divided and the ventricles are then laid out flat. The base of the heart with the atria removed is at the top of the figure and the apex (electrodes A1 through A8) is at the bottom. It is not that critical to analyze each point but rather to realize that the entire epicardial surface of the ventricle is activated relatively quickly. (See Color Plate 1.)

disturbances. In Fig. 1-9, first-degree AV block is demonstrated by a PR interval of 220 ms (0.22 s) and conduction of every P wave. The QRS duration is 90 ms, which is normal. The cause of first-degree block is noted in the His bundle electrogram. The AH interval measured 155 ms, which is markedly prolonged. However, in Fig. 1-10, the prolonged PR interval in a patient with first-degree AV block and left bundle branch block is due to a severe conduction abnormality in the His-Purkinje system, as demonstrated by an HV interval of 165 ms. This latter situation represents a more critical cardiac

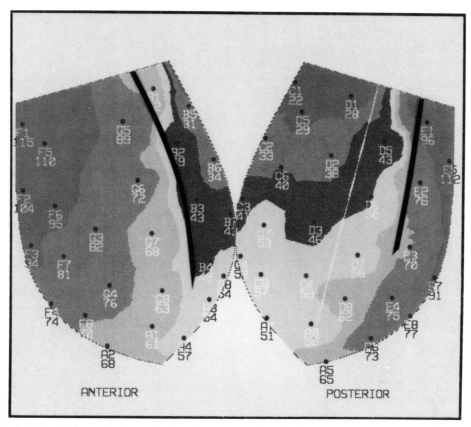

*Figure 1-4*   Epicardial ventricular activation during right bundle branch block. (See Fig. 1-3 for details of mapping methods.) Note that the left ventricle, represented by electrodes B through D, is activated in a normal fashion and relatively quickly. However, the right ventricle, represented by electrodes E through G, is activated late, as would be expected in right bundle branch block. Point $F_1$ is activated 115 ms after the initiation of the surface QRS complex. Compare this activation with that noted in Fig. 1-3. (See Color Plate 2.)

conduction disturbance, as discussed in more detail in Chap. 10. A third example of first-degree AV block is shown in Fig. 1-11. This patient has a PR interval of 210 ms and left bundle branch block. However, the HV interval is only moderately prolonged to 65 ms, but a combination of all conduction times still yields an ECG pattern of first-degree AV block. Finally, first-degree AV block can be due to conduction abnormalities in both the AV node and His-Purkinje system (Fig. 1-12).

The PR interval recorded during sinus rhythm usually demonstrates minimal variability unless marked changes in autonomic tone occur (see "Auto-

nomic Nervous System Effects," p. 14). Thus, the appearance of two distinctly different stable PR intervals during electrocardiographic recording strongly suggests the existence of two functionally separate anterograde conduction pathways, both presumably in the AV node (Fig. 1-13). The PR interval in panel A is 180 ms and in panel B 400 ms. This patient had dual AV nodal physiology, as illustrated in Fig. 1-14.[12–16] In this figure, the first three PR intervals represent AV nodal conduction over the slowly conducting pathway, and the AH interval is 290 ms. A premature atrial stimulus ($S_2$) was introduced into the high right atrium and blocked in the

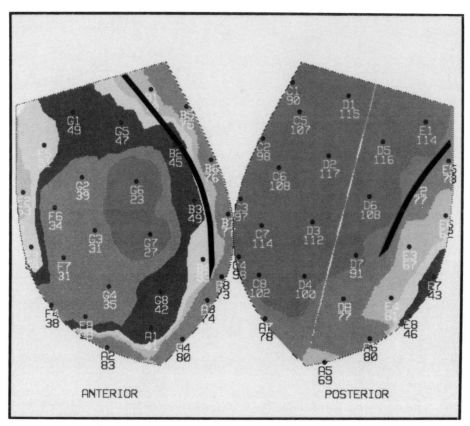

*Figure 1-5*　Epicardial ventricular activation in left bundle branch block. (See Fig. 1-3 for details of mapping.) In contrast to Fig. 1-4, the earliest activated sites in this patient are on the right ventricle and the latter activated points on the left ventricle, as expected with left bundle branch block. Right ventricular points are primarily noted by G and E, which are left of the LAD in the anterior view and right of the PDA in the posterior view. Note that the last area to be activated is on the left ventricle at D2 (117 ms), in contrast to the last area activated during right bundle branch block, which is on the right ventricular epicardial surface (see Fig. 1-4). (See Color Plate 3.)

AV node (no His depolarization after atrial premature complex). Atrioventricular nodal conduction resumed over the fast conducting pathway, as shown in the last three complexes on this tracing and demonstrated by a normal PR interval and an AH conduction time of 80 ms.

**ATRIOVENTRICULAR NODAL BLOCK**　Incremental atrial pacing is used to evaluate AV nodal function in the electrophysiology laboratory. Atrial pacing is started at a rate slightly faster than the spontaneous sinus rate. The pacing rate is progressively increased until AV nodal block occurs. The AH interval increases with faster-paced rates as shown schematically in Fig. 1-15. This is an example of 3:2 Wenckebach block. Complex 1 conducts with relatively minimal AV nodal delay, complex 2 shows a substantial increase in the AH interval, and complex 3 fails to conduct to the His bundle. Records from a patient are demonstrated in Fig. 1-16. Note in ECG lead II a progressive increase in the PR interval for the first three paced beats, followed by a P wave

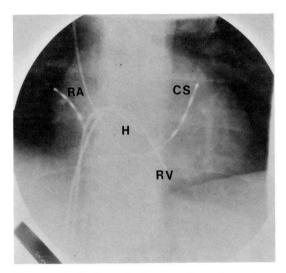

*Figure 1-6*   Radiograph of endocardial catheter placement. (Key: RA = right atrium; CS = coronary sinus; RV = right ventricle; H = His bundle area.)

*type I second-degree, AV block*. The changes in PR interval in this example occur within the AV node, as demonstrated by the progressive increase in the AH interval from 70 to 110 ms without change in the HV interval. Note that in the fourth paced beat the atrial depolarization in the HBE tracing is not followed by a His bundle deflection, confirming block within the AV node. Conduction resumes with an AH interval of 70 ms.

In unusual instances it is very difficult to detect a measurable increase in the PR interval prior to block. An example of this is noted in Fig. 1-17. This patient has spontaneous episodes while awake of nonconducted P waves with minimal or no prior PR prolongation. Figure 1-17A was recorded upon electrophysiologic study at a routine ECG paper speed of 25 mm/s. There is only a minimal change in the PR interval measurable in this example. Analysis of the intracardiac electrograms reveals conduction block in the AV node, with a mere 10 to 15 ms increase in the AH interval prior to the nonconducted P wave (Fig. 1-17B). This recording was done at a 100-mm/s paper speed, where more precise measurements can be obtained. The normal QRS complex strongly suggests that block will be in the AV node, although some patients will demonstrate intra-His block, as discussed in Chap. 10.

without conduction to the ventricle; conduction resumes with the last paced beat, and the PR interval is shorter than the PR interval of the last conducted beat prior to block. This pattern of conduction abnormality is referred to as *Wenckebach, or Mobitz*

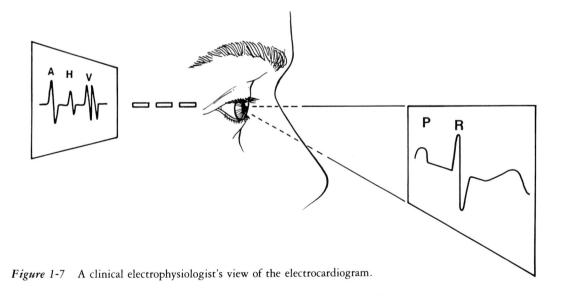

*Figure 1-7*   A clinical electrophysiologist's view of the electrocardiogram.

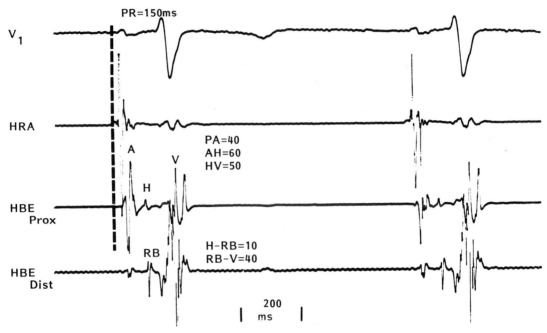

*Figure 1-8*  Intracardiac electrophysiologic conduction intervals during the PR interval. (See text for further details.) (Key: HRA = high right atrium; HBE (Prox) = proximal His bundle electrode pair; HBE (Dist) = distal His bundle electrode pair; A = atrial; H = His; V = ventricle; RB = right bundle.)

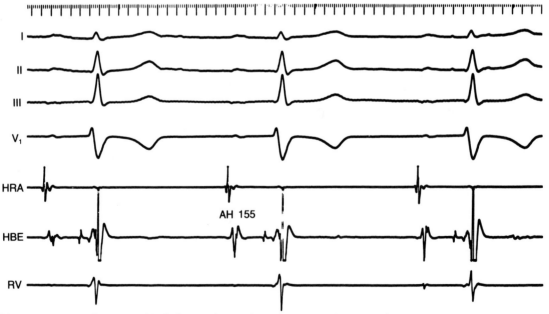

*Figure 1-9*  First-degree AV block due to abnormal conduction in the AV node. (Key: RV = right ventricle. See Fig. 1-8 for other abbreviations. Time lines: each major division = 50 ms.)

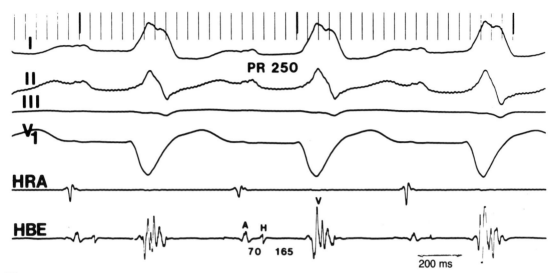

*Figure 1-10*   First-degree AV block and left bundle branch block with a markedly prolonged HV interval. (See text for details.)

On rare occasions a Wenckebach conduction pattern can occur in the His-Purkinje system (Fig. 1-18). At electrophysiologic study during incremental atrial pacing, there was a progressive increase in the PR interval, as noted in ECG lead II. Analysis of conduction times in the His bundle electrogram shows a progressive increase in the HV interval from 130 to 165 ms prior to a nonconducted P wave. The AH interval remained constant. Note that the fifth paced atrial complex demonstrates activation of the His bundle but no conduction beyond this point. Thus, conduction block is infra-His, which repre-

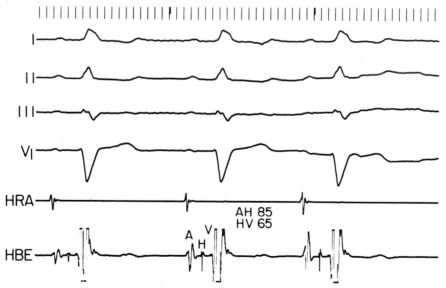

*Figure 1-11*   First-degree AV block with left bundle branch block and minimal intracardiac conduction abnormalities.

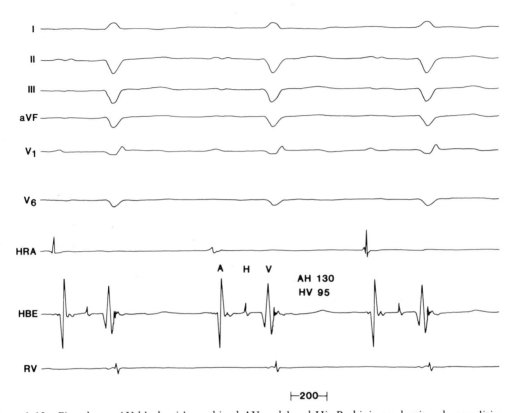

*Figure 1-12*    First-degree AV block with combined AV nodal and His-Purkinje conduction abnormalities.

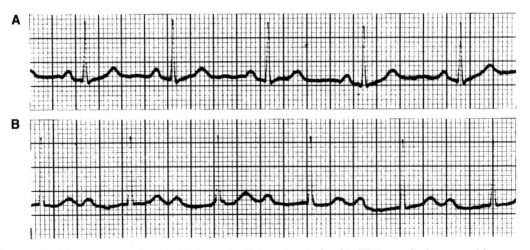

*Figure 1-13*    Two separate and stable PR intervals. This patient had stable PR intervals that were either normal (A) or long (B). *(Reproduced with permission from Kelley WN (ed), Textbook of Internal Medicine. Lippincott, Philadelphia, PA, 1989.)*

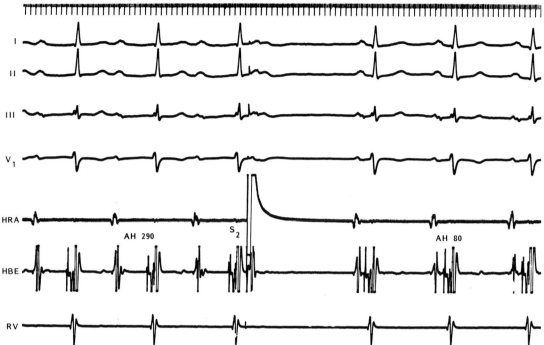

*Figure 1-14* Dual AV nodal physiology demonstrated at electrophysiologic study. (See text for details.) *(Reproduced with permission from Prystowsky EN, Page RL, Electrophysiology of the Sino-Atrial and Atrioventricular Nodes. Alan R. Liss, New York, 1988.)*

sents a severe form of conduction disturbance. Note that the patient has a right bundle branch block pattern. Even with a bundle branch block pattern, a Wenckebach conduction sequence most commonly implies conduction delay and block in the AV node.

Testing of the AV nodal conduction system with incremental atrial pacing in the electrophysiology laboratory yields a wide range of atrial paced cycle lengths at which Wenckebach AV nodal block occurs. In the resting state during electrophysiologic testing, we consider AV nodal conduction to be normal if 1:1 conduction is present to a right atrial paced cycle length of less than 505 ms.[17] Of particular interest is that even though Wenckebach block may occur at a wide range of cycle lengths, the AV nodal function curve is physiologically similar for all patients. This is demonstrated in Fig. 1-19, which shows the lengthening of the AH interval, noted on the ordinate, as a function of shortening of the atrial pacing

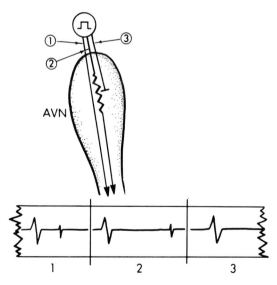

*Figure 1-15* Schematic of Wenckebach AV nodal block during incremental atrial pacing.

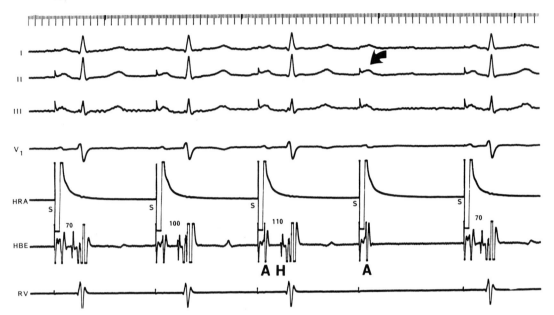

*Figure 1-16*   Wenckebach AV nodal block. (See text for details.) Arrow points to nonconducted P wave.

cycle length (increased heart rate), noted on the abscissa. Each line represents a group of patients with Wenckebach block occurring at different cycle lengths. For example, the curve on the far right includes patients in whom Wenckebach block occurs at cycle lengths greater than 500 ms, whereas the curve on the far left represents patients in whom Wenckebach occurs at paced cycle lengths less than 300 ms. Each curve is divided into separate segments, with the most distal segment represented by *A*. Analysis of these data showed that the curves were progressively shifted to the left as shorter atrial paced cycle lengths were required to yield Wenckebach block, but the slopes of each part of the curves were similar for all curves. In essence, only minimal to moderate prolongation of the AH interval occurs until the Wenckebach cycle length is approached. As a corollary, drugs that demonstrate negative dromotropic effects, that is, depress conduction, on the AV node—such as verapamil or beta-adrenergic blockers—minimally affect condition on the flat portion of these curves but have a marked effect on the stressed portion (part *A*) of the curve.

### Autonomic Nervous System Effects

#### Sinus Node

The sinus node is richly supplied with nerves from the parasympathetic and sympathetic nervous systems.[1] At rest, humans are "vagal animals" with regard to sinus nodal behavior. That is, although the sympathetic nervous system affects the sinus node tonically, the parasympathetic nervous system is prepotent. Experimental studies, including those in humans, demonstrate that when both sympathetic and parasympathetic inputs to the sinus node are blocked, the resultant sinus nodal rate substantially increases.[19,20] Since sympathetic blockade decreases and parasympathetic blockade increases sinus rate, a faster rate during autonomic blockade confirms the predominant effect of vagal tone.

The interaction of parasympathetic and sympathetic influences on the sinus node is often quite complex; these influences act in concert to alter the sinus rate. For example, the change to a standing from a reclining position or from relaxation to exercise results in parasympathetic withdrawal as well as

25mm/s

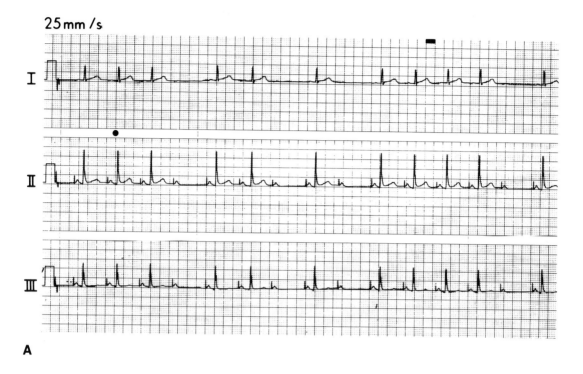

**A**

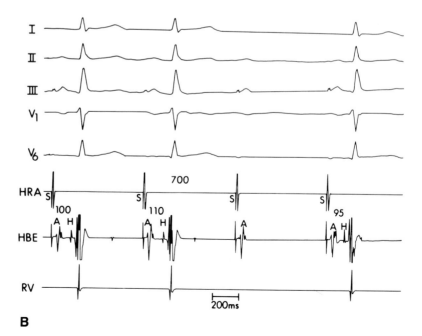

*Figure 1-17* Wenckebach AV nodal block with minimal PR prolongation prior to block. *A.* Wenckebach block during routine ECG recording. *B.* Wenckebach AV nodal block demonstrated at electrophysiologic study. (See text for details.)

**B**

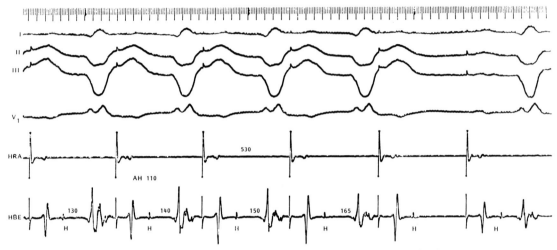

*Figure 1-18*    Wenckebach block conduction pattern with infra-His block. (See text for details.)

increased sympathetic tone. Figure 1-20 shows the resultant sinus rate after a variety of maneuvers that affect the autonomic nervous system. Note that sinus tachycardia occurs in the resting supine state, which was usual for this patient but is a decidedly abnormal

finding. Even though this patient had a persistent sinus tachycardia, he still responded appropriately to a variety of maneuvers with an increased rate while standing; an increased sinus rate during phase two of the Valsalva maneuver, with subsequent sinus

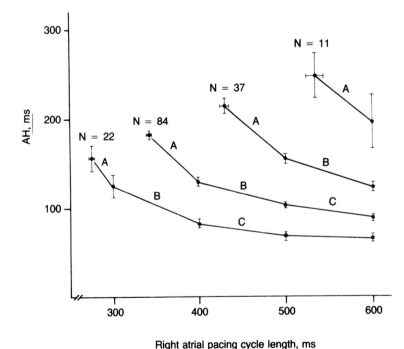

*Figure 1-19*    Family of AV nodal function curves obtained during electrophysiologic testing. From top to bottom the curves represent patients who had shortest 1:1 atrial pacing cycle length <600 ms but ≥500 ms; <500 ms but ≥400 ms; <400 ms but ≥300 ms; and <300 ms. (*Reproduced with permission from Jackman WM et al. Circulation 67:441, 1983.*)

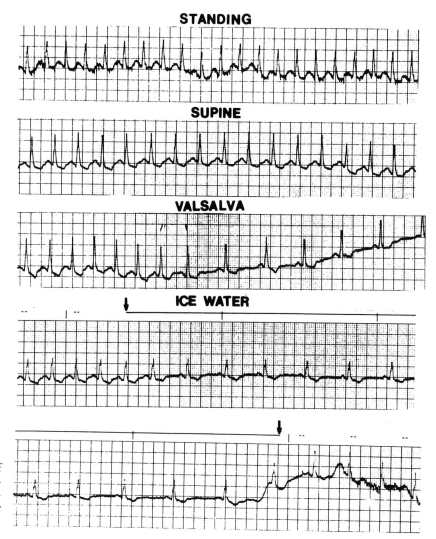

**Figure 1-20** Effect of various autonomic maneuvers on sinus nodal automaticity. (See text for details.)

slowing during phase four; and sinus nodal slowing during immersion of his face in ice water—a situation that markedly enhances vagal tone.

The sinus rate results from an interplay of the individual's intrinsic sinus nodal automaticity, the background tonic influences of the autonomic nervous system, and perturbations in the environment that reflexly change the autonomic input to the sinus node. An example of the effects of a brief increase in systolic blood pressure on sinus nodal automaticity

is demonstrated in Fig. 1-21. The left-hand portion of this figure demonstrates a resting sinus cycle length of 675 ms (89/min). The bottom half of the figure shows the blood pressure, which is approximately 91 mmHg systolic at rest. A 200-$\mu$g intravenous bolus of phenylephrine was given to increase systolic pressure, which was approximately 116 mmHg at its peak. The increase in systolic blood pressure results in a short period of enhanced vagal tone that prolongs the sinus cycle length to a

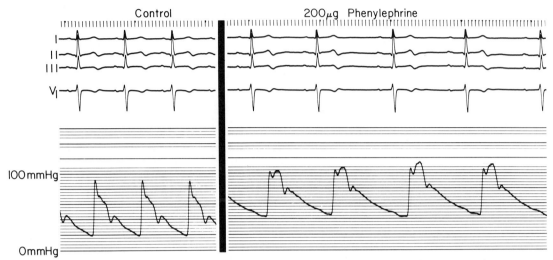

**Figure 1-21**    Slowing of sinus rate as result of enhanced vagal tone following an increase in systolic blood pressure during phenylephrine infusion. (See text for details.)

maximum of 1110 ms (54/min), but this effect soon dissipates and sinus rate returns to control values shortly thereafter. Sinus rate also varies with respiration; it typically increases with inspiration and slows with expiration—an effect modulated by the parasympathetic nervous system.[21-23] In fact, lack of respiratory variability in sinus rate has been noted in patients with long-standing diabetes mellitus who have autonomic dysfunction.[24] It has also been correlated with a worse prognosis after acute myocardial infarction,[25,26] presumably because of the beneficial effects of vagal tone on preventing the emergence of life-threatening ventricular arrhythmias. The preceding hypothesis has yet to be proven.

An interesting arrhythmia seen in patients with variable degrees of heart block is ventriculophasic sinus arrhythmia (Fig. 1-22). Note the characteristically shorter P-P intervals that surround a QRS complex compared with the longer P-P intervals without an intervening QRS complex. The explanation for this phenomenon stems at least in part from alterations in sinus nodal automaticity resulting from changes in blood pressure. For example, ventricular electrical systole is followed by a rise in systolic blood pressure that would tend to slow the sinus cycle length, as demonstrated in Fig. 1-21. However,

if the systolic rise in blood pressure occurs too late to affect the next sinus-generated P wave, it may still slow the subsequent sinus impulse. In Fig. 1-22, this would cause the P wave immediately following the QRS complex to occur on time but the next P wave to be delayed, yielding a longer P-P interval without an intervening QRS complex. Since the effect of heightened blood pressure is short-lived, the P wave immediately after the QRS complex is not delayed and therefore the P-P interval surrounding the QRS complex is relatively short. That this mechanism is operative is strengthened by the observation noted in Fig. 1-23.

The data in Fig. 1-23 were generated from a patient undergoing autonomic testing by means of neck-collar suction.[27,28] With the patient in a supine position, this is accomplished by the placement of a malleable lead collar, resembling an ordinary neck brace, around the patient's neck with an airtight seal. The collar has two ports, one for intracollar pressure readings and the other to be connected to a vacuum source. Negative intracollar pressure of −60 mmHg for a duration of 600 ms is initiated at various points throughout the sinus cycle, and the resultant increase in P-P interval is plotted as a function of the time that neck suction is initiated

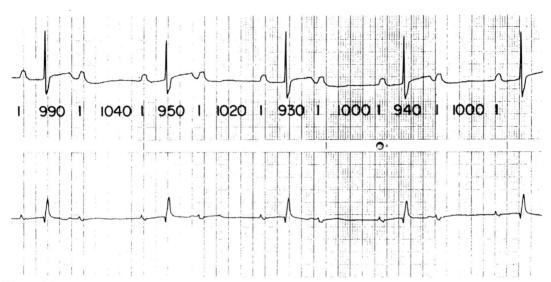

**Figure 1-22**   Ventriculophasic sinus arrhythmia in a patient with 2:1 AV block. (See text for details.)

prior to the anticipated onset of the sinus P wave. The neck suction imposed through the collar creates a deformation of the carotid sinus, mimicking a sudden increase in blood pressure and thus producing increased vagal tone. This technique can be used to determine the earliest time possible prior to an anticipated sinus impulse at which a sudden increase in vagal tone can affect sinus nodal automaticity. It can also be used to demonstrate for that individual the timing of the peak effect and when the vagal

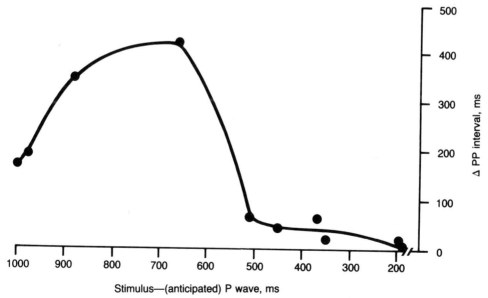

**Figure 1-23**   Example of a baroreflex inhibition curve of the sinus node obtained during pulses of neck collar suction of $-60$ mmHg for 600 ms throughout the cardiac cycle. (See text for details.)

tone will dissipate. In this 22-year-old patient, the latency—that is, the time before the anticipated P wave when the imposed vagal tone did not affect sinus nodal automaticity—was approximately 200 ms. A substantial effect was seen only after 500 ms prior to the onset of the P wave. The latency tends to increase with age, and it is not uncommon for patients in their fifth and sixth decades to have latencies of 400 to 500 ms.[29] Reevaluation of Fig. 1-22 reveals an approximate 500 ms interval between the QRS complex and P wave immediately following this complex. It is quite possible in this older individual that the expected enhanced vagal tone following cardiac contraction fell within the latency period of the next sinus impulse and thus produced no effect on the sinus rate. However, the increased vagal tone could clearly have depressed automaticity of the subsequent sinus impulse, producing a prolonged P-P interval.

### AV Node

Unlike the sinus node, the AV node in humans at rest appears to have a relatively balanced input from the parasympathetic and sympathetic nervous systems.[20] But in patients who have abnormal AV nodal conduction, a preponderance of vagal effect may be noted at rest.[17] An increase in sympathetic tone or withdrawal of vagal tone can shorten AV nodal conduction time and, in the electrophysiology laboratory, yield a shorter atrial paced cycle length maintaining 1:1 AV nodal conduction. However, spontaneous changes in autonomic tone may alter the heart rate, producing rate-related changes in AV

nodal conduction, as discussed previously; but the direct autonomic influence on the AV node may offset the rate-related effects. For example, during pacing of the atrium at electrophysiologic study, the AH interval progressively increases at faster-paced rates. This effect is usually not observed with increases in heart rate that occur spontaneously, for example, during exercise. Under these conditions, the sinus rate accelerates because of decreased parasympathetic and increased sympathetic tone, both of which enhance conduction in the AV node. Thus, if one were to measure the PR interval during exercise, not only would there be continued 1:1 conduction at rates likely to cause block when the atrium is paced at rest during electrophysiologic evaluation, but the PR interval would be minimally changed or even shorter at these faster rates. In summary, the overall result of autonomic perturbations on AV nodal conduction will depend on the interaction of rate-related and direct changes on AV nodal physiology.

A common observation noted at times of expected high vagal tone—for example, during sleep—is Wenckebach AV nodal block in the presence of a relatively slow rate (Fig. 1-24). This figure is from a patient with normal sinus and AV nodal function. Note the telltale finding of a progressive increase in the length of the sinus cycle prior to the nonconducted P wave. A combination of sinus slowing and Wenckebach AV block strongly suggests the mechanism to be enhanced parasympathetic tone, a normal physiologic event that tends to occur during sleep. We stress that this is not an abnormal finding and, by itself, should never be an indication for permanent pacemaker implantation.

**5:08 AM**

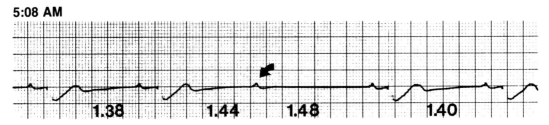

*Figure 1-24*    Wenckebach AV nodal block during sleep. Arrow points to nonconducted P wave. The intervals represent the timing between P waves. (See text for details.)

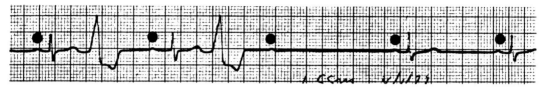

*Figure 1-25* Wenckebach AV nodal block during carotid sinus massage. The dots signify each P wave.

In some patients, carotid sinus massage can produce Wenckebach block at rest, although this observation is uncommon enough to suggest an abnormality of AV nodal conduction or the presence of hypersensitive carotid sinus reflex. In the patient demonstrated in Fig. 1-25, two interesting events occur. This patient has baseline sinus bradycardia at a rate of 45/min (1320 ms) and ventricular bigeminy is present. Carotid sinus massage was applied, slowing the sinus rate, and the third P wave was not conducted. Note also the lack of ventricular ectopic activity after the third P wave, which suggests that the generation of ventricular extrasystoles in this patient was linked to the normal conducted QRS complex. Alternatively, the absence of ventricular extrasystoles could also have occurred partly because of the increase in parasympathetic activity, which can affect the ventricles and His-Purkinje system. It is possible that both of these mechanisms play a role in this particular patient.

Another manifestation of disturbed AV nodal conduction, at least in part related to autonomic perturbations, is high-degree heart block during sleep apnea (Fig. 1-26).[30,31] Experimental data have shown that conduction disturbances and sinus nodal abnormalities during apnea can be ameliorated with supplemental oxygen delivery but can also be prevented with atropine. This suggests that the effect on the AV node during this pathophysiologic state is mediated via the parasympathetic nervous system.

As noted earlier, increased sympathetic tone or decreased parasympathetic tone can facilitate conduction through the AV node. In some patients, we have noted that administration of intravenous isoproterenol or atropine can alter automaticity in junctional tissue prior to affecting sinus nodal automaticity (Fig. 1-27). This patient was given an intravenous infusion of 3 μg/min of isoproterenol. Note in the left-hand portion of the figure a junctional tachycardia, with a His bundle deflection occurring before each QRS complex and retrograde atrial activity. The sinus rate accelerates and the sixth QRS complex is generated by the sinus node and not the junction. Thus, although the primary effects of increased sympathetic and decreased parasympathetic tone on the AV node are usually manifest through changes in AV nodal conduction, on occasion enhanced automaticity may predominate.

### His-Purkinje System

Most data suggest that normal His-Purkinje conduction is minimally affected by sympathetic and parasympathetic input. However, recent observations suggest that abnormal His-Purkinje conduction—for example, Mobitz type II block—can be worsened with beta-adrenergic blockade and improved with atropine.[32] The mechanism for these effects is still unclear. However, as with AV nodal physiology, changes in autonomic tone can have a direct effect

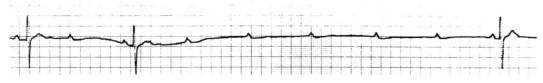

*Figure 1-26* High-grade AV block during sleep apnea. (See text for details.)

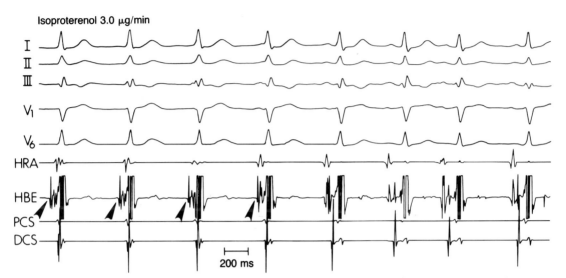

*Figure 1-27*    Accelerated junctional tachycardia during isoproterenol infusion. The first four complexes demonstrate a junctional tachycardia with a His deflection (*arrowhead*) preceding each QRS complex and with atrial activation being retrograde and noted first in the His bundle lead followed by the high right atrial lead. There are no P waves identified on the surface ECG. In beat 4 there appears to be some activation of the atria by the sinus node, although the QRS complex is generated by the junctional focus. Note the slight alteration of the beginning of the QRS complex, representing atrial activity that is different from the first three beats. Beat 5 demonstrates capture of the atrium primarily by the sinus focus, but the QRS complex is most likely still generated from the junctional focus. The sixth QRS complex is generated by the sinus node, which results in the high right atrium being activated first, followed by His bundle (septal) atrial activation and then conduction through the AV node and His-Purkinje system. The proximal coronary sinus (PCS) and distal coronary sinus (DCS) represent left atrial activation that occurs after that of the right atrium.

on His-Purkinje conduction and an indirect effect mediated by a change in sinus rate. An example of this is shown in Fig. 1-28. In the top tracing (panel A), during sinus rhythm at rest in the electrophysiology laboratory, the HV interval is 70 ms, which is prolonged in a patient with underlying left bundle branch block and 1:1 AV conduction. In panel B, the sinus rate has substantially increased during atropine infusion from a cycle length of 1175 ms (51/min) to 770 ms (78/min) but 1:1 AV conduction is still present, although the HV interval has increased to 80 ms. Note, however, the shortening of AH interval from 100 to 60 ms, demonstrating that the predominant effect of atropine on AV nodal function was a direct one that countered the expected lengthening of AH interval due to the increased heart rate. In panel C, Mobitz-type II AV block is present after an increased amount of atropine was given that shortens the sinus cycle length to 550 ms

(109/min) and results in a rate fast enough to cause infra-His block. Thus, atropine has been shown to improve diseased His-Purkinje conduction during electrophysiologic study;[32] however, when the sinus rate increases to a critical point during atropine administration, Mobitz type II block will occur because of the overriding stressful influence of increased heart rate on tenuous conduction in the His-Purkinje system.

A clinical counterpart of this phenomenon is heart block that occurs during exercise testing, usually in patients with bundle branch block. This is almost invariably due to block in the His-Purkinje system and implies a markedly abnormal situation that often requires pacemaker implantation. On rare occasions we have noted this phenomenon in patients with a narrow QRS complex, and block in these individuals has usually been within the His bundle itself. When heart block is noted during exercise

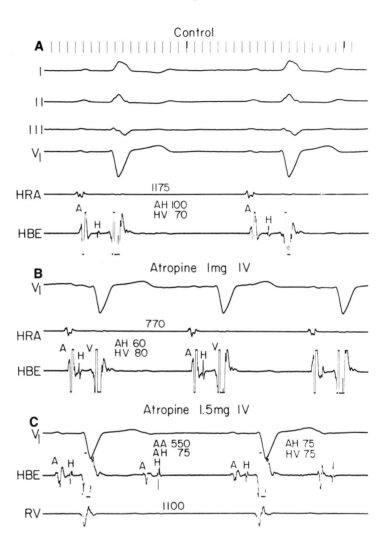

**Figure 1-28** The effects on His-Purkinje conduction of increased heart rate due to atropine infusion. (See text for details.)

testing and the mechanism is unclear, electrophysiologic evaluation is indicated. However, AV nodal block would be distinctly uncommon during exercise, because the autonomic alterations of both vagal withdrawal and enhanced sympathetic activity have a salutary effect on AV nodal conduction.

### Atrium and Ventricle

Both the atrium and ventricle receive input from the parasympathetic and sympathetic nervous systems. In general, increased vagal tone has a more marked effect on atrial tissue than on ventricular

tissue in humans. In our experience, increased parasympathetic tone shortens atrial refractoriness but may lengthen ventricular refractoriness.[20,33] Increased sympathetic tone tends to shorten refractoriness in both types of tissue. In the absence of antiarrhythmic drug therapy, changes in autonomic tone minimally affect the rate of sustained monomorphic ventricular tachycardia, although exceptions do occur (Fig. 1-29).

### Vasovagal Phenomenon

In most situations, alterations in autonomic tone provide a fine-tuning effect on cardiac electrophysiologic properties. The potential magnitude of

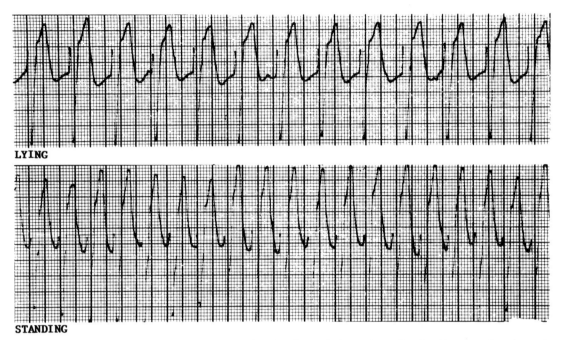

LYING

STANDING

*Figure 1-29*    The effects of posture on the cycle length of ventricular tachycardia. In this unusual patient, the rate of ventricular tachycardia substantially increased when the patient rose from the supine position. It is unclear whether this was due primarily to changes in autonomic activity, such as parasympathetic withdrawal and increased sympathetic tone, changes in ventricular filling, or both. Most patients with ventricular tachycardia have minimal changes in ventricular tachycardia rate with changes in body position.

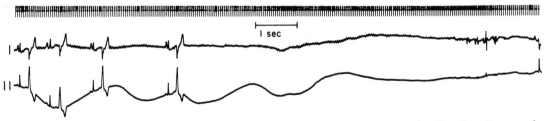

I sec

*Figure 1-30*    Vasovagal episode with no evidence of sinus nodal or subsidiary pacemaker function. (See text for details.)

the effects of increased parasympathetic tone can be observed during a vasovagal episode, a period of imposition of immense vagal tone on the heart that can have devastating results, such as total asystole and syncope (Fig. 1-30). During a vasovagal episode in this patient, there was no sinus nodal activity or any junctional or His-Purkinje escape rhythm for over 7 s; we have seen asystolic episodes last longer than 15 s. The lack of automaticity in any subsidiary

pacemaker during one of these episodes should remove any doubt that the parasympathetic nervous system can have a significant effect on His-Purkinje and ventricular tissue.

## References

1.    Strauss HC et al: Sino-atrial and atrial electrogenesis. *Prog Cardiovasc Dis* 14:5, 385, 1977.

2. Durrer D et al: Total excitation of the isolated human heart. *Circulation* 41:899, 1970.

3. VanDam RTh, Janse MJ: Activation of the heart, in Macfarlane PW, Lawrie TDV (eds): *Comprehensive Electrocardiology: Theory and Practice in Health and Disease.* Pergamon Press, New York, pp 101–127.

4. Spach MS et al: Excitation sequence of the atrial septum and AV node in isolated hearts of the dog and the rabbit. *Circ Res* 29:156, 1971.

5. Paes de Carvalho A, de Almeida DF: Spread of activity through the atrioventricular node. *Circ Res* 8:801, 1960.

6. Anderson RH et al: A combined morphological and electrophysiological study of the atrioventricular node of the rabbit heart. *Circ Res* 35:909, 1974.

7. Billette J et al: Cycle-length dependent properties of AV nodal activation in rabbit hearts. *Am J Physiol* 231:1129, 1976.

8. Tawara S: *Das Reizleitungssystem des Saügetierherzens: Eine Anatomisch-Histologische Studie über das Atrioventrikurbündel und die Purkinjeschen Fäden.* Jena, Fischer, 1906.

9. Demoulin JC, Kulbertus HE: Histopathological examination of the concept of left hemiblock. *Br Heart J* 34:807, 1972.

10. Scherlag BJ et al: Catheter technique for recording His bundle activity in man. *Circulation* 39:13, 1969.

11. Prystowsky, EN: Electrophysiologic testing, in Kelley WN (ed): *Textbook of Internal Medicine.* Lippincott, Philadelphia, 1989, pp 344–353.

12. Prystowsky EN, Page RL: Electrophysiology and autonomic influences of the human atrioventricular node, in, *Electrophysiology of the Sino-Atrial and Atrioventricular Nodes.* New York, Alan R. Liss, 1988, pp 259–277.

13. Moe GK et al: Physiologic evidence of a dual A-V transmission system. Circ Res 6:357, 1956.

14. Rosenblueth A: Ventricular "echoes." *Am J Physiol* 195:53, 1958.

15. Mendez C, Moe GK: Demonstration of a dual A-V nodal conduction system in the isolated rabbit heart. *Circ Res* 19:378, 1966.

16. Denes P et al: Demonstration of dual A-V nodal pathways in patients with paroxysmal supraventricular tachycardia. *Circulation* 48:549, 1973.

17. Rahilly GT et al: Autonomic blockade in patients with normal and abnormal atrioventricular nodal function. *Am J Cardiol* 49:898, 1982.

18. Jackman WM et al: Reevaluation of enhanced atrioventricular nodal conduction: Evidence to suggest a continuum of normal atrioventricular nodal physiology. *Circulation* 67:441, 1983.

19. Levy MN, Zieske H: Autonomic control of cardiac pacemaker activity and atrioventricular transmission. *J Appl Physiol* 27:465, 1969.

20. Prystowsky EN et al: Effect of autonomic blockade on ventricular refractoriness and atrioventricular nodal conduction in humans. *Circ Res* 49:511, 1981.

21. Katona P, Jih F: Respiratory sinus arrhythmia: Noninvasive measure of parasympathetic cardiac control. *J Appl Physiol* 39:801, 1975.

22. Katona PG et al: Cardiac vagal efferent activity and heart period in the carotid sinus reflex. *Am J Physiol* 218:1030, 1970.

23. Coker R et al: Does the sympathetic nervous system influence sinus arrhythmia in man? Evidence from combined autonomic blockade. *J Physiol* 356:459, 1984.

24. Ewing DJ et al: New method for assessing cardiac parasympathetic activity using 24 hour electrocardiograms. *Br Heart J* 52:396, 1984.

25. Wolf MM et al: Sinus arrhythmia in acute myocardial infarction. *Med J Aust* 2:52, 1978.

26. Kleiger RE et al: Heart rate variability: A variable predicting mortality following acute myocardial infarction. *J Am Coll Cardiol* 3:547A, 1984.

27. Prystowsky EN, Zipes DP: Postvagal tachycardia. *Am J Cardiol* 55:995, 1985.

28. Eckberg DL et al: A simplified neck suction device for activation of carotid baroreceptors. *J Lab Clin Med* 85:167, 1975.

29. Prystowsky EN et al: Carotid baroreflex abnormalities and end-organ responsiveness in patients with diabetes mellitus. *J Am Coll Cardiol* 7:126A, 1986.

30. Prystowsky EN, Klein GJ: Arrhythmias in chronic lung disease, in Rubin LJ (ed): *Pulmonary Heart Disease.* Martinus Nijhoff Publishing, Boston/The Hague/Dordrecht/Lancaster, 1984, pp 273–283.

31. Zwillich C et al: Bradycardia during sleep apnea—characteristics and mechanism. *J Clin Invest* 69:1286, 1982.

32. Markel ML et al: Parasympathetic and sympathetic alterations of Mobitz type II heart block. *J Am Coll Cardiol* 11:271, 1988.

33. Prystowsky EN et al: Enhanced parasympathetic tone shortens atrial refractoriness in man. *Am J Cardiol* 51:96, 1983.

# Chapter 2

# Electrocardiographic Consequences of Atrial and Ventricular Ectopy

Ectopic complexes arise from areas other than the sinus node and, when manifest, disturb the normal sequence of automaticity and conduction in the heart. Premature complexes most commonly originate in the ventricles (PVC) and atria (PAC) but may also occur in the atrioventricular (AV) junction. Regarding terminology, *ectopic* does not refer to a mechanism but to the origin of the complex outside the sinus nodal area. Mechanisms include automaticity and reentry and are discussed in more detail in Chap. 5. These abnormal complexes are often referred to as *beats*, although technically a beat suggests a stroke or pulsation of the pulse or heart, whereas PVCs and PACs are actually electrical events and may not be coupled with contraction. Regardless, *premature beats* is a term so ingrained in the literature that is is not worth altering merely for semantics. This chapter discusses the electrocardiographic (ECG) consequences of premature complexes.

## Premature Atrial Complexes

### Effects on Sinus Nodal Function

Premature atrial complexes can affect sinus nodal automaticity and conduction. The ECG events are a result of conduction from the PAC that is "concealed" but the results of which are manifest.[1-4] Figure 2-1 is a schematic illustrating some of these general principles. Premature atrial complexes may result in a compensatory pause, reset, or are interpolated (Fig. 2-1).[5,6] A compensatory pause occurs when an atrial complex fails to conduct retrogradely into the sinus node and does not allow the regular sinus impulse to manifest itself because of refractoriness of the tissue after the PAC. The subsequent sinus impulse is on time and conducts normally to the atrium (Fig. 2-1, I). Thus, the interval from the spontaneous atrial complex ($A_1$) preceding the PAC ($A_2$) plus the time from the PAC to the subsequent sinus beat ($A_3$) after the PAC ($A_1A_2 + A_2A_3$) equals twice the spontaneous sinus interval ($2 \times A_1A_1$). Further, the return cycle length ($R_1$), or $A_2A_3$, in this example is greater than the spontaneous sinus cycle length. The second return cycle ($R_2$), or $A_3A_4$, will equal the basic (B) sinus cycle length if there has been no disturbance of sinus nodal automaticity and the sinus rate has minimal normal variability. An example of a compensatory pause produced at electrophysiologic testing is shown in Fig. 2-2.

Reset occurs when a PAC conducts through the atriosinus junction and depolarizes the sinus nodal pacemaker (Fig. 2-1, II).[5,6] In unusual circumstances, a PAC can cause reset without actual capture of the sinus nodal pacemaker.[7-9] Reset tends to happen with a PAC that occurs at 70 percent or less of the spontaneous sinus cycle length. Mathematically, reset is defined as the sum of $A_1A_2$ plus $A_2A_3$ being less than twice $A_1A_1$ with the $A_2A_3$ interval greater than $A_1A_1$. Reset is an excellent example of concealed conduction. The PAC is manifest but its conduction into the sinus nodal region is not apparent on the ECG. However, reset demonstrates that the PAC

### I. Compensatory Pause

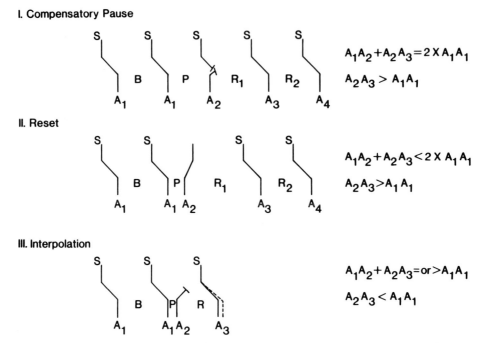

$$A_1A_2 + A_2A_3 = 2 \times A_1A_1$$

$$A_2A_3 > A_1A_1$$

### II. Reset

$$A_1A_2 + A_2A_3 < 2 \times A_1A_1$$

$$A_2A_3 > A_1A_1$$

### III. Interpolation

$$A_1A_2 + A_2A_3 = or > A_1A_1$$

$$A_2A_3 < A_1A_1$$

*Figure 2-1*   Schematic of effects of premature atrial complexes on sinus nodal automaticity. The ladder diagram represents conduction from the sinus node (S) to the atrium (A) showing conduction time by the diagonal line connecting S with A. Block is represented by a small horizontal line perpendicular to the normal conduction line. With interpolation, the third sinus impulse conducts without increased anterograde delay from the sinus node to atrium, as represented by the solid line, or with some additional conduction delay shown by the dotted line. (Key: Basic cycle length = B; premature cycle length = P; first return cycle = $R_1$; second return cycle length = $R_2$.) (See text for further details.)

affected the sinus nodal pacemaker, yielding an earlier-than-expected return complex ($A_3$). Assuming no change in sinus nodal automaticity caused by the PAC, $A_3A_4$ will approximately equal $A_1A_1$ (Fig. 2-3).

Interpolation is present when a PAC neither enters the sinus node to reset the pacemaker nor prevents the spontaneous sinus depolarization from activating the atrium (Fig. 2-1, III). Complete interpolation, which is relatively rare, occurs when the PAC has no influence on sinus nodal automaticity or sinoatrial conduction and therefore the $A_1A_2$ plus $A_2A_3$ interval equals the spontaneous sinus interval, $A_1A_1$. The $A_2A_3$ interval necessarily must be less than $A_1A_1$ in this instance. More commonly, a PAC

will affect automaticity, conduction, or both, and the $A_1A_2$ plus $A_2A_3$ interval is greater than $A_1A_1$; this is referred to as *incomplete interpolation* (Fig. 2-4). In Fig. 2-4, the second return cycle ($A_3A_4$) is substantially longer than expected, presumably due to depression of sinus nodal automaticity by the PAC—another manifestation of concealed conduction.[10,11] Sinus node reentry may also occur when a very early PAC conducts into the sinus node and produces one or more reentrant complexes.[12-16] With one reentrant complex, the $A_1A_2$ plus $A_2A_3$ interval is less than the basic $A_1A_1$ sinus cycle length. Spontaneous sinus node echo beats are rarely observed on a routine 12-lead ECG or even during 24-h ambulatory recordings. Sinus node echo beats and

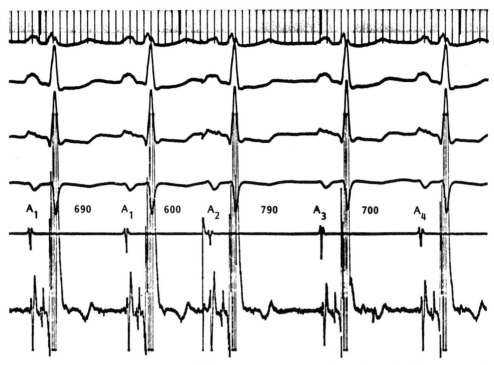

*Figure 2-2* Complete compensatory pause following a premature atrial complex. Simultaneous recordings of surface ECG and intracardiac electrograms from the right atrium and His bundle area (*top to bottom*). The sinus cycle length ($A_1A_1$) is 690 ms with a premature atrial complex ($A_2$) introduced at an $A_1A_2$ interval of 600 ms. The return sinus complex ($A_3$) has an $A_2A_3$ interval of 790 ms, yielding a complete compensatory pause (790 + 600 = 1390 ms). The second return cycle ($A_3A_4$) essentially equals $A_1A_1$, demonstrating no effect on sinus nodal automaticity from $A_2$. (See text for further details.)

short runs of sinus node reentry are occasionally initiated at electrophysiologic study, but sinus node reentry is rarely a significant clinical problem.

### Effects on Atrioventricular Conduction

Premature atrial complexes can conduct to the ventricles with or without prolongation of the PR interval or may be blocked in the AV node or less commonly the His-Purkinje system (HPS). Conduction of a PAC over the AV conduction system depends on several factors, including the prematurity of the ectopic complex, the sinus cycle length, and conduction characteristics of the AV node and HPS. Bundle branch block and aberrancy are discussed in greater

detail in Chap. 3. In general, only PACs that occur late in diastole are able to conduct with no increase in the PR interval. When conduction delay occurs, it is usually in the AV node (Fig. 2-5). In this example, the P wave of the PAC is inscribed on the preceding T wave (P on T). Note that AV nodal conduction time represented by the AH interval is longer in the PAC than the normal sinus complexes. In this example, the actual PR interval of the PAC is difficult to determine from the surface electrocardiogram because the P wave is obscured by the preceding T wave. AV nodal delay with a PAC is clearly identified from the intracardiac His bundle electrogram (HBE) recording.[17-19] One measurement that is sometimes useful to identify AV delay with

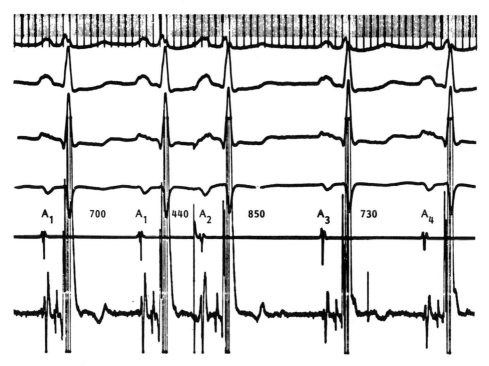

*Figure 2-3*  Sinus nodal reset with premature atrial complex in same patient noted in Fig. 2-2. An earlier PAC with an $A_1A_2$ interval of 440 ms is followed by an $A_2A_3$ return cycle of 850 ms demonstrating sinus nodal reset. The interval $A_1A_3$ = 1290 ms, considerably shorter than 1,400 ms expected with a complete compensatory pause. $A_3A_4$ is essentially unchanged.

a PAC is a comparison of the isoelectric segment between the end of the T wave and the beginning of the QRS complex of the PAC with the isoelectric segment of the PR interval of the preceding sinus complex. Although the end of the P wave is not certain in many of these instances, a longer isoelectric interval of the PAC compared with the normal PR interval certainly suggests AV conduction delay as seen in Fig. 2-5. Examples of conducted and blocked premature atrial complexes in the same patient are shown in Fig. 2-6. In ECG strip A, PACs are responsible for the fifth and eighth QRS depolarizations. A blocked PAC occurs in ECG strip B, as noted by the arrowhead. Electrocardiographic recording C is complex and demonstrates Mobitz type I second-degree AV block with a blocked PAC noted by the arrow. In this example, there are two consecutively nonconducted P waves, the first due

to AV nodal Wenckebach block and the second caused by a PAC. Of note, the interval between the sinus P wave and PAC in ECG strip C is similar to the PAC interval in ECG recording A (Fig. 2-6).

In some instances block may occur in the HPS. This can be physiologic, for example, in a patient with excellent AV nodal conduction who has a slow heart rate in which a relatively early PAC conducts through the AV node but blocks in or below the His bundle (see Chap. 3). In some patients with abnormal His-Purkinje conduction, a PAC can block within the HPS at a relatively long premature interval even in the presence of a normal or accelerated supraventricular rate (Fig. 2-7).[19-21] A relatively rare example of infra-His block in a patient during atrial fibrillation is shown in Fig. 2-8.

Concealed conduction can also occur with a blocked PAC (Fig. 2-9). In this example, taken from

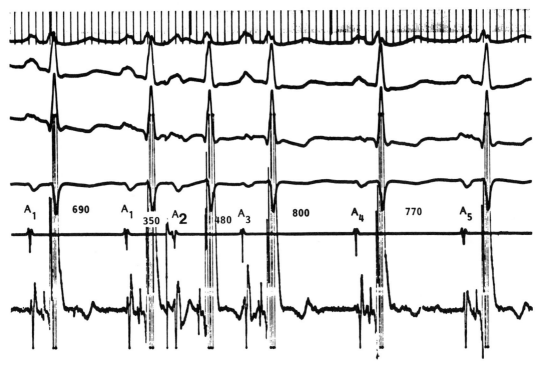

*Figure 2-4*  Interpolated premature atrial complex in same patient demonstrated in Fig. 2-2. A premature atrial complex is introduced with an $A_1A_2$ interval of 350 ms and the subsequent sinus impulse occurs with an $A_2A_3$ interval of 480 ms. The combined $A_1$ to $A_3$ interval of 830 ms is greater than the baseline cycle length of 690 ms, demonstrating incomplete interpolation. This is probably due to depression of sinus nodal automaticity with some delay in the sinus nodal impulse following $A_2$, and sinus nodal depression is demonstrated by the prolonged $A_3A_4$ and even $A_4A_5$ intervals compared with $A_1A_1$. Some contribution from an increase in sinoatrial conduction time might also have contributed to the greater-than-expected $A_2A_3$ interval had this been completely interpolated.

an electrophysiologic study, the right atrium is initially paced at cycle length 400 ms (150/min) and 2:1 AV nodal block is present. Note on the HBE that the second and fourth atrial impulses are not followed by a His bundle depolarization, indicating block in the AV node. The conducted beats have an AV node conduction time of 100 ms. The last two paced complexes are at cycle length 800 ms, or twice that of the preceding cycle length. Conduction of each atrial complex occurs, and the AH interval is now 80 ms, or 20 ms shorter than conducted atrial beats during the 2:1 conduction pattern on the left-hand side of this figure. The prolonged AH interval in the presence of 2:1 block is due to penetration of the nonconducted atrial complex into the AV node,

resulting in a wake of refractoriness that is encountered by the next conducted beat, causing a prolongation of AV nodal conduction time. This is a classic example of anterograde concealed AV nodal conduction.[3,21,22] Concealed conduction of a PAC into an accessory pathway is noted in Fig. 2-10.[23]

## Premature Junctional Complexes

Premature junctional complexes originate from areas of the AV node and His bundle that are capable of automaticity. In a given patient, it is not possible

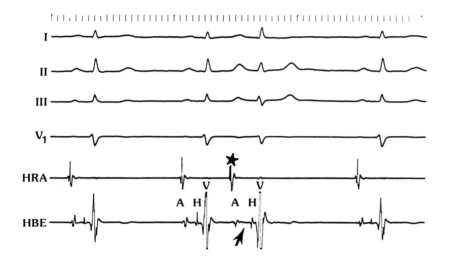

*Figure 2-5* Prolonged AV nodal conduction time with a premature atrial complex. The star represents the PAC and the arrow demonstrates an increase in AH interval (AV nodal conduction time) bcompared with the preceding two complexes. (Key: HRA = high right atrium; HBE = His bundle electrogram.)

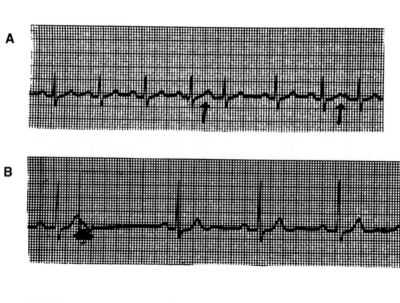

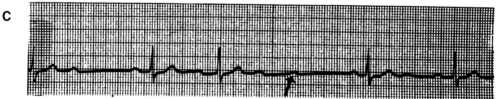

*Figure 2-6* Electrocardiographic rhythm strips in a patient with conducted and blocked premature atrial complexes. The arrows in *A* demonstrate conducted PACs. The arrowhead in *B* shows a nonconducted PAC. In *C* a PAC (*arrow*) follows a nonconducted P wave that is the culmination of an AV nodal Wenckebach sequence.

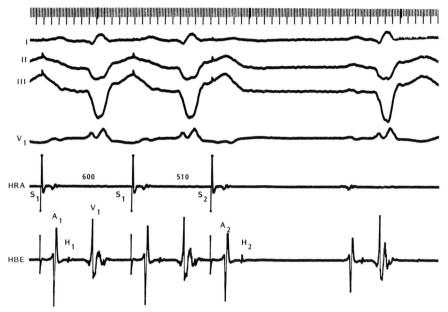

***Figure 2-7***   Premature atrial complex with block below the recorded His potential. This patient had baseline right bundle branch block with left anterior fascicular block and the high right atrium (HRA) was paced for 8 beats at 600 ms (100/min). A PAC was introduced at an interval of 510 ms and on the HBE block is noted after His depolarization ($H_2$). Block below the His bundle at this heart rate and with such a long premature interval is abnormal and identifies pathology in the HPS.

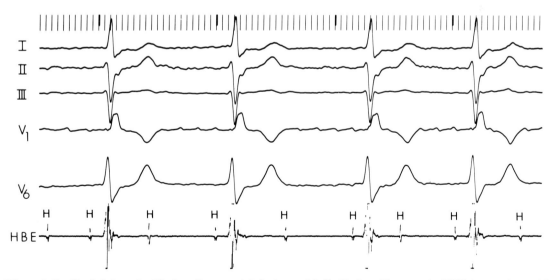

***Figure 2-8***   Block below the His bundle potential during atrial fibrillation. Note on the HBE in a patient with right bundle branch block with left anterior fascicular block that conduction block occurs below some His potentials. This relatively rare observation signifies marked abnormality of the HPS. Of note, this patient had a history of syncope and required permanent ventricular pacing.

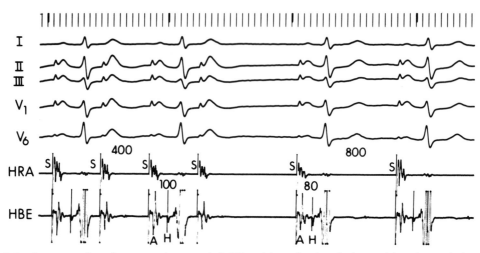

***Figure 2-9***    Demonstration of anterograde concealed AV nodal conduction during atrial pacing techniques. (See text for details.)

to identify the precise origin of these complexes even with intracardiac electrograms. Most junctional premature beats are manifest and produce a retrograde P wave, QRS complex, or both. Concealed junctional premature complexes can occur and produce many interesting ECG phenomena.[24,25]

Figure 2-11 shows two ECG abnormalities resulting from junctional premature beats. The arrow points to a retrograde P wave occurring near the end of the T wave. It would not be possible to diagnose this deflection conclusively as a P wave unless other areas of the ECG strip demonstrated normal T-wave morphology, as noted in QRS complexes four and five on the right. Under most circumstances, one would designate these as PACs, but an alternative explanation should be considered after analysis of the entire ECG recording. Note the sudden, unexpected PR prolongation (*arrowhead*) in the fifth conducted QRS complex. There is no sudden change in the sinus rate, and autonomic influences rarely cause such a sudden isolated change in the PR interval without affecting the sinus rate (see Chap. 1).[26,27] Thus, a likely diagnosis for both phenomena is junctional premature complexes with retrograde conduction to the atrium manifesting as P waves on the ECG (first three QRS complexes) and a concealed junctional premature complex that does not conduct

to the ventricle or atrium but causes conduction delay in the AV node with sudden PR prolongation (fifth QRS complex). Confirmation of this diagnosis is shown with His bundle electrocardiography (Fig. 2-12).

Junctional premature complexes often occur in patients with underlying His-Purkinje disease and can simulate Mobitz type II second-degree AV block (Fig. 2-13). In this simultaneously recorded 12-lead ECG, note that the fourth P wave does not conduct to the ventricles and the preceding PR intervals are constant. This is consistent with Mobitz type II second-degree AV block, but further analysis of this ECG shows that the fifth QRS complex is a junctional premature beat. Thus, a reasonable alternative diagnosis is AV block due to a concealed junctional premature complex, confirmed by His bundle electrocardiography (Fig. 2-14).

## *Premature Ventricular Complexes*

Premature ventricular complexes (PVCs) are ubiquitous and increase in frequency with age and the presence and degree of heart disease. We do not recommend therapy to suppress PVCs unless they

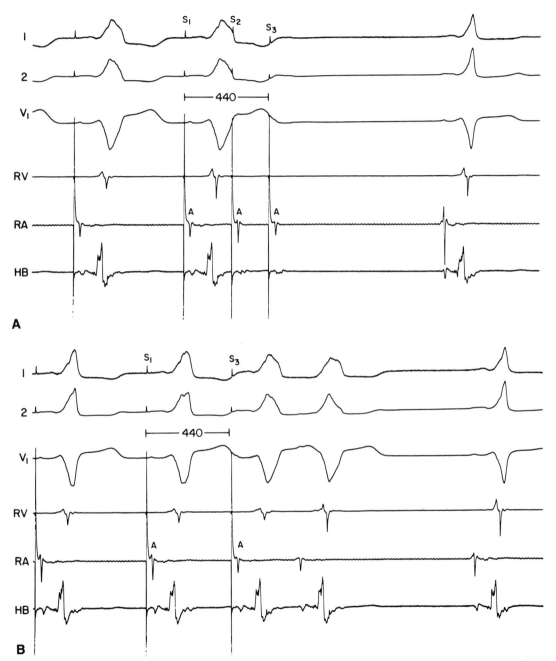

*Figure 2-10*   Anterograde concealed conduction into an accessory pathway. *A.* An atrial premature complex (S₂) after the basic drive beat (S₁) is blocked. A second premature complex (S₃) with a S₁S₃ interval of 440 ms is also blocked. Note the marked preexcitation on the drive beats. *B.* The S₂ is omitted, and now the S₃ with the same S₁S₃ interval of 440 ms conducts over the accessory pathway. This finding suggests concealed conduction of S₂ into the accessory pathway in panel *A.* *(Reproduced with permission from Ref. 23).*

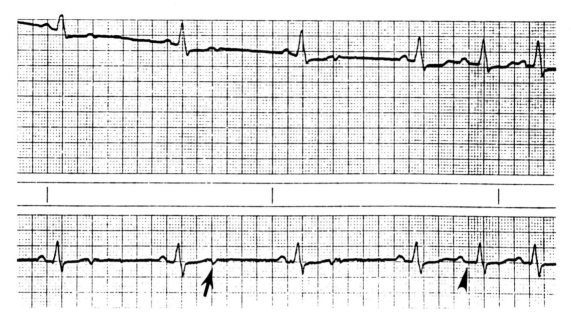

***Figure 2-11***   Junctional premature complexes with retrograde atrial activation (*arrow*) and concealed conduction with manifest prolonged PR interval (*arrowhead*). (See text for details.)

produce intolerable symptoms, which is unusual. A PVC can conduct retrogradely over the ventriculoatrial conduction system to the atrium or can be blocked in the AV node or, less commonly, in the HPS. Even when a PVC activates the atrium

retrogradely, it is uncommon to have reset of the sinus node. Thus, under most circumstances a PVC yields a compensatory pause, as noted below. The inability of a PVC to reset the sinus node is due to the conduction times involved. As an example,

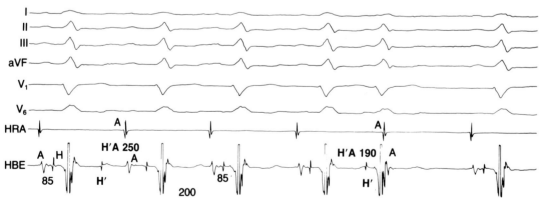

***Figure 2-12***   Junctional premature complexes diagnosed at electrophysiologic study. Same patient as in Fig. 2-11. The first complex conducts with a normal AH interval of 85 ms. A junctional premature complex (H′) conducts neither to the atrium or ventricle but prolongs AV nodal refractoriness with a sudden prolongation of the PR interval and AH interval of the next sinus-conducted complex. A second junctional premature complex is noted, with anterograde conduction yielding the fifth QRS complex in this tracing. The H′A interval of 190 ms is too short to allow recovery of AV nodal conduction such that the next sinus impulse blocks in the AV node. Note that only anterograde conduction occurred with this premature beat.

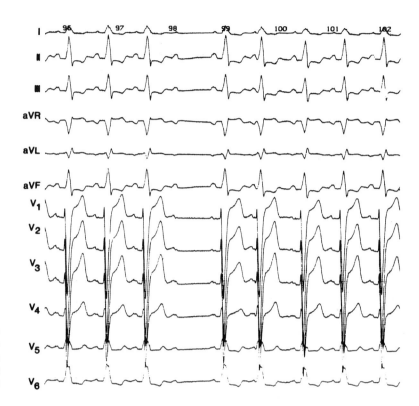

*Figure 2-13* Twelve-lead simultaneous ECG demonstrating sudden loss of conduction and a junctional premature complex. (See text for details.)

suppose a PVC occurs 400 ms after the last conducted QRS complex in a patient with a sinus cycle length of 840 ms (71/min). If the PR interval of the beat prior to the PVC is 160 ms, then a total of 560 ms have already elapsed and the next sinus impulse is expected in approximately 280 ms. Retrograde conduction times are highly variable, but for this example we will allow 120 ms for the PVC to activate the atrial septum and another 30 ms to reach the high right atrium near the sinus node. By these calculations, the atrium near the sinus node is prematurely activated approximately 130 ms prior to activation of this area by the next sinus complex. It would be highly unlikely for an atrial depolarization this late to effect reset in the sinus node, and therefore a complete compensatory pause would ensue. Depending on the circumstances, it would certainly be possible for some PVCs to produce a noncompensatory pause.

Figure 2-15 demonstrates the effect of PVCs on

subsequent AV conduction. When a PVC blocks retrogradely in the AV node, interpolation is uncommon but concealed conduction is often present. Concealed conduction occurs when the PVC enters the HPS and AV node retrogradely but does not conduct to the atrium.[4,21,28–30] There is an increase in refractoriness of these tissues and the next sinus impulse either does not conduct to the ventricle or conducts with PR prolongation. Without doubt, the most common area of anterograde block following a PVC is in the AV node (Fig. 2-16). Note in this example that the PVC does not conduct to the atrium and the next sinus impulse blocks without depolarization of the His bundle, confirming block in the AV node. Very uncommonly in our experience, anterograde block following a PVC occurs below the recorded His bundle potential (Fig. 2-17). Note that in this example the nonconducted second sinus complex has an increase in the AH interval (*arrow*), demonstrating concealed conduction of the PVC not

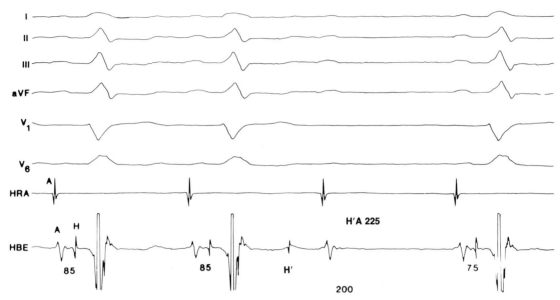

*Figure 2-14*   Electrophysiologic correlation of apparent heart block seen in Fig. 2-13. Note that following the second sinus conducted beat, a "concealed" premature junctional complex (H′) is present without conduction retrograde to the atrium or anterograde to the ventricles. The H′A interval of 225 ms is too short to allow recovery of anterograde AV nodal conduction and thus the next sinus P wave blocks in the AV node. This simulates Mobitz type II second-degree heart block. The last AH interval of 75 ms is slightly shorter than the baseline AH interval of 85 ms. This was probably due to some recovery of AV nodal conduction after the prolonged pause, but one cannot rule out with certainty a junctional complex that occurred fortuitously 10 ms earlier than when normal conduction would have been expected. The former explanation is more likely.

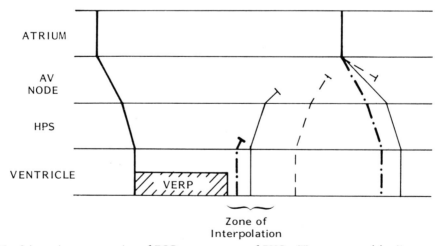

*Figure 2-15*   Schematic representation of ECG consequences of PVCs. These are noted by lines starting in the ventricle with retrograde conduction block in the HPS (*dash-dot*) and AV node (*solid and dashed lines*). Block is represented by a short perpendicular line. (Key: VERP = ventricular effective refractory period.) Each retrograde line is paired with a subsequent similar line denoting anterograde conduction. (See text for details.)

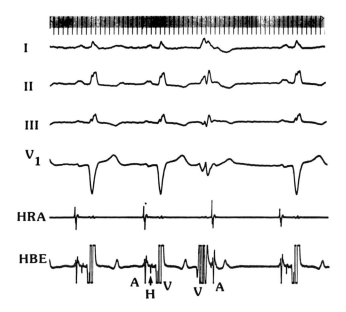

*Figure 2-16*   Premature ventricular complex with complete compensatory pause. Following the PVC, the sinus complex does not conduct to the His bundle, demonstrating increased refractoriness in the AV node and block due to concealed conduction from the PVC into this structure.

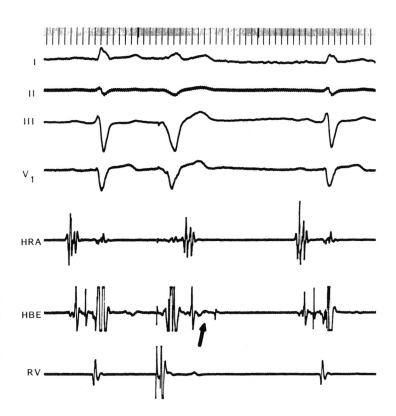

*Figure 2-17*   Premature ventricular complex with complete compensatory pause. A PVC introduced at electrophysiologic study is followed by a sinus impulse that conducts through the AV node with an increase in the AH interval (*arrow*) but subsequent block below the His potential. (Key: RV = right ventricle electrogram.) (See text for details.)

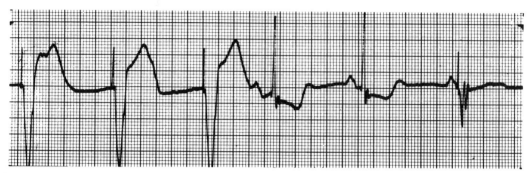

*Figure 2-18*    Concealed conduction during ventricular paced rhythm. (See text for details.)

only into the HPS but also into the AV node. Another demonstration of concealed conduction is shown in Fig. 2-18. The initial three QRS complexes are ventricular paced beats. Note that the PR interval after the third paced QRS complex is prolonged, compared with the subsequent PR interval. The presumption is that the paced ventricular complex conducted into the AV node and HPS system retrogradely, which is concealed, and the subsequent prolonged PR interval is a manifestation of the concealed conduction. The concept of concealed conduction is very important and explains many

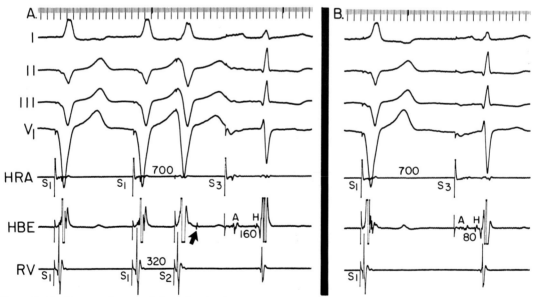

*Figure 2-19*    Retrograde concealed conduction demonstrated by electrophysiologic pacing techniques. Simultaneous tracings from top to bottom are ECG leads I, II, III, and VI, with intracardiac tracings from the HRA, HBE, and RV. In panel *A*, the right atrium and right ventricle are paced simultaneously for an 8-beat drive train and a premature ventricular complex ($S_2$) is introduced at an interval of 320 ms. The PVC is followed by a atrial paced complex ($S_3$) with an interval from $S_1$ to $S_3$ of 700 ms. The arrow points to retrograde His activation and undoubtedly subsequent conduction into the AV node. The $S_3$ complex has an AH interval of 160 ms. In panel *B* the last beat of the drive train is noted but $S_2$ was deleted. The $S_1S_3$ interval was kept constant and the AH interval of $S_3$ is now 80 ms, 80 ms shorter than noted when $S_2$ is present (panel *A*). The only difference in panel *B* is the lack of the PVC, and this demonstrates conclusively that the PVC did conduct into the AV node.

ECG phenomena. It can be studied in detail at electrophysiologic study,[30] an example of which is shown in Fig. 2-19.

As previously stated, interpolated PVCs are uncommon, as explained by a more in-depth analysis of Fig. 2-15. Several requisite conditions must be present for interpolation to occur. These include retrograde block of the PVC, a close-coupled PVC, a relatively slow sinus rate, and reasonably good anterograde AV conduction. As noted in Fig. 2-15, there is a relatively narrow potential zone of interpolation, with ventricular refractoriness defining the inner limits and concealed conduction with subsequent anterograde block closing the outer limits (*dashed line*). Slower heart rates will prolong ventricular refractoriness by a small amount, disallowing earlier PVCs; in our experience, however, the increase in ventricular refractoriness is relatively minor compared with the resultant longer time for recovery of anterograde AV refractoriness and subsequent interpolation during slower rates. For these reasons it is unusual to observe interpolated PVCs in the presence of

relatively fast sinus rates. In fact, we have observed this many times in the electrophysiology laboratory when induced PVCs are interpolated with relatively slow but not faster sinus rates.

Incomplete interpolation is shown in Fig. 2-20. Sinus arrhythmia is present with the first $A_1A_1$ interval of 1350 ms (44/min). Note that the AH interval after the PVC is 225 ms, compared with 165 ms for the normal sinus complex. The increase in AH interval is a manifestation of concealed conduction of the PVC into the AV node and would be represented schematically by the solid line in Fig. 2-15. For complete interpolation to occur, there would have to be full recovery of AV node and His-Purkinje refractoriness, which is represented by the dot-dashed line of Fig. 2-15. This is very uncommon in our experience.

It has been known for decades that an inverse relationship exists between the interval from the PVC to the next P wave (RP) and the subsequent PR interval. Thus, the shorter the RP interval, the longer the next PR interval. The prolongation of the

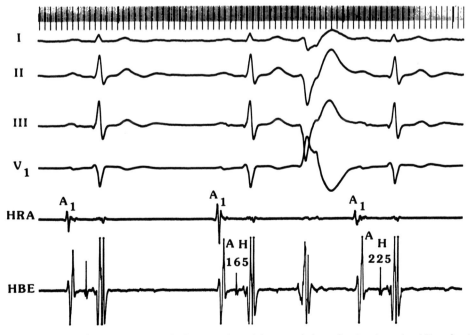

*Figure 2-20*   Interpolated premature ventricular complex with concealed conduction into the AV node. (See text for details.)

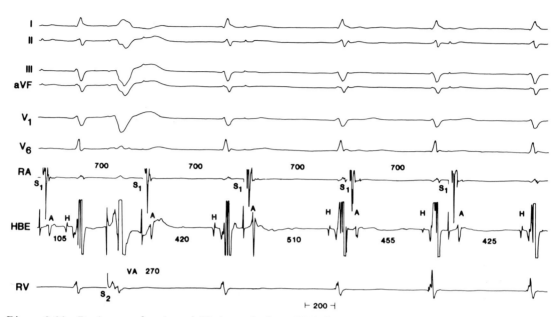

*Figure 2-23*   Persistence of prolonged PR interval after a PVC demonstrating dual AV nodal physiology. (See text for details.)

while pacing the atrium at a constant cycle length of 700 ms ($S_1$). The AH interval is 105 ms during baseline pacing, as noted by the first complex. A PVC ($S_2$) was introduced, with a VA interval of 270 ms measured to the next atrial depolarization in the His bundle lead. The subsequent AH interval markedly increased to 420 ms and remained long,

with some variation between 420 and 510 ms, until atrial pacing was discontinued. In our experience, this persistence of marked AH or PR prolongation is diagnostic of dual AV nodal physiology. Concealed retrograde conduction into the AV node fast pathway from the slow anterograde pathway is a likely explanation for this finding.

## References

1. Engelmann TW: Beobachtungen und Versuche am suspendirten Herzen. *Pflügers Arch* 56:149, 1894.
2. Erlanger J: On the physiology of heart-block in mammals, with especial reference to the causation of Stokes-Adams disease. *J Exp Med* 7:676, 1905.
3. Lewis T, Master AM: Observations upon conduction in the mammalian heart. *Heart* 12:209, 1925.
4. Langendorf R: Concealed A-V conduction: The effect of blocked impulses on the formation and conduction of subsequent impulses. *Am Heart J* 35:542, 1948.
5. Langendorf R et al: Atrial parasystole with interpolation. Observations on prolonged sinoatrial conduction. *Am Heart J* 63:649, 1962.
6. Strauss HC et al: Premature atrial stimulation as a key to the understanding of sinoatrial conduction in man. Presentation of data and critical review of the literature. *Circulation* 47:86, 1973.
7. Prystowsky EN et al: An analysis of the effects of acetylcholine on conduction and refractoriness in the rabbit sinus node. *Circ Res* 44:112, 1979.
8. Miller HC, Strauss HC: Measurement of sinoatrial conduction time by premature atrial stimulation in the rabbit. *Circ Res* 35:935, 1974.
9. Steinbeck G et al: Sinus node response to premature atrial stimulation in the rabbit studied with multiple microelectrode impalements. *Circ Res* 43:695, 1978.

10. Bonke FIM et al: Effect of an early atrial premature beat on activity of the sinoatrial node and atrial rhythm in the rabbit. *Circ Res* 29:704, 1971.

11. Breithardt G, Seipel L: The effects of premature atrial depolarization on sinus node automaticity in man. *Circulation* 53:920, 1976.

12. Barker PS et al: The mechanism of auricular paroxysmal tachycardia. *Am Heart J* 26:435, 1943.

13. Han J et al: Sinoatrial reciprocation in the isolated rabbit heart. *Circ Res* 22:355, 1968.

14. Paulay KL et al: Sinus node re-entry: An in vivo demonstration in the dog. *Circ Res* 32:455, 1973.

15. Narula OS: Sinus node re-entry. *Circulation* 50:1114, 1974.

16. Allessie MA, Bonke FIM: Direct demonstration of sinus node reentry in the rabbit heart. *Circ Res* 44:557, 1979.

17. Damato AN et al: Study of heart block in man using His bundle recordings. *Circulation* 39:297, 1969.

18. Narulo OS et al: Localization of A-V conduction defects in man by recording of the His bundle electrogram. *Am J Cardiol* 25:228, 1970.

19. Damato AN et al: A study of atrioventricular conduction in man using premature atrial stimulation and His bundle recordings. *Circulation* 40:61, 1969.

20. Wit AL et al: Patterns of atrioventricular conduction in the human heart. *Circ Res* 27:345, 1970.

21. Prystowsky EN, Page RL: Electrophysiology and autonomic influences of the human atrioventricular node, in *Electrophysiology of the Sino-atrial and Atrioventricular Nodes.* New York, Liss, 1988, p 259.

22. Steinman RT, Lehmann MH: Beat-to-beat changes in atrioventricular nodal excitability and its modulation by concealed conduction during functional 2:1 block in man. *Circulation* 76:759, 1987.

23. Klein GJ et al: Concealed conduction in accessory pathways: An important determinant of the expression of arrhythmias in patients with Wolff-Parkinson-White syndrome. *Circulation* 70:402, 1984.

24. Langerdorf R, Mehlman JS: Blocked (non-conducted) A-V nodal premature systoles imitating first and second degree A-V block. *Am Heart J* 34:500, 1947.

25. Rosen KM et al: Pseudo A-V block secondary to premature non-propagated His bundle depolarizations: Documentation by His bundle electrocardiography. *Circulation* 42:367, 1970.

26. Prystowsky EN et al: Effect of autonomic blockade on ventricular refractoriness and atrioventricular nodal conduction in humans: Evidence supporting a direct cholinergic action on ventricular muscle refractoriness. *Circ Res* 49:511, 1981.

27. Page RL et al: Effect of continuous enhanced vagal tone on atrioventricular nodal and sinoatrial nodal function in humans. *Circ Res* 68:1614, 1991.

28. Moe GK et al: Aberrant A-V impulse propagation in the dog heart: A study of functional bundle branch block. *Circ Res* 16:261, 1965.

29. Moore EN: Microelectrode studies on retrograde concealment of multiple premature ventricular responses. *Circ Res* 10:88, 1967.

30. Schuilenburg RM: Patterns of V-A conduction in the human heart in the presence of normal and abnormal A-V conduction, in Wellens HJJ, Lie KI, Janse MJ (eds): *The Conduction System of the Heart.* Philadelphia, Pennsylvania, Lea and Febiger, 1976, p 485.

31. Moe GK et al: An appraisal of "supernormal" A-V conduction. *Circulation* 38:5, 1968.

32. Meijler FL et al: Comparative atrioventricular conduction and its consequences for atrial fibrillation in man, in Kulbertus HE, Olsson SB, Schlepper M (eds): *Atrial Fibrillation.* Mölndal, Sweden, Hassle, 1981, p 72.

33. Langendorf R, Pick A: Concealed conduction in the A-V junction, in Dreifus and Likoff (eds): *Mechanism and Therapy of Cardiac Arrhythmias.* New York, Grune & Stratton, 1966, p 395.

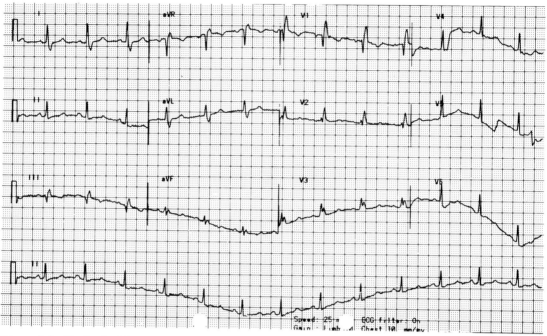

*Figure 3-1*    Twelve-lead ECG of right bundle branch block.

interventricular septum and is therefore prone to mechanical trauma—for example, catheter-induced right bundle branch block during electrophysiologic study or passage of a Swan-Ganz catheter.[4] Anatomic damage to the right bundle branch has been demonstrated at pathologic examination of the conduction system in patients with ECG evidence of right bundle branch block.[4,5] In one study of patients with ECG documentation of right bundle branch block, significant lesions of the right bundle branch were demonstrated in all patients but, interestingly, total anatomic disruption was not demonstrated in most.[5] Whether this represents very slow conduction of the right bundle branch with the inability to activate the right ventricle prior to activation of the ventricles by the left bundle branch system, as stated earlier, or indeed complete conduction disruption is not known.

Right bundle branch block is usually associated with organic heart disease. However, it can occur in apparently normal individuals, and Hiss et al.[6] reported an incidence of right bundle branch block of 1.8 per 1000 in seemingly normal U.S. Air Force personnel. In this study, the incidence of right bundle branch block increased with age.[6] The prognosis with right bundle branch block depends on the presence or absence of associated cardiovascular disease. Rotman and Triebwasser[7] reported on 394 people with right bundle branch block at the U.S. School of Aerospace Medicine; during a mean follow-up period of 10.8 years, new cases of coronary heart disease and hypertension occurred in 6 percent of these patients, and 4 percent died. Similar observations were reported by Fleg et al.[8] The Framingham Study evaluated 70 people who developed complete right bundle branch block during an 18-year follow-up.[9] In this study, the mean age at the onset of right bundle branch block was 60 years, and in 70 percent of cases at least one cardiovascular abnormality preceded the onset of right bundle branch block.

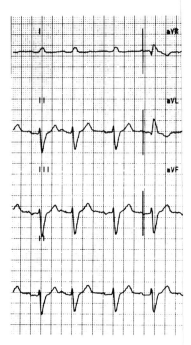

*Figure 3-5*   Twelve-lead ECG of le

left bundle branch at slower hea
reverse occurs at faster heart rat
some instances, right and left bur
aberrancy may occur at a similar h
bundle branch block aberrancy alm
with prolongation of the HV int
concomitant conduction delay in
branch. Figure 3-9 shows right bur
aberrancy and left bundle branch b
a patient with minimal change in
first two QRS complexes are condu
a premature atrial depolarization i:
right bundle branch block aberrancy
of the premature complex is 220
interval is 420 ms. Later in the rhy
premature atrial complex occurs w
coupling interval. However, this
conducted with left bundle branch
with a PR interval of 280 ms. The
PR interval most likely reflects cor

Cardiovascular mortality was approximately three times greater in the patients who developed right bundle branch block than in age-matched persons without right bundle branch block. In summary, it appears that mortality is related to the development of organic heart disease and not specifically to the conduction defect of the right bundle branch.

### Left Bundle Branch Block

The sequence of initial ventricular activation is significantly altered in left bundle branch block, and activation occurs first on the right septal surface near the base of the anterior papillary muscle of the right ventricle. Therefore, activation overall will primarily proceed from right to left, explaining the absence of the normal "septal" Q wave in ECG leads I, $V_5$, and $V_6$.[2] As noted in Table 3-1, the duration of the QRS complex is 120 ms or more and terminal activation of the epicardial surface of the left ventricle occurs near the posterolateral base (Fig. 1-5, Chap. 1).

A 12-lead ECG in a patient with complete left bundle branch block is illustrated in Fig. 3-2. Endocardial catheter mapping data from 18 patients with left bundle branch block who had either (1) no obvious organic heart disease, (2) cardiomyopathy or (3) coronary artery disease revealed the left ventricular endocardial activation sequence to be variable.[10] However, most of the endocardial surface of the left ventricle was not mapped in this study, thus precluding more precise determination of left ventricular endocardial activation. The observation of variable activation sequences may explain the differences noted in the ECG manifestations of left bundle branch block in patients.

Pathology studies in patients with complete left bundle branch block demonstrate destruction of a substantial proportion of the septal fibers of the left

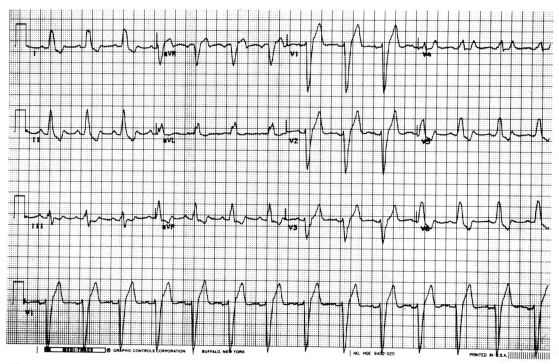

*Figure 3-2*   Twelve-lead ECG of left bundle branch block.

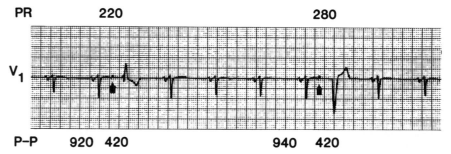

**Figure 3-9**   Premature atrial complexes with a fixed P-P interval, producing both right and left bundle branch block aberrancy. (See text for details.)

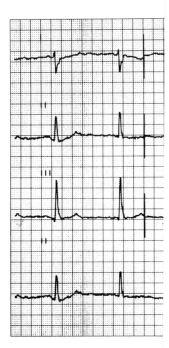

*Figure 3-4*   Twelve-lead ECG patient has 2:1 heart block, de pacemaker was required.

occurs during supraventricular able cycle lengths.[25,26] Figure bundle branch block aberrar tachyarrhythmia initiated at ele The first two QRS complexes a to the ventricles. A relatively to persistence of AV nodal blo on His bundle lead), and the closes the long pause. The r conducted with incomplete block aberrancy due to the l which increased right bundle and the subsequent relatively s val between the third and fc (long-short sequence or Ashm though left bundle branch bl occur with a long-short sequ rates refractoriness of the left b shorter than that of the right

*tion-dependent* for block that appears during slowing of heart rate because the actual heart rates at which block happens may be in the range of normal sinus rates or only relative bradycardia or tachycardia, as noted below.

Denes et al.[29] evaluated 15 patients at electrophysiologic study who demonstrated acceleration-dependent bundle branch block. Of these, 10 had left bundle branch block and 5 right bundle branch block. Of note, complete left bundle branch block occurred at a range of cycle lengths from 429 to 800 ms and complete right bundle branch block was noted at cycle lengths from 450 to 1000 ms. These

ranges of cycle lengths clearly demonstrate that block can occur in a particular patient at a relatively fast rate but one that is still considered normal sinus rhythm. A typical finding demonstrated by these authors was a hysteresis curve for the occurrence and disappearance of bundle branch block during atrial pacing. In other words, as the atrial paced rate is progressively increased, bundle branch block appears (e.g., at 100/min); but as the atrial paced rate gradually slows, disappearance of bundle branch block occurs at a paced rate *slower* than the rate required to produce block initially (e.g., at 90/min). Similar findings have been noted by others.[30,31] The

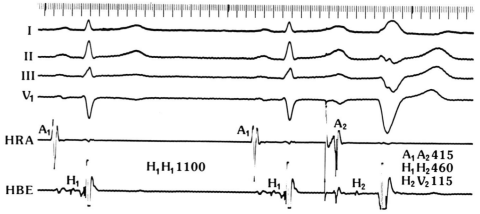

**Figure 3-10**   Premature atrial stimulus with left bundle branch block aberrancy and prolonged His-Purkinje conduction time. Note that the $H_2V_2$ interval of the premature complex is markedly prolonged at 115 ms, representing conduction delay below the His bundle deflection. It is not possible in this example to diagnose whether conduction delay occurred solely in the distal His bundle or in the His bundle and right bundle branch system, but right bundle branch conduction delay was most likely present.

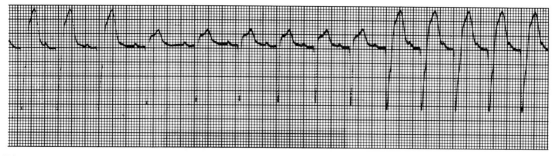

***Figure 3-11***    Acceleration-dependent left bundle branch block. The first QRS complexes in this tracing demonstrate left bundle branch block aberrancy. Carotid sinus massage was performed and the sinus rate slowed, with concomitant narrowing of the QRS complex. As the sinus rate increased, left bundle branch block aberrancy reemerged at the end of the rhythm strip.

reason that bundle branch block disappears at slower rates than it occurs is not definitely known, but several explanations have been proposed, including "fatigue" of the bundle branch during the faster-paced rates that requires some recovery for normal conduction to occur, or possibly disappearance of concealed transseptal conduction that was necessary for perpetuation of the bundle branch block at the faster rates (see below). The exact electrophysiologic mechanism for this hysteresis loop is not known.

Acceleration-dependent bundle branch block appears to occur much more commonly in the left bundle branch system.[29–31] Also, although not universal, the presence of heart disease is common in this situation.[31] Examples of acceleration-dependent bundle branch block are shown in Figs. 3-11 through 3-13. In our experience, deceleration-dependent bundle branch block is relatively rare compared with acceleration-dependent bundle branch block.

In 40 patients with rate-related intermittent bundle branch block aberrancy, four different patterns of recovery from block were characterized by Nau et al.[32] These authors[32] evaluated multiple R-R intervals during bundle branch block aberrancy and resumption of normal QRS complex conduction. Type A recovery was considered normal and demonstrated a 30- to 50-ms time period as the heart rate slowed where incomplete bundle branch block occurred. Type B recovery showed a greater range of heart rates over which complete bundle branch block persisted compared with type A, but there was still

a short time period of incomplete bundle branch block prior to recovery of the normal QRS morphology. Type C was noted to have an extension of heart rates with complete bundle branch block, but no intermittent bundle branch block was seen prior to normalization of the QRS complex. Type D was characterized by a prolonged range of heart rates for both complete bundle branch block and incomplete bundle branch block. In other words, there appeared to be a critical range of heart rates at which bundle branch block would occur, and this range could be prolonged either due to complete bundle branch block alone or to both complete bundle branch block and incomplete bundle branch block. Importantly, the clinical significance of this observation remains to be determined. In another study from these investigators,[33] it was shown that intermittent bundle branch block per se is not predictive of development of complete irreversible bundle branch block. In fact, the authors present one patient with 18 years of intermittent bundle branch block without development of complete bundle branch block. Likewise, identification of bundle branch block at one point in time at a specific heart rate does not confirm that bundle branch block will subsequently be present, and the presence of fixed bundle branch block can only be confirmed with multiple ECG observations over a substantial period of time.

The mechanism of acceleration-dependent bundle branch block aberrancy probably does not correlate in most patients with the actual duration of the

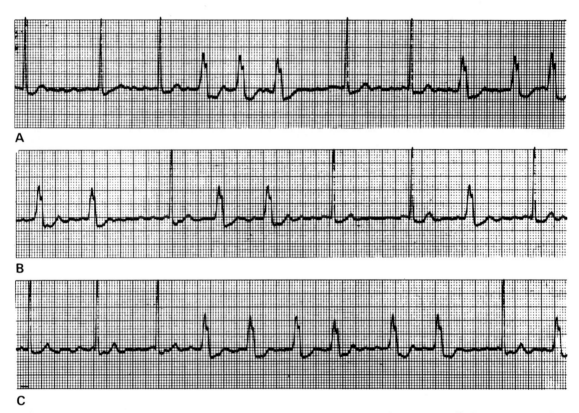

**A**

**B**

**C**

*Figure 3-12* Acceleration-dependent left bundle branch block aberrancy during atrial fibrillation. In rhythm strips *A*, *B*, and *C*, whenever the R-R interval shortens sufficiently, bundle branch block aberrancy occurs and normal ventricular conduction resumes when the pause is long enough after the last bundle branch block aberrant complex. One must differentiate this observation from premature ventricular complexes or nonsustained ventricular tachycardia. Analysis of long ECG rhythm strips usually enables one to do this, and there will be a range of heart rates over which the bundle branch block aberrancy will emerge. Further, there is no consistent coupling interval between the narrow QRS complex and the first bundle branch block complex, and grossly irregular R-R intervals are apparent between the aberrantly conducted R-R complexes. All of these strongly favor aberrancy over ventricular ectopy.

bundle branch action potential. Rather, it may represent postrepolarization refractoriness—that is, refractoriness that outlasts the duration of the action potential that can occur in diseased Purkinje tissue.[35] If one postulated that acceleration-dependent block was due only to a prolonged duration of the action potential, then this duration would have to be enormously lengthened in some patients, since block can occur at relatively slow rates—for example, 60/ min (1000 ms). Evidence supporting postrepolarization refractoriness as the mechanism for acceleration-

dependent block was presented by Davidenko and Antzelevitch.[35] These investigators examined Purkinje fibers in a sucrose gap model in which a piece of the Purkinje fiber was made progressively inexcitable. They noted in this model that greater degrees of conduction impairment yielded prolonged refractoriness, called postrepolarization refractoriness, that extended considerably beyond the end of the action potential duration. As rate increased, postrepolarization refractoriness increased, and this was due mainly to changes in membrane resistance. These

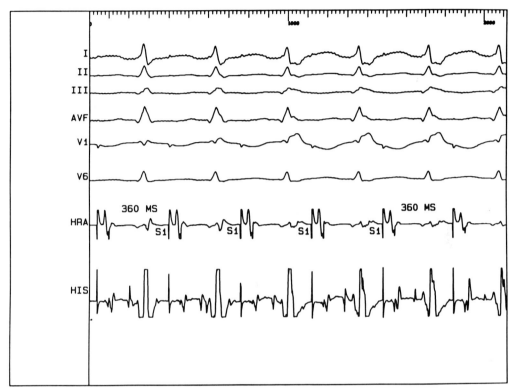

*Figure 3-13*   Acceleration-dependent right bundle branch block during atrial pacing at cycle length 360 ms. Note that the first QRS complex in this tracing represents incomplete right bundle branch block that becomes complete by the third conducted complex. Not shown on this figure are normal QRS complexes that occurred at slightly slower-paced rates. As the pacing rate progressively increased, right bundle branch block aberrancy emerged.

observations are consistent with the clinical findings in humans.

The mechanism for deceleration-dependent block is controversial. Singer et al.[36] considered block due to slow diastolic depolarization during phase four of the action potential that led to inexcitability. More recent observations of Antzelevitch et al.[37] suggest that alternative mechanisms exist, and they showed that slow diastolic depolarization is not a prerequisite for deceleration-dependent block and in certain circumstances may even facilitate conduction. Although the precise mechanism for deceleration-dependent block may differ among patients and may be multifactorial, Fisch and Miles[34] evaluated two patients who demonstrated complete and incomplete

left bundle branch block at variable heart rates; they considered these observations to support the concept of slow diastolic depolarization as the cause of block.[36]

### Repetitive Bundle Branch Block Aberrancy

Bundle branch block aberrancy that occurs after a long-short sequence can be repetitive or persistent, and this has been known for many years.[25] Figure 3-14 is a reproduction of Fig. 251 from Ref. 25 and is a recording of an atrial tachycardia in a child with an atrial rate of 290/min. In this figure, both ECG rhythm strips are displayed on top of a "Lewis" ladder diagram. In the top strip, the atrial tachycardia undergoes progressive AV conduction delay until the

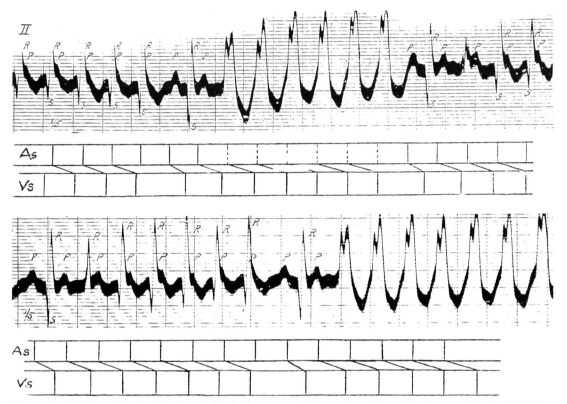

*Figure 3-14*   Repetitive bundle branch block aberrancy during atrial tachycardia. (See text for details.) *(From Lewis.*[25] *Reproduced by permission.)*

fifth P wave does not conduct to the ventricle. The subsequent P wave conducts with a relatively narrow QRS complex, but the next P wave conducts with a wide QRS complex, presumably because of the preceding relatively long R-R interval closed by a short R-R interval (long-short sequence). Each subsequent P wave is conducted with a wide QRS complex that is due to bundle branch block aberrancy, and this persists until a P wave fails to conduct to the ventricle. A similar sequence is noted on the bottom ECG rhythm strip. One needs to explain both the onset of bundle branch block aberrancy and its persistence. As noted earlier in this chapter, the long R-R interval produces a prolongation of bundle branch refractoriness due to slowing of heart rate, and the subsequent atrial complex blocks over one of the bundle branches because it falls within its

absolute refractory period. Persistence of bundle branch block aberrancy may be explained by two different mechanisms (Fig. 3-15).

One potential mechanism for persistence of aberrancy is repetitive transseptal retrograde concealed conduction from the nonblocked bundle into the blocked bundle at a site distal to anterograde block (Fig. 3-15A-2). In this example, proximal anterograde block occurs in the right bundle branch and the impulse proceeds to the ventricle over the left bundle branch system. The impulse then conducts transseptally left to right through the interventricular septum and is able to enter the distal right bundle branch and conduct up to the point of refractoriness. When this occurs, the right bundle branch refractory period will be prolonged compared with the left bundle branch because the distal portion of the right

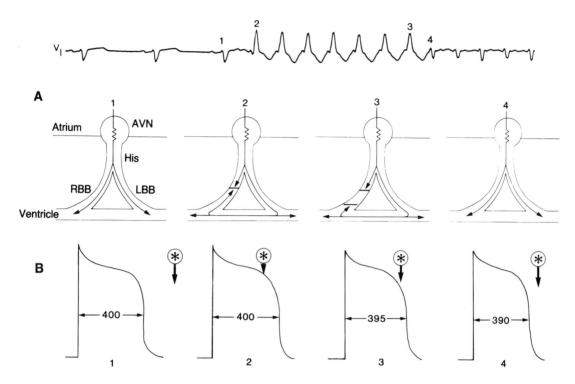

***Figure 3-15*** Potential mechanisms for repetitive bundle branch block aberrancy. In the top tracing, the first three sinus-conducted complexes demonstrate normal QRS morphology. Rapid atrial pacing was then initiated and right bundle branch block aberrancy occurred for several beats; then normalization of the QRS complex became evident. (See text for details.)

bundle branch is activated later in time than the left bundle branch. If the next anterograde impulse comes soon enough, it will conduct normally over the left bundle branch but will block once again over the right bundle branch. This pathophysiologic state can last for long periods of time and is probably the mechanism in most patients for persistent bundle branch block aberrancy during sustained supraventricular tachycardia. Transseptal concealed conduction causing repetitive bundle branch block was demonstrated by Moe and colleagues[19] in a detailed study of this phenomenon. Transseptal concealed conduction can also be responsible for persistent left bundle branch block aberrancy, but in this situation the circuit is reversed, with the initial block occurring in the proximal left bundle branch.

An alternative mechanism is depicted in Fig.

3-15*B*. The first aberrant QRS complex (number 2) occurs because of the relatively slow heart rate preceding the premature atrial complex, with prolongation of the right bundle branch action potential duration and refractoriness. Continued bundle branch block aberrancy is due to persistence of the prolonged action potential duration. Although we favor transseptal concealed conduction as the cause of sustained bundle branch block aberrancy during supraventricular tachycardia, we think that prolongation of action potential duration is the cause of block in those instances in which bundle branch block aberrancy persists for only several beats. This reasoning is supported by observations on normalization of QRS conduction.

The transition from bundle branch block aberrancy to a normal QRS complex due to loss of

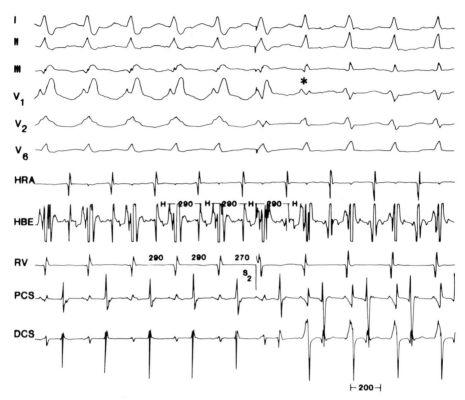

*Figure 3-16*  Termination of transseptal concealed conduction with a premature ventricular complex introduced during atrioventricular reentrant tachycardia. The first six QRS complexes demonstrate right bundle branch block aberrancy. A premature ventricular complex ($S_2$) is introduced after activation of the ventricular septum but prior to activation of the right ventricular apex. This premature ventricular complex prevents penetration into the right bundle branch retrogradely from transseptal concealed conduction and allows for a greater recovery from excitability of the right bundle branch by the time the next atrial impulse conducts to the His bundle. The seventh QRS complex (*) has minimal right bundle branch block aberrancy, and the rest of the QRS complexes are normal. (See Fig. 3-17 for a schematic representation of this phenomenon.)

transseptal concealed conduction is demonstrated in Fig. 3-15A and supported by the observations of Moe et al.[19] and Wellens and Durrer.[38] In this figure, conduction to the ventricle from atrial impulses for QRS complexes 1, 2, 3, and 4 is represented schematically below the actual ECG tracing. QRS complex 1 is conducted normally, and in this schematic the ventricle is activated over both the right bundle branch and left bundle branch to yield a narrow QRS complex. Right bundle branch block in QRS complex 2 is caused by a relatively long right bundle branch refractory period that results from the preceding slow heart rate. The schematic

shows anterograde conduction to the ventricle over the left bundle branch with subsequent transseptal conduction that penetrates into the distal right bundle branch. This mechanism persists, resulting in continued right bundle branch block aberrancy. QRS complex 3 is the last one with aberrancy, and the schematic demonstrates sudden retrograde block into the right bundle branch, which allows for earlier recovery from refractoriness in the right bundle branch. The next atrial complex can now activate the ventricles over both the right and left bundle branches; therefore no bundle branch block aberrancy occurs in QRS complex 4. We do not think this is the mechanism for short runs of bundle branch block aberrancy as noted in $V_1$, but persistent transseptal concealed conduction as the mechanism for sustained bundle branch block aberrancy is supported by the observation in Figs. 3-16 and 3-17.

Figure 3-16 is an example of atrioventricular reentry with right bundle branch block aberrancy. Note that on the right ventricular tracing a premature complex ($S_2$) is introduced simultaneously with anterograde activation of the His bundle. The next QRS complex is minimally aberrant and the subsequent complexes demonstrate normal QRS conduction, although the heart rate is unchanged. This observation supports transseptal concealed conduction for the mechanism for aberrancy, as shown schematically in Fig. 3-17. The left-hand panel represents persistent right bundle branch block aberrancy due to transseptal concealed conduction, with a consequence of continued prolongation of refractoriness of the right bundle branch due to late activation of the distal right bundle (b) from retrograde invasion. In the right-hand panel, a premature ventricular complex is introduced after anterograde block occurs in the right bundle branch but prior to transseptal conduc-

tion from the left bundle branch to the distal right bundle branch. In Fig. 3-16, the ventricular extrastimulus was introduced rather late in diastole; therefore the QRS complex still showed right bundle branch block aberrancy. In the schematic, an even earlier ventricular extrastimulus is introduced that activates the right ventricle first with a left bundle branch block morphology, and transseptal activation occurs from the right to left with even possible retrograde invasion into left bundle branch system (Fig. 3-17). Regardless, the premature ventricular complex will prevent the transseptal concealed conduction that would have occurred, and this now allows ample time for recovery of refractoriness in the right bundle branch. This "peeling" back of the refractoriness of the right bundle branch due to earlier activation from the right ventricular extrastimulus ends the perpetual sequence of transseptal concealed conduction; thus normalization of subsequent QRS complexes will occur. In almost all patients in whom a long-short pacing sequence in the electrophysiology laboratory initiates bundle branch block that persists, introduction of one or sometimes two ventricular extrastimuli can normalize

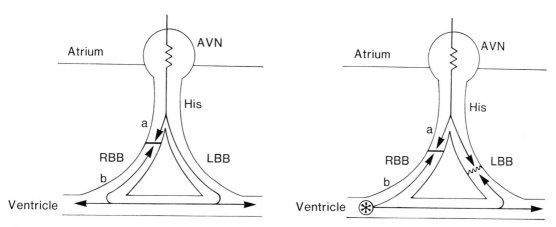

*Figure 3-17*  Schematic representation of a right ventricular extrastimulus introduced during transseptal concealed conduction into right bundle branch retrogradely that results in "peeling" back of refractoriness of the right bundle branch with subsequent normalization of conduction. In the figure, the proximal right bundle branch is represented by "a" and the distal right bundle branch by "b." The left-hand panel shows anterograde block in "a," followed by retrograde activation of the distal right bundle noted by "b." In the right-hand panel, earlier activation of "b" occurs with the right ventricular extrastimulus; therefore recovery from excitability occurs sooner, resulting in a "peeling" of refractoriness of the right bundle branch. (See text for details.)

the QRS complex, with continuation of tachycardia strongly suggesting that transseptal concealed conduction is the mechanism in these cases.

Normalization of the QRS complex due to progressive shortening of action potential duration is illustrated in Fig. 3-15*B*. QRS complex 2 demonstrates right bundle branch block aberrancy because the atrial premature complex arrives at the right bundle branch during the absolute refractory period. A progressive shortening of action potential duration occurs at the newly established faster heart rate, and there is enough shortening from QRS complex 3 to QRS complex 4 for the atrial impulse to conduct over the right bundle branch, normalizing QRS morphology. Evidence to support progressive shortening of action potential duration as the mechanism for disappearance of aberrancy noted in this figure is shown in Fig. 3-18, reproduced from Miles and Prystowsky.[39] In this study, the effect of the duration of the atrial drive train at a new faster heart rate on right bundle branch refractoriness was studied. Figure 3-18 demonstrates the mean cumulative shortening of the right bundle branch refractory period at the new faster heart rate. As can be seen from this figure, the right bundle branch refractory period progressively shortened by a mean duration of approximately 15 ms, and one-third of the shortening occurred within the first eight complexes at the new heart rate. Thus, it is easy to understand how bundle branch block aberrancy can disappear after several beats at a faster heart rate due to progressive shortening of the action potential duration in lieu of transseptal concealed conduction suddenly failing for one complex.

In summary, bundle branch block aberrancy that occurs with a premature interval that follows a preceding relatively long interval is due to prolonged refractoriness of the blocked bundle because of the preceding slow heart rate. Sustained aberrant conduction is explained best in our opinion by transseptal concealed conduction in most instances, whereas normalization of aberrancy within several complexes at the new faster rate is most likely due to progressive shortening of action potential duration.

## Mechanisms to Convert Wide QRS Complex to Narrow QRS Complex

In most instances, the ECG observation that requires explanation is the mechanism for the sudden appearance of a wide QRS complex. Just as important, although not as frequently encountered, is the differential diagnosis for sudden and seemingly unexpected normalization of the QRS complex in a patient with preceding wide QRS conduction. Table 3-2 lists many of the mechanisms that explain the sudden transition from wide to narrow QRS complex conduction. The first three mechanisms—change in heart rate, peeling back of refractoriness, and rate-dependent progressive shortening of bundle branch refractoriness—have been explained in detail in this chapter; the fourth and fifth mechanisms, dealing with gap phenomenon and supernormality, are described in Chap. 4.

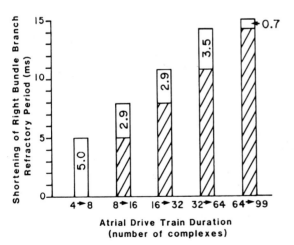

*Figure 3-18*  Demonstration of progressive shortening of bundle branch refractoriness over time at a newly established faster heart rate. (See text for details.) *(From Miles and Prystowsky.[39] Reproduced by permission.)*

*Table 3-2   Mechanisms to Convert Wide QRS Complex to Narrow QRS*

Change in heart rate
   Increase rate (deceleration-dependent block)
   Decrease rate (acceleration-dependent block)

"Peel" back refractoriness (transseptal concealed conduction)

Rate-dependent progressive shortening of bundle branch refractoriness

Gap phenomenon

Supernormality

Loss of preexcitation

PVC ipsilateral to bundle branch block

Equal conduction delay in both bundle branches

Intermittent ventricular preexcitation is demonstrated in Fig. 3-19. In this patient, during a constant atrial paced rate, the first and fourth QRS complexes are conducted with a narrow QRS morphology, but the second, third, and fifth QRS complexes are wide due to conduction over an accessory pathway. Note in the His bundle lead the easily identifiable His bundle depolarization between the atrial and ventricular deflections with narrow QRS complexes, which is obscured within the ventricular electrogram during conduction over the accessory pathway. Another mechanism is the occurrence of a premature ventricular complex ipsilateral to the bundle branch block. This is demonstrated in Fig. 3-20 in a patient with right bundle branch block in whom right ventricular pacing is initiated. The first

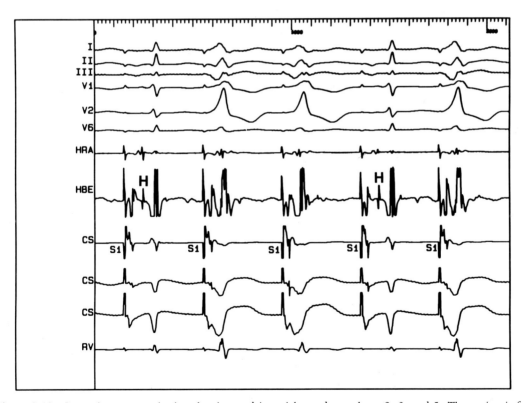

*Figure 3-19*   Intermittent preexcitation that is noted in atrial paced complexes 2, 3, and 5. The pacing is from the coronary sinus (CS). His bundle depolarization (H). (See text for details.)

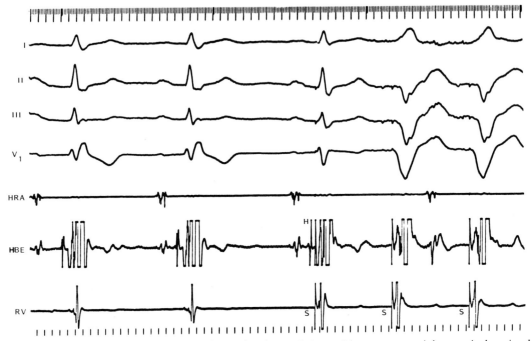

***Figure 3-20***   Normalization of right bundle branch block morphology with a premature right ventricular stimulus (S) that activates the ventricle almost simultaneously with depolarization of the left ventricle by the left bundle branch system. The last two QRS complexes demonstrate left bundle branch block morphology due to right ventricular apical pacing that captures both ventricles.

paced complex results in early activation of the right ventricle at a time nearly equal to arrival of the sinus complex through the left bundle branch to activate the left ventricle.

Thus, the third QRS complex "normalizes" (pseudonormalization), but the mechanism for this is clearly evident in the last two ventricular paced beats that demonstrate a left bundle bundle branch block QRS morphology consistent with the right ventricular pacing site. Similarly, in a patient with left bundle branch block a left ventricular premature complex critically timed could normalize QRS morphology for that complex.

A more complex mechanism for normalization of the QRS complex, equal conduction delay in both bundle branches, is illustrated in Figs. 3-21 and 3-22. In Fig. 3-21*A*, a premature atrial complex ($S_1S_2$) is introduced with a coupling interval of 380 ms with a corresponding $H_1H_2$ interval of 426 ms, which is

the premature interval for the bundle branch system. There is a very slight alteration of QRS conduction of the premature complex, associated with a minimal increase in the His-Purkinje conduction time from a baseline of 44 ms ($H_1V_1$) to 46 ms ($H_2V_2$). A closer-coupled premature complex at 340 ms is associated with an $H_1H_2$ interval of 390 ms and left bundle branch block morphology with marked prolongation of His-Purkinje conduction time noted by an $H_2V_2$ interval of 100 ms (Fig. 3-21*B*). The prolonged $H_2V_2$ interval implies concomitant conduction delay in the His bundle, right bundle branch, or both. An even more premature atrial complex of 320 ms conducts with an even shorter $H_1H_2$ interval of 372 ms, but the premature complex nearly normalizes (Fig. 3-21*C*). Inspection of the His bundle electrogram of the premature complex reveals a slightly more prolonged $H_2V_2$ interval of 102 ms with the emergence of a right bundle potential. The $H_2RB_2$

interval of 68 ms is substantially prolonged, demonstrating conduction delay between the His bundle recording and the right bundle branch recording. Further, the $RB_2V_2$ interval of 34 ms is also somewhat delayed. Thus, normalization of the QRS complex with an even closer-coupled atrial premature interval is probably due to both gap phenomenon as well as progressive conduction delay in the right bundle branch, which allows enough time for conduction over the left bundle branch to reach the ventricle, with resultant normalization of the QRS complex. This concept is illustrated in Fig. 3-22.

In Fig. 3-22, a schematic of a premature atrial complex with right bundle branch block is shown in panel *A*. The right bundle branch block could be due to either complete "block" (*A*-1) over the right bundle branch or slowing of conduction (*A*-2) over the right bundle branch with initial activation of the

ventricle from the left bundle branch. It would be impossible to know which mechanism produced the right bundle branch block pattern on the surface ECG. In panel *B*, a premature atrial complex causes sudden normalization of the QRS complex. In *B*-1, the mechanism depicted for QRS normalization is gap caused by proximal slowing of conduction in the His bundle that allows recovery of excitation in the right bundle branch and subsequent conduction to the ventricles over both bundle branches with a normal QRS complex. In *B*-2, the premature atrial complex conducts without gap to both bundle branches, but marked slowing of conduction now occurs in the left bundle branch, enabling ventricular activation to occur nearly simultaneously over both bundle branches, which results in a narrow QRS complex. In both of these situations, one would expect a prolonged PR interval, and it would be

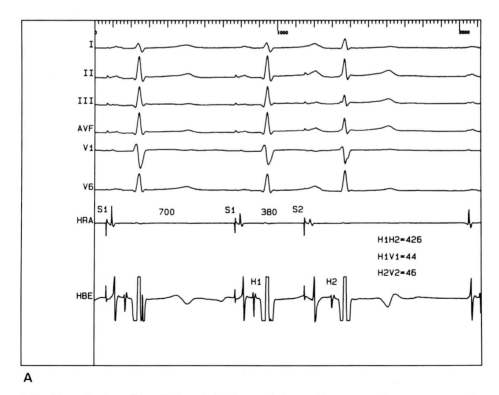

**A**

*Figure 3-21*   Normalization of bundle branch block morphology with a very early premature atrial complex because of equal conduction delay in both bundle branches and possibly gap physiology. (See text for details.)

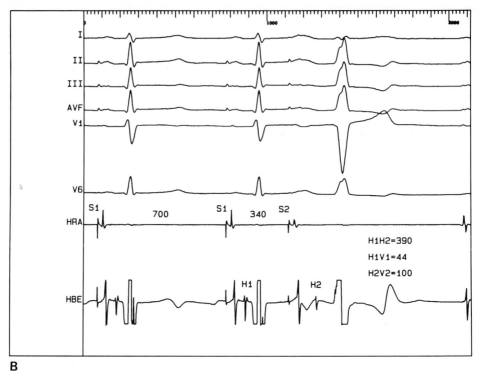

**B**

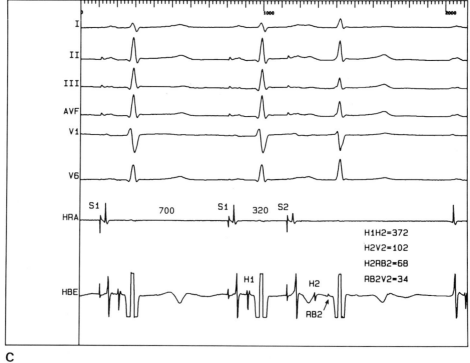

**C**

*Figure* 3-21 (*Continued*)

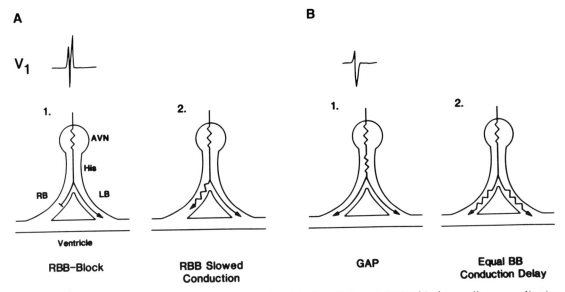

*Figure 3-22*   Schematic demonstrating mechanisms for right bundle branch (RBB) block as well as normalization of QRS complex due to gap or equal bundle branch (BB) conduction delay. (See text for details.)

nearly impossible to identify whether one or both mechanisms were in part responsible for normalization of the QRS complex from examination of the ECG only.

In summary, there are many potential mechanisms to explain the sudden and unexpected normalization of a QRS complex in a patient with a baseline wide QRS complex. However, knowledge of the potential mechanisms responsible for this phenomenon should allow a correct diagnosis in most instances.

## References

1.  Durrer D. et al: Total excitation of the isolated human heart. *Circulation* 41:899, 1970.

2.  Willems JL et al: Criteria for intraventricular conduction disturbances and pre-excitation. *J Am Coll Cardiol* 5:1261, 1985.

3.  Kastor JA et al: Intraventricular conduction in man studied with an endocardial electrode catheter mapping technique. *Circulation* 51:786, 1975.

4.  Davies MJ, Anderson RH, Becker AE: *The Conduction System of the Heart.* London, Butterworths, 1983, p 281.

5.  Lev M et al: Pathology of the conduction system in acquired heart disease: Complete right bundle branch block. *Am Heart J* 61:593, 1961.

6.  Hiss RG et al: Electrocardiographic findings in 122,043 individuals. *Circulation* 25:947, 1962.

7.  Rotman M, Triebwasser JH: A clinical and follow-up study of right and left bundle branch block. *Circulation* 51:477, 1975.

8.  Fleg JL et al: Right bundle branch block: Long-term prognosis in apparently healthy men. *J Am Coll Cardiol* 1:887, 1983.

9.  Schneider JF et al: Newly acquired right bundle-branch block: The Framingham Study. *Ann Intern Med* 92:37, 1980.

10. Vassallo JA et al: Endocardial activation of left bundle branch block. *Circulation* 69:914, 1984.

11. Lev M et al: The anatomic substrate of complete left bundle branch block. *Circulation* 50:479, 1974.

12. Johnson RP et al: Prognosis in bundle branch block: II. Factors influencing the survival period in left bundle branch block. *Am Heart J* 41:225, 1951.

13. Scott RC: Left bundle branch block: A clinical assessment: Part I. *Am Heart J* 70:535, 1965.

14. Schneider JF et al: Newly acquired left bundle-branch block: The Framingham Study. *Ann Intern Med* 90:303, 1979.

15. Denes P et al: Sudden death in patients with chronic bifascicular block. *Arch Intern Med* 137:1005, 1977.

16. McAnulty JH et al: A prospective study of sudden death in "high risk" bundle-branch block. *N Engl J Med* 299:209, 1978.

17. Rosenbaum MB: The hemiblocks: Diagnostic criteria and clinical significance. *Mod Concepts Cardiovasc Dis* 39:141, 1970.

18. Mendez C et al: Influence of cycle length upon refractory period of auricles, ventricles, and A-V node in the dog. *Am J Physiol* 184:287, 1956.

19. Moe GK et al: Aberrant A-V impulse propagation in the dog heart: A study of functional bundle branch block. *Circ Res* 16:261, 1965.

20. Moore EN et al: Durations of transmembrane action potential and functional refractory periods of canine false tendon and ventricular myocardium: Comparison in single fibers. *Circ Res* 17:259, 1965.

21. Denes P et al: The effects of cycle length on cardiac refractory periods in man. *Circulation* 49:32, 1974.

22. Prystowsky EN et al: Electrophysiologic assessment of the atrioventricular conduction system after surgical correction of ventricular preexcitation. *Circulation* 59:789, 1979.

23. Chilson DA et al: Functional bundle branch block: Discordant response of right and left bundle branches to changes in heart rate. *Am J Cardiol* 545:313, 1984.

24. Schuilenburg RM, Durrer D: Rate-dependency of functional block in the human His bundle and bundle branch–Purkinje system. *Circulation* 48:526, 1973.

25. Lewis T: *The Mechanism and Graphic Registration of the Heart Beat*, 3rd ed. London, Shaw and Sons, 1925, p 256.

26. Gouax JL, Ashman R: Auricular fibrillation with aberration simulating ventricular paroxysmal tachycardia. *Am Heart J* 34:366, 1947.

27. Denker S et al: Effects of abrupt changes in cycle length on refractoriness of the His-Purkinje system in man. *Circulation* 67:60, 1983.

28. Lewis T: Certain physical signs of myocardial involvement. *Br Med J* 1:484, 1913.

29. Denes P et al: Electrophysiological observations in patients with rate dependent bundle branch block. *Circulation* 51:244, 1975.

30. Neuss H et al: Electrophysiological findings in frequency-dependent left bundle-branch block. *Br Heart J* 36:888, 1974.

31. Fisch C et al: Rate dependent aberrancy. *Circulation* 48:714, 1973.

32. Nau GJ et al: Recovery of impulse propagation in the bundle branches of the human heart. The different varieties of phase 3 bundle branch block, in Rosenbaum MB, Elizari MV (eds): *Frontiers of Cardiac Electrophysiology*. Boston, Martinus Nijhoff, 1983, p 416.

33. Lazzari JO et al: The "making" of a bundle branch block, in Rosenbaum MB, Elizari MV (eds): *Frontiers of Cardiac Electrophysiology*. Boston, Martinus Nijhoff, 1983, p 657.

34. Fisch C, Miles WM: Deceleration-dependent left bundle branch block: A spectrum of bundle branch conduction delay. *Circulation* 65:1029, 1982.

35. Davidenko JM, Antzelevitch C: Electrophysiological mechanisms underlying rate-dependent changes of refractoriness in normal and segmentally depressed canine Purkinje fibers. *Circ Res* 58:257, 1986.

36. Singer DH et al: Inter-relationship between automaticity and conduction in Purkinje fibers. *Circ Res* 21:537, 1967.

37. Antzelevitch C et al: Frequency-dependent alterations of conduction in Purkinje fibers. A model of phase-4 facilitation and block, in Rosenbaum MB, Elizari MV (eds): *Frontiers of Cardiac Electrophysiology*. Boston, Martinus Nijhoff, 1983, p 397.

38. Wellens HJJ, Durrer D: Supraventricular tachycardia with left aberrant conduction due to retrograde invasion into the left bundle branch. *Circulation* 38:474, 1968.

39. Miles WM, Prystowsky EN: Alteration of human right bundle branch refractoriness by changes in duration of the atrial drive train. *Circulation* 73:244, 1986.

# Chapter 4

# *Apparent Paradoxical Conduction*

Conduction of premature atrial complexes (PACs) is usually predictable in a patient with a relatively constant heart rate. A late (i.e., long atrial coupling interval) PAC will conduct to the ventricle and a relatively early (i.e., short atrial coupling interval) PAC often blocks in the atrioventricular (AV) conduction system. In some instances, however, apparent paradoxical conduction can occur in the AV conduction system. This happens when a late PAC conducts to the ventricle, an earlier PAC blocks, but—unexpectedly—a PAC with even a shorter coupling interval again conducts to the ventricle. Various electrophysiologic phenomena can explain these conduction patterns, but they are often very difficult to diagnose by surface electrocardiography only. Resumption of conduction may occur because of supernormal excitability and conduction, which is probably relatively rare, but more commonly can be explained by other mechanisms, especially the gap phenomenon. Specific issues related to the bundle branch conduction system are presented in detail in Chap. 3.

## Gap Phenomenon

Moe and colleagues[1] noted in a series of canine experiments that a PAC that did not conduct to the ventricle could occur in timing between a later and earlier PAC that did conduct to the ventricle. The unexpected conduction of the earliest PAC was referred to as a *gap* in AV transmission. The gap phenomenon was studied by many investigators

and several subdivisions of gap were identified.[2-5] However, the basic underlying electrophysiologic principle for all varieties of gap is the same and can be described as follows. A relatively late-coupled PAC that conducts to the ventricle involves transmission through the atria, AV node, His bundle, and all or part of the bundle branch system (Fig. 4-1). When the PAC occurs early enough, it may fail to conduct to the ventricle due to block either in the AV node or His-Purkinje system (areas B, C, and D in Fig. 4-1). In essence, the effective refractory period of the tissue at the site of block is greater than the functional refractory period of tissue proximal to the site of block. In other words, an electrical impulse can be conducted through areas proximal to but not distal to the site of block because of the longer refractory period at that point. Gap occurs when a PAC with an even earlier premature atrial interval undergoes *slowing of conduction in tissue proximal to the previous area of block* such that this site of previous block has time to recover excitability and allow the electrical impulse to conduct to the ventricle.

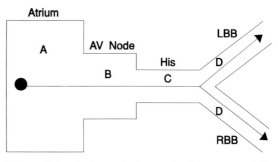

*Figure 4-1* Atrioventricular conduction system with levels of potential block and conduction delay.

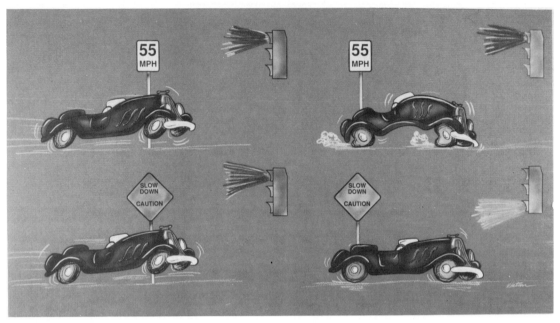

*Figure 4-2*    Analogy for gap phenomenon (see text). (See Color Plate 4.)

This seemingly complex electrophysiologic event may be simplified by considering an analogy that occurs during everyday driving of an automobile (Fig. 4-2). In this figure, the red traffic light represents the distal site of block and the automobile the conducting impulse. In the top panel, as the automobile approaches the red light, there is no decrease in speed, or slowing of conduction; consequently the car must come to an abrupt stop when it reaches the red light, or distal site of block. In the bottom panel of Fig. 4-2, the driver of the automobile, recognizing a red light ahead, slows down so that more time is allowed to elapse before the automobile, or electrical impulse, reaches the red light. In this instance the car does not need to stop when it reaches the traffic light, or site of previous block, because the slower speed has allowed time for the light to turn green or, in electrophysiologic terms, the slower conduction velocity enabled recovery of excitability at the previous distal site of block. Importantly, a PAC may encounter slow conduction in any tissue proximal to the site of block including atrium, AV node, and His-Purkinje system, and gap was originally subdivided by the tissue involved in the proximal delay and distal block site. In our opinion, differentiation into specific types of gap is artificial, serves no useful purpose, and belies the underlying fundamental electrophysiologic property common to all forms of gap phenomenon.

An example of gap physiology with proximal conduction delay in the atrium is shown in Fig. 4-3. In panel $A$, a premature ($S_1S_2$) stimulus with an interval of 250 ms is introduced into the right atrium after eight paced atrial complexes ($S_1$) at 500 ms (120/min). This PAC results in conduction to the ventricle with some conduction delay in the left bundle branch system. Note that although the $S_1S_2$ is 250 ms, there is considerable atrial conduction delay between the $S_2$ stimulus and the next atrial electrogram, yielding an $A_1A_2$ interval of 285 ms as measured on the His bundle lead. In panel $B$, the $S_1S_2$ interval is shortened by 10 ms with a corresponding $A_1A_2$ of 275 ms, and the PAC conducts through the AV node with an atrio-His (AH) interval of 110 ms, but block occurs after the recorded His potential. Thus, distal block in this instance is in the His-Purkinje system (level C or D in Fig. 4-1). A further shortening of the premature interval to 230 ms (panel *C* of Fig. 4-3) results in resumption of conduction of the PAC to the ventricle. This apparent paradoxical conduction is explained by proximal conduction delay from the site of the premature stimulus ($S_2$) to the atrial tissue near the AV node (level A in Fig. 4-1). Even though the $S_1S_2$ interval is shortened to 230 ms, the resultant $A_1A_2$ interval is 285 ms, comparable to that noted in panel A, and conduction can resume because the proximal delay of conduction in the atrium allows recovery of excitability in the His-Purkinje system.

Another type of gap is noted in Fig. 4-4. In this example, the site of distal block is in the His-Purkinje system (Fig. 4-4A; level C or D in Fig. 4-1). The right atrium is paced at a cycle length of 700 ms (86/min) and a premature atrial complex is introduced at a coupling interval of 360 ms. The resultant $H_1H_2$ interval is 396 ms and block occurs below the recorded His potential ($H_2$). A closer-coupled PAC with an $S_1S_2$ interval of 330 ms conducts to the ventricle (Fig. 4-4B). The $H_1H_2$ interval remained the same at 396 ms, but there was a marked delay in His-Purkinje conduction, with the premature complex, resulting in an $H_2V_2$ interval of 124 ms (normal $\leq$55 ms). As is usually the case in these instances, the QRS complex demonstrates some form of aberrant conduction, left bundle in this

instance. Thus, the site of proximal delay for gap to occur in this example is somewhere distal to the recorded His potential but still within the His-Purkinje system (level D or lower part of C in Fig. 4-1).

The AV node is often the proximal site of conduction delay in gap physiology. Although subtle changes in vagal tone imposed on the AV node may account for a sudden prolongation in AV nodal conduction time, as demonstrated by Mazgalev et al.,[6] we think this is not necessary to explain AV nodal gap in most instances. Typical AV nodal behavior is for closer-coupled premature atrial complexes to engender more AV nodal conduction delay. Thus, if a PAC produced block in some part of the His–Purkinje system, an earlier PAC would be expected to prolong AV nodal conduction time; if the resultant slowed conduction was sufficient to allow recovery of excitability in the His-Purkinje system, gap would occur ,without any alteration in autonomic tone. Regardless, it is still possible in certain instances for autonomic influences to play a role in gap physiology. Examples of gap in the AV node are shown in Figs. 4-5 and 4-6.

Figure 4-5A is taken from a patient with left bundle branch block who underwent pacing of the right atrium at cycle length 600 ms (100/min), and a premature atrial interval of 350 ms demonstrates block below the recorded His potential. The $H_1H_2$ interval is 362 ms. Premature atrial stimuli were initiated at progressively shorter coupling intervals,

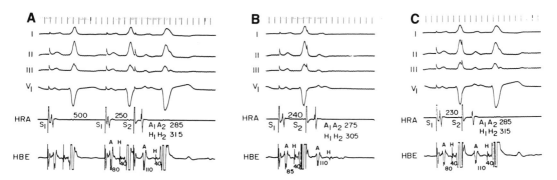

*Figure 4-3*   Gap with distal block in the His-Purkinje system and proximal delay in the atrium. (See text for details.)

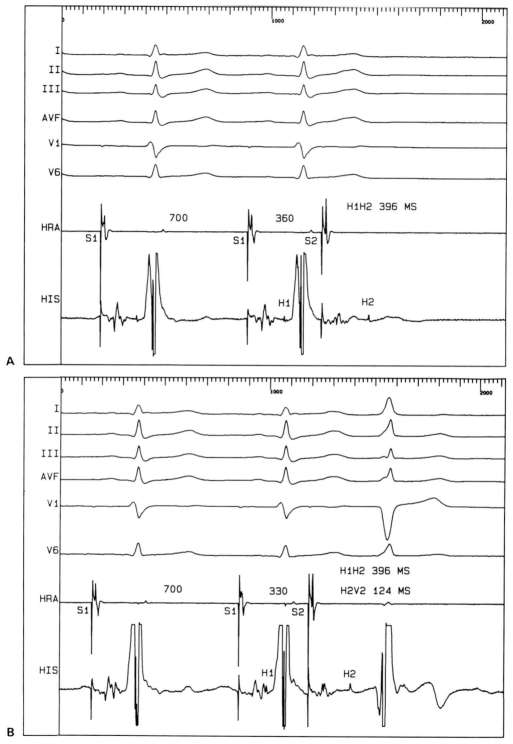

*Figure 4-4*   Gap with distal block in the His-Purkinje system and proximal delay also in the His-Purkinje system. (See text for details.)

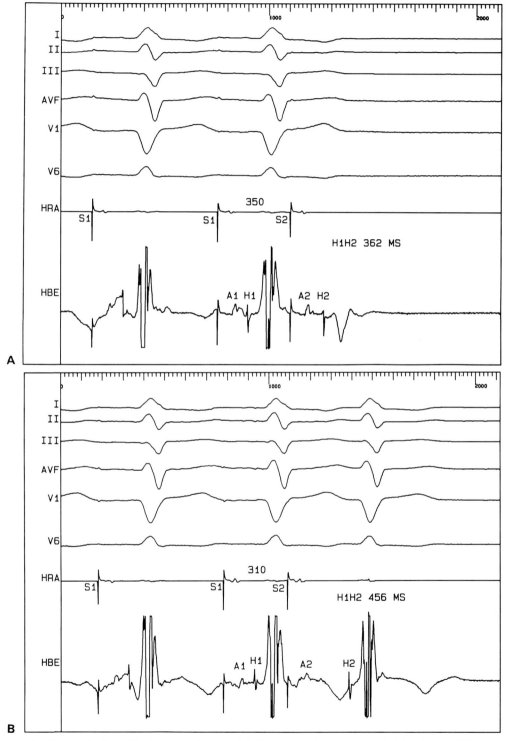

*Figure 4-5*  Gap with distal block below the recorded His potential and proximal delay in the AV node. (See text for details.)

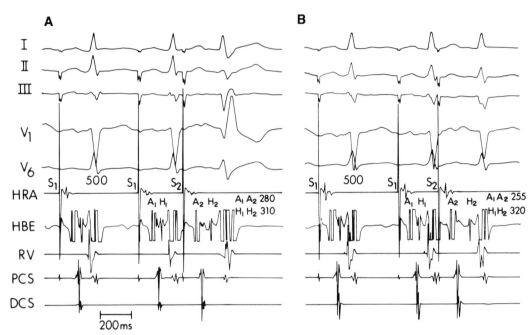

*Figure 4-6*    Gap with distal block in the right bundle branch and proximal delay in the AV node. (See text for details.)

and at an $S_1S_2$ of 310 ms, conduction of the PAC to the ventricle suddenly reappeared (Fig. 4-5B). In this example, AV nodal conduction delay of the PAC is substantial, with an $A_2H_2$ interval of 200 ms and a subsequent $H_1H_2$ interval of 456 ms. This marked increase in AV nodal conduction delay of the PAC allows for a longer $H_1H_2$ interval, and recovery of excitability has occurred in the His-Purkinje system (level D or lower C in Fig. 4-1). Figure 4-6 demonstrates a variant of this type of gap physiology. In panel *A*, the PAC with an $A_1A_2$ interval of 280 ms conducts to the His bundle with an $H_1H_2$ interval of 310 ms, but block occurs in the right bundle branch. A closer-coupled PAC with an $A_1A_2$ interval of 255 ms (panel *B*) produced AV nodal delay, noted by the increase in $A_2H_2$ interval and subsequent increase in $H_1H_2$ interval to 320 ms. At this $H_1H_2$ interval, which is greater than that noted in panel *A*, conduction through the right bundle branch occurs with normalization of the QRS complex.

Gap phenomena have also been described during retrograde conduction through the ventriculoatrial

conduction system.[7] In our experience of introducing premature ventricular complexes as part of the routine electrophysiologic study of patients, we have rarely encountered this phenomenon in the absence of *pacing* the ventricle and introducing extrastimuli. Thus, although retrograde gap occurs as noted in Fig. 4-7, its spontaneous occurrence is probably rare. In contrast, we have often noted gap physiology during introduction of premature atrial complexes during sinus rhythm.

## Supernormal Conduction

Supernormal conduction has been studied in detail by analysis of action potential characteristics in vitro as well as in some in vivo canine experiments.[8–11] These basic investigations demonstrated a brief time period of improved tissue conduction and excitability that occurs near the end of the transmembrane

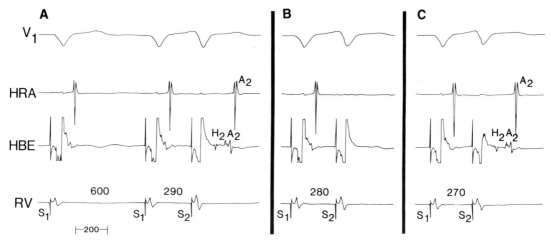

*Figure 4-7*    Retrograde gap physiology during right ventricular pacing and premature stimulation. In panel *A*, the right ventricle is paced at a cycle length of 600 ms and a premature interval of 290 ms yields retrograde conduction to the atrium with a retrograde His potential ($H_2$) followed by an atrial potential ($A_2$). In panel *B*, shortening of the premature interval to 280 ms results in retrograde block to the His bundle and atrium. A shorter premature interval of 270 msec (panel *C*) is associated with resumption of conduction to the atrium. Careful measurement of the interval from the premature stimulus to the $H_2$ deflection reveals prolongation of the $S_2H_2$ interval compared with the $S_1S_2$ of 290 ms noted in panel *A*. Since there is no measurable delay between the stimulus and local ventricular recording, this most likely represents retrograde conduction delay in the His-Purkinje system proximal to the previous site of block, which allows resumption of conduction to the His bundle and subsequently to the atrium.

action potential repolarization, or phase 3, and the mechanism appears to be voltage-dependent, occurring when the threshold potential has recovered more completely than the membrane potential. Such findings cannot be discerned in analyzing electrocardiographic tracings or even intracardiac electrograms. Thus, in clinical terms, supernormal conduction may be defined as *propagation of an electrical impulse at a time when the tissue would be expected to be refractory to conduction*.

The mechanism for supernormal conduction in humans is unclear, and it most likely represents many possible electrophysiologic events at the basic level. For example, when it has been identified in His-Purkinje tissue, abnormalities of baseline His-Purkinje conduction are usually present, and it is often demonstrated after long intervals when repolarization of the tissue would have been expected to be complete.[12] Similar observations occur with supernormal conduction over accessory pathways in

patients with Wolff-Parkinson-White syndrome.[13-14] In addition to electrophysiologic events that occur during phase 3 repolarization of an action potential, the mechanism for supernormal conduction in some individuals might be linked to discontinuous propagation of an impulse through anisotropic cardiac tissue—that is, muscle in which fiber orientation occurs in more than one direction.[15] Importantly, there are many other electrophysiologic mechanisms in humans that can account for most cases of apparent supernormal conduction—for example, gap physiology—and these should always be considered when entertaining this diagnosis.[16-17]

An example of supernormal conduction over an accessory pathway is demonstrated in Fig. 4-8. In this patient, the right atrium was paced for eight beats at cycle length 600 ms (100/min). In panel *A*, a premature atrial complex with a coupling interval of 560 ms conducts to the ventricle over the accessory pathway, which also conducts during the

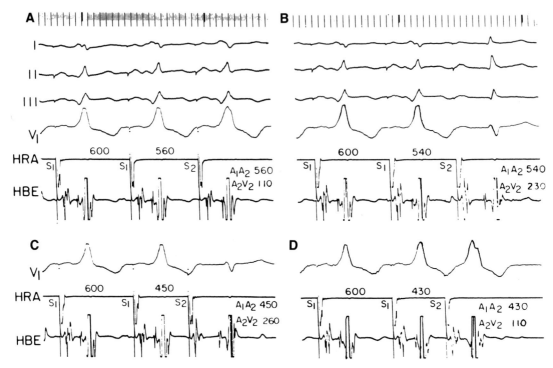

**Figure 4-8**   Supernormal conduction over an accessory pathway. (See text for details.) *(Reproduced with permission from The American Journal of Cardiology, 59:852, 1987.)*

basic pacing drive train. Note that the QRS complex in the surface electrocardiographic leads is wide, and the intracardiac His potential recording occurs after the onset of the surface ECG delta wave. Further, the His bundle electrogram advances into the QRS complex with the PAC without any change in the interval between the atrium and QRS complex ($A_2V_2$). These findings are typical for conduction over an accessory pathway that connects the atrium and ventricle. As the coupling interval of the premature stimulus is shortened to 540 ms (panel *B*), the PAC conducts to the ventricle with block over the accessory pathway, as can be identified by the narrow QRS complex in the electrocardiogram and the His bundle deflection that now precedes the QRS complex by a normal interval. In panel *C*, a closer-coupled interval continues to block over the accessory pathway, but in panel *D*, with a PAC interval of 430 ms, conduction over the accessory pathway suddenly and unexpectedly resumes. There is no measurable slowing of proximal conduction as occurs in gap physiology, and the $A_2V_2$ intervals in panel *A* and panel *D* are identical. Thus, the most likely explanation is supernormal conduction, although the exact electrophysiologic mechanism for this cannot be determined. A graph of conducted and nonconducted atrial impulses over the accessory pathway is shown in Fig. 4-9. Note that all preexcited QRS complexes have an identical $A_2V_2$ interval and there is a distinct window of block over the accessory pathway interposed between earlier and later PACs that conduct over the accessory pathway.

An example of supernormal conduction in the ventricle is demonstrated in Fig. 4-10. This is a patient with an implanted permanent ventricular demand pacemaker that has a sensing malfunction. During long periods of observation, a repetitious pattern of ventricular capture by the pacemaker

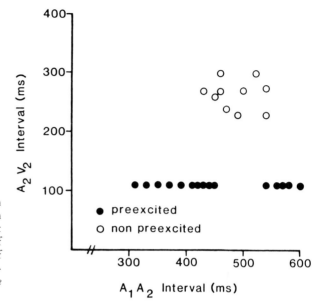

*Figure 4-9*   Graph of atrioventricular conduction over the accessory pathway with preexcitation or over the normal conduction system without preexcitation. Note the constant $A_2V_2$ intervals of preexcited complexes. There is some overlap of supernormal conduction with block over the accessory pathway. *(Reproduced with permission from The American Journal of Cardiology  59:852, 1987.)*

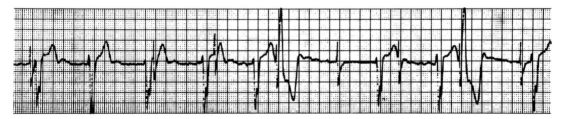

*Figure 4-10*   Possible supernormal excitability and conduction in the ventricle. Note that the sixth and ninth QRS complexes are ventricular-paced and capture of the ventricle only occurs when the stimulus is positioned near a critical point on the descending limb of the T wave. (See text for further details.)

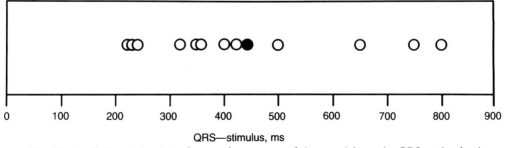

*Figure 4-11*   Graph of the relationship of pacemaker capture of the ventricle to the QRS—stimulus interval of the pacemaker spike. QT = 480. (Key: ○, no capture; ●, capture.)

occurred (Fig. 4-11). The QT interval in this patient was approximately 480 ms, and the pacemaker captured the ventricle only during a very distinct QRS to stimulus interval near the end of the T wave of the QRS complex (Figs. 4-10 and 4-11). This portion of the QRS complex occurs during phase 3 repolarization, and this observation is consistent with supernormal conduction, although other mechanisms are not totally excluded.

## References

1. Moe GK et al: Aberrant A-V impulse propagation in the dog heart: A study of functional bundle branch block. *Circ Res* 16:261, 1965.

2. Wit AL et al: Phenomenon of the gap in atrioventricular conduction in the human heart. *Circ Res* 27:679, 1970.

3. Akhtar M et al: Unmasking and conversion of gap phenomenon in the human heart. *Circulation* 49:624, 1974.

4. Agha AS et al: Type I, type II, and type III gaps in bundle-branch conduction. *Circulation* 47:325, 1973.

5. Wu D et al: Nature of the gap phenomenon in man. *Circ Res* 34:682, 1974.

6. Mazgalev T et al: A new mechanism for atrioventricular nodal gap—Vagal modulation of conduction. *Circulation* 79:417, 1989.

7. Akhtar M et al: The gap phenomena during retrograde conduction in man. *Circulation* 49:811, 1974.

8. Weidmann S: Effects of calcium ions and local anesthetics on electrical properties of Purkinje fibers. *J Physiol (London)* 129:568, 1955.

9. Dominguez G, Fozzard HA: Influence of extracellular K + concentration on cable properties and excitability of sheep cardiac Purkinje fibers. *Circ Res* 26:556, 1970.

10. Spear JF, Moore EN: Supernormal excitability and conduction in the His Purkinje system of the dog. *Circ Res* 35:782, 1974.

11. Childers RW et al: Supernormality of Bachmann's bundle: An in vivo and vitro study. *Circ Res* 22:363, 1968.

12. Levi RJ et al: A reappraisal of supernormal conduction, in Rosenbaum MB, Elizari MV (eds): *Frontiers of Cardiac Electrophysiology.* Boston: Martinus Nijhoff, 1982, p 427.

13. Chang MS et al: Supernormal conduction in accessory atrioventricular connections. *Am J Cardiol* 59:852, 1987.

14. Przybylski J et al: Supernormal conduction in the accessory pathway of patients with overt or concealed ventricular preexcitation. *J Am Coll Cardiol* 9:1269, 1987.

15. Spach MS, Dolber PC: The relation between discontinuous propagation in anisotropic cardiac muscle and the "vulnerable period" of reentry, in Zipes DP, Jalife J (eds): *Cardiac Electrophysiology and Arrhythmias.* Orlando, Florida, Grune & Stratton, 1985, p 241.

16. Moe GK et al: An appraisal of "supernormal" AV conduction. *Circulation* 38:5, 1966.

17. Gallagher JJ et al: Alternative mechanisms of apparent supernormal atrioventricular conduction. *Am J Cardiol* 31:362, 1973.

# Chapter 5

# Mechanisms of Tachycardia

Although it is possible to treat patients who have rhythm disorders with empiric drug therapy, a fundamental understanding of arrhythmia mechanisms facilitates a more successful approach. Indeed, the advent of operative and catheter ablative approaches to arrhythmia management is facilitated by a reasonable understanding of the arrhythmia mechanism so that the procedure may be planned and executed in the intended fashion. The basic scientist is able to explore mechanisms in tissue preparations in a controlled and rigorous fashion that can never be duplicated by the clinical electrophysiologist. On the other hand, the clinician is dealing with the actual pathologic entity and does not have to be concerned with the clinical relevance of the model. Basic and clinical information are complementary to the student of arrhythmias. The following will attempt to summarize basic tachycardia mechanisms, emphasizing highlights of interest to clinicians. The intent is to emphasize phenomenology without enumerating the fundamental ionic events.

## Classification of Tachycardia Mechanisms

Tachycardia mechanisms have been traditionally classified as due to disorders of impulse formation, impulse conduction, or combinations of the two (Table 5-1).[1]

### Abnormal Impulse Formation

#### Normal Automaticity[2-3]

All impulse formation results from localized changes in ionic currents that traverse cell membranes. The natural pacemaker cells exhibit a phasic, spontaneous depolarization during diastole (phase 4), which results in an action potential when threshold potential is reached (Figs. 5-1 and 5-2). These cells are found in the sinus node, parts of the atria, the atrioventricular (AV) junctional region, and the His-Purkinje system. In the normal heart, the sinus node is the dominant pacemaker, since it depolarizes most rapidly and remains dominant due to "overdrive suppression" of the subsidiary pacemakers.[4] Subsidiary pacemakers may become dominant under certain conditions, such as sympathetic stimulation. Digitalis may enhance the automaticity of subsidiary pacemakers by inhibiting extracellular $Na^+$ transport that promotes $Ca^{2+}$ entry into cells. Automaticity can neither be initiated nor terminated by pacing techniques.

#### Abnormal Automaticity

Normal working muscle remains at a high negative resting membrane potential in the range of $-90$ mV, depolarizing only when stimulated. Under certain conditions (such as electrolyte imbalance or ischemia), the action potential is transformed to one

*Table 5-1  Mechanisms of Tachycardia*

| Impulse Formation | Conduction | Combined Abnormality |
|---|---|---|
| Normal automaticity | Reentry | Conduction and automaticity (e.g., parasystole) |
| Abnormal automaticity | Reflection | |
| Triggered activity | | |

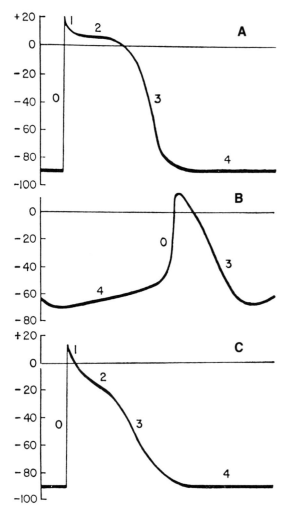

***Figure 5-1*** Action potentials from typical ventricular (*A*), sinoatrial node (*B*), and atrial (*C*) cells. Cells with intrinsic automaticity show clear spontaneous depolarization during phase 4, typical of the SA node. (*From Hoffman et al.[2] Reproduced by permission.*)

with a reduced membrane potential (range of −60 mV), resembling a "slow response" action potential typical of natural pacemaker cells (Fig. 5-3). Such cells may exhibit spontaneous phase 4 depolarization[5] and have been demonstrated experimentally—for example, in canine Purkinje fibers surviving myocardial infarction. Like normal automaticity, abnormal automaticity cannot be induced by programmed

stimulation. In contrast to normal automaticity, abnormal automaticity does not tend to be suppressed by overdrive stimulation, and this provides a useful clinical distinction of the two mechanisms. This may be related to the fact that abnormal automaticity tends to involve more $Ca^{2+}$-dependent action potentials not affected by activation of the $Na^+/K^+$ pump felt to be causative in overdrive suppression of normal automaticity.[6]

### Triggered Activity—Early after-Depolarizations (EADs)

Triggered activity is defined as pacemaker activity that requires at least one preceding impulse or action potential.[7] Triggered activity is caused by after-depolarizations—subthreshold depolarizations occurring during repolarization (early after-depolarization or EAD) or after repolarization is complete (delayed after-depolarization or DAD).

EADs occur during repolarization of action potentials from a normal resting membrane potential (approximately −90 mV).[3,4] They appear as a positive deflection during repolarization (Fig. 5-4). They may reach threshold potential for activation of the slow inward current and result in a second action potential. Repetitive rhythmic activity may occur, continuing until repolarization is completed to a point where the initiating action potential is nearer to its normal resting potential. Thus, single ("fixed coupled"), repetitive, or sustained activity can occur. A variety of experimental conditions including hypoxia, mechanical injury, ischemia, hypokalemia, aconitine, cesium, catecholamines, and antiarrhythmic drugs (sotalol, quinidine, N-acetylprocainamide) have been associated with EAD. The unifying theme in many of these experimental preparations is the increase in the time course of repolarization which favors occurrence of EAD.

It is difficult to prove EADs as a mechanism in clinical arrhythmias. They may be suspected in arrhythmias associated with prolonged repolarization (long QT), especially if they are bradycardia-dependent.[8] Pacing at more rapid rates should diminish or abolish EAD-dependent arrhythmias, since this usually decreases action potential duration. Arrhyth-

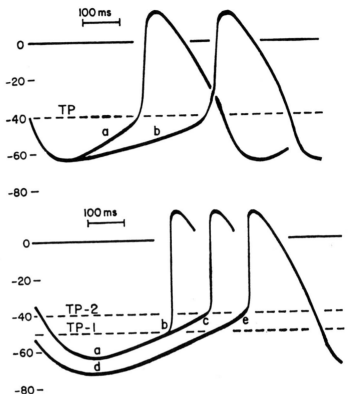

*Figure 5-2* Representation of the major mechanisms responsible for changes in frequency of depolarization of a fiber with normal automaticity. A decrease in the slope of phase 4 (a to b) in the upper trace reduces frequency. A lowering (less negative) of threshold potential, TP-1 to TP-2, in the lower trace also prolongs cycle length, as does an increase in resting potential from a to d. *(From Hoffman et al.[2] Reproduced by permission.)*

mias resulting from EAD would be expected to exhibit slowing of the heart rate prior to spontaneous termination, since this is usually observed in experimental preparations. There is some evidence that the syndrome of QT prolongation and polymorphic ventricular tachycardia (torsade de pointes) initially described by Dessertenne is related to EADs, especially the bradycardia-dependent variety associated with many antiarrhythmic agents, such as quinidine.[9] Arrhythmias associated with this syndrome "fit" the experimental model in their behavior, and potentials resembling EAD have been recorded by monophasic action potentials in individuals.[10]

### Triggered Activity—Delayed after-Depolarizations (DADs)

Delayed after-depolarizations are oscillatory depolarizations that are dependent on a preceding action potential and occur after completion of repolariza-

tion.[4,11,12] Triggered activity may be seen in atrial, ventricular, or Purkinje cells. A unifying mechanism in experimental models is a buildup and oscillation of intracellular calcium concentration (for example, digitalis toxicity, potassium-free environment, or high-catecholamine environment). Delayed after-depolarizations have also been recorded in disease models such as human atrial myocardium and surviving Purkinje fibers in infarcted canine myocardium.[4] Delayed after-depolarizations may be subthreshold and initiate a triggered impulse only when their amplitude reaches threshold. The response of DADs to stimulation techniques is variable, but a few generalizations can be made.[13,14] Increasing the rate of stimulation or the prematurity of extrastimuli will increase the amplitude of DADs, increasing the probability of inducing tachycardia (Fig. 5-5). The time to the emergence of the first triggered response decreases as the cycle length of the drive shortens (faster drive, earlier coupling of first tachycardia

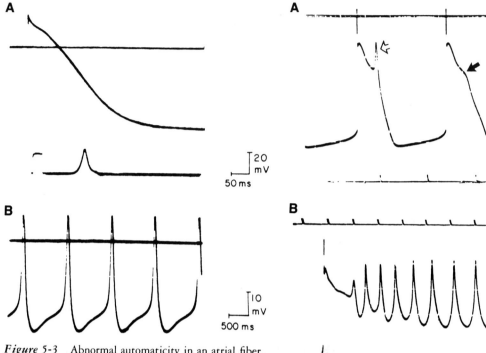

**A**

**B**

$\boxed{\phantom{x}}$ 20 mV

50 ms

$\boxed{\phantom{x}}$ 10 mV

500 ms

*Figure* 5-3    Abnormal automaticity in an atrial fiber. Panel *A* shows an action potential and the first derivative (dv/dt) from a normal atrial fiber. It has a high ( − 80 mV) resting potential and no spontaneous depolarization. Panel *B* is a record from diseased human atrium. Spontaneous diastolic depolarization is occurring from an abnormally low ( − 40 mV) resting potential. (*From Rosen et al.*[5] *Reproduced by permission.*)

**A**

**B**

*Figure* 5-4    Early after-depolarizations in canine Purkinje fibers exposed to 4 mM K$^+$ Tyrode's solution. Panel *A* shows a second upstroke arising from an EAD (*unfilled arrow*) and a second EAD during repolarization (*solid arrow*) after a brief exposure to norepinephrine. Panel *B* shows another preparation where the EAD gives rise to repetitive rhythmic activity from a low membrane potential. The maximum diastolic potential was − 84 mV in panel *A* and − 87 mV in panel *B*. Time lines occur every second. (*From Wit AL, Cranefield PF, Gadsby DG: Triggered activity, in Zipes DP, Bailey JC, Elharrar V (eds): The Slow Inward Current and Cardiac Arrhythmia. The Hague, Martinus Nijhoff, 1980. Reproduced by permission.*)

beat). The cycle length of the first triggered beat after an *extrastimulus* is, in contrast, more variable. In some preparations, the cycle length of tachycardia rate varies directly with the cycle length of the inducing drive.

Triggered rhythms will terminate reproducibly with overdrive pacing at a sufficiently rapid rate but will frequently persist for several cycles after cessation of pacing. Delayed after-depolarizations have been implicated though not proven in clinical arrhythmias due to digitalis toxicity,[15] torsade de pointes associated with adrenergic-dependent QT syndrome,[10] and some types of idiopathic VT in patients with "normal" hearts, especially "right ventricular outflow" VT induced by exercise.[16,17]

### Abnormal Conduction

#### Classic Reentry

Normally, a cardiac impulse is transmitted from the sinus node to its final destination, leaving a wake of refractoriness, and is then extinguished. Under specific circumstances, the propagating impulse may detour from its destined path and return to a

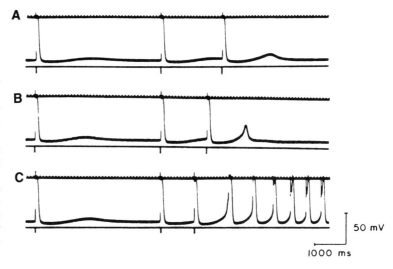

*Figure 5-5* Effect of prematurity on after-depolarization amplitude. The preparation is canine coronary sinus superfused with Tyrode's solution containing norepinephrine. Panels *A* to *C* show progressive prematurity of an extrastimulus after a drive. Progressive prematurity results in increasing amplitude of the after-depolarization (delayed) until repetitive activity is triggered in panel *C*. *(From Wit and Cranefield.*[12] *Reproduced by permission.)*

previously depolarized area to reexcite it (reenter) if it has recovered excitability. An autonomous rhythm can then result if this sequence is repetitive.

It is useful to classify reentry into two categories. The first is *classic reentry* as described by Mines;[18] it is also called *ordered reentry* by Hoffman and Rosen[19] or reentry utilizing an anatomic obstacle. The second is *random reentry,*[19] or *leading circle* reentry,[20] that does not involve a fixed pathway and will be described further below.

Classic reentry involves a relatively constant anatomic pathway, a concept described lucidly by

Mines[18] in studying isolated strips of cardiac muscle cut into rings. The frequently reproduced hypothetical circuit (Fig. 5-6) illustrates the fundamental features. Establishment of reentry in this model requires unidirectional block, slow conduction in an alternate pathway, and return of the impulse to the original pathway after it has recovered excitability. The established circuit may be thought of as a revolving wave with an advancing "head" and a "tail" with relatively refractory and absolutely refractory portions. A "gap" (excitable gap) between the head and tail reflects a "margin of safety" for the circuit

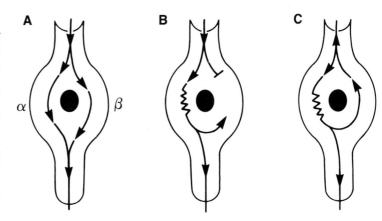

*Figure 5-6* Traditional model of classic reentry with an anatomic obstacle. The impulse passes through a hypothetical conduit via two pathways, α and β, which meet at a common exit point (panel *A*). Since α and β have different refractory properties, a hypothetical extrasystole could be blocked in β pathway (unidirectional block), conduct slowly over α pathway, and "reenter" β pathway retrogradely (panel *B*). This could result in sustained circus movement (panel *C*).

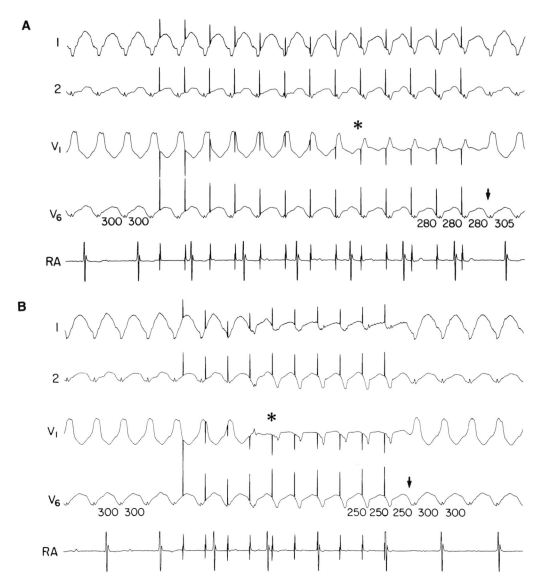

*Figure* 5-8    Entrainment of VT. Ventricular tachycardia in this patient was stable with a cycle length of 300 ms. In panel *A*, right ventricular apical pacing is initiated at a slightly shorter cycle length than the VT cycle length (280 ms). By the ninth paced beat (*asterisk*), a stable fusion pattern has been established and the tachycardia has been accelerated to the paced rate (cycle length, 280 ms). After pacing is discontinued (*arrow*), the first nonpaced cycle is entrained and the subsequent cycle is again at the VT cycle length. In panel *B*, ventricular pacing is initiated at a slightly shorter cycle length (250 ms). By the fifth paced beat (*asterisk*) a stable fusion pattern has been established and the tachycardia rate has been accelerated to the paced rate. The fusion pattern is progressive (i.e., greater contribution from ventricular pacing than VT) as compared to panel *A*. The first nonpaced cycle after cessation of pacing (*arrow*) occurs at cycle length 250 ms which is the cycle length of pacing. This indicates clearly that this first nonpaced cycle has been entrained. That is, the excitable gap was clearly penetrated by the last paced stimulus, resulting in acceleration of the next cycle to the paced rate.

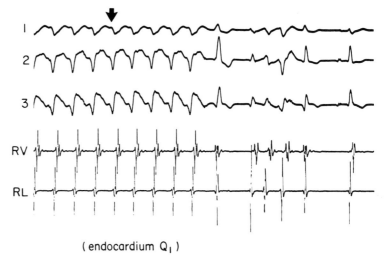

*Figure 5-9*  Ice mapping of VT circuits. This record was obtained during operative ablation of VT associated with remote MI. Endocardial mapping suggested a reentrant circuit, and a cryoprobe was placed on the narrowest part of the circuit between the scar and the mitral valve ring. When this region was cooled to $-10°C$ (*at the arrow*), VT terminated reproducibly, almost instantly.

## Mechanisms of Tachycardia: Clinician's Viewpoint

Basic scientists using controlled experimental conditions and sophisticated cellular and subcellular techniques have provided a comprehensive framework for understanding the many potential mechanisms resulting in arrhythmia. The clinical electrophysiologist faces the formidable challenge of relating these concepts to clinical settings. The clinician dealing with "natural" arrhythmias in patients is constrained by logistic and technical limitations and must depend heavily on inference. Even different experimental models of a given mechanism (for example, DADs in ouabain-superfused Purkinje fibers versus DADs in catecholamine superfused coronary sinus[14] differ sufficiently to complicate the exercise of applying the experimental template to a clinical arrhythmia. For these reasons, a clinician proclaiming a "mechanism" for an unknown arrhythmia does so with appropriate reservations and humility. The following discussion is intended to facilitate a mental framework for approximating an arrhythmia mechanism in a clinical setting, appreciating that the generalizations to follow can always be challenged in specific circumstances (Tables 5-2 and 5-3).

Following below are the principal methods by which an arrhythmia mechanism may be approximated clinically.

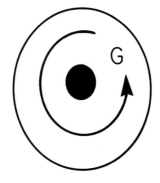
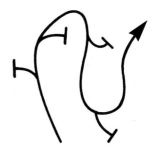

*Figure 5-10*  Graphic representation of "ordered" reentry (*left panel*) and "random" reentry (*right panel*). Ordered reentry has a relatively fixed anatomic route with an excitable gap (G). In reentry without an anatomic obstacle, the pathways are fluid, with the advancing circuit constantly seeking nonrefractory tissue.

*Table 5-2   Characteristics of Tachycardia by Different Mechanisms*

|  | Normal Automaticity | Abnormal Automaticity | Triggered (EAD) | Triggered (DAD) | Reentry (Anatomic Obstacle) |
|---|---|---|---|---|---|
| Initiation by basic drive | No | No | Enhanced by decrease in drive rate | Enhanced by increase in drive rate | Enhanced by increase in drive rate; usually highly reproducible |
| Initiation by extrastimulus | No | No | No | Enhanced by shorter coupling interval; less reproducible | Range of critical coupling intervals; highly reproducible |
| Sustained tachycardia | May "warm up" | May "warm up" | Variable | Often initial "warmup" and terminal "slow down" | Usually stable but may oscillate or slow down before termination |
| Response of tachycardia to overdrive | No termination; overdrive suppression | No termination; may accelerate; no overdrive suppression | No termination | Terminates with critical rate; reproducible | Terminates with critical rate; entrainment demonstrable |
| Response of tachycardia to single extrastimulus | No termination | No termination | Unlikely termination | Unlikely termination; not reproducible | Terminates within a defined range; may "reset" (stimulus must penetrate excitable gap) |

**ELECTROCARDIOGRAPHIC OBSERVATION OF SPONTANEOUS ARRHYTHMIAS**   This is most useful when the arrhythmia occurs frequently and one is fortunate enough to record a particularly illuminating episode. Autonomic and pharmacologic maneuvers during a sustained arrhythmia may cause changes in arrhythmia upon which specific hypotheses regarding mechanism can be formulated. Early electrocardiographers created an impressive body of knowledge using deductive reasoning and these simple techniques (Fig. 5-11).[29] These methods have obvious limitations in arriving at a specific mechanism. The record obtained may be brief, or multiple hypotheses may fit the observations. The effect of certain drugs and autonomic maneuvers can be useful, but none is absolutely specific for a given mechanism. Facilitation

or induction with catecholamines is compatible with multiple mechanisms.[30] Termination of a supraventricular tachycardia with the $Ca^{2+}$ blocker verapamil usually suggests that the AV node is a critical part of a reentrant circuit causing tachycardia. However, an uncommon type of ventricular tachycardia has been described[31] that terminates with verapamil (Fig. 5-12; see Chap. 12). It has been suggested that this represents VT due to triggered activity suppressed by verapamil. However, entrainment has been demonstrated, strongly implicating reentry as the mechanism in these patients.

**EFFECT OF PROGRAMMED STIMULATION**  Programmed stimulation and intracardiac recording is arguably the single most useful technique for deter-

*Table 5-3   Clinical Algorithm for Arrhythmia Mechanism*

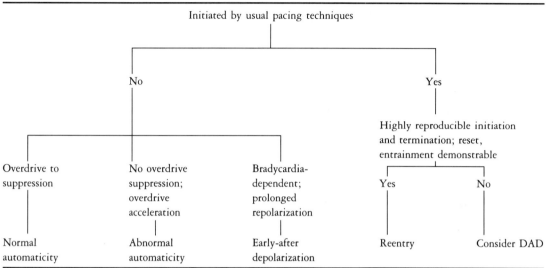

mining mechanisms of arrhythmias (Chap. 17). Failure to induce a given tachycardia after a rigorous protocol of stimulation including isoproterenol suggests that the suspect arrhythmia may not be due to classic reentry with a stable substrate. It is possible that conditions at that time of spontaneous arrhythmia (such as acute ischemia or heart failure) provided a reentrant substrate no longer present at the time of study, and this must be considered. One should also consider that the observed tachycardia was due to alternate mechanisms, such as abnormal automaticity, enhanced "normal" automaticity, or after-depolarizations. Arrhythmias due to EADs would be expected to occur in conditions resulting in prolonged repolarization[8] and relative bradycardia.

Arrhythmias inducible by programmed stimulation may be considered to be reentrant or triggered (DADs). The features of triggered activity vary according to the experimental preparation, but those of classic reentry are relatively more constant and independent of a specific preparation. Thus, it may be useful to consider how closely the given arrhythmia resembles typical reentry and to consider triggered activity as an alternative possibility when such is not the case. Features favoring reentry include highly

reproducible (in an individual) initiation and termination by extrastimuli within a given range, an inverse relationship between prematurity of an initiating extrastimulus and the first beat of tachycardia, the demonstration of an excitable gap using rapid pacing (entrainment) or extrastimuli (reset), the requirement of slow conduction in the circuit, the presence of a relatively stable rate independent of induction mode, and sudden termination of the tachycardia with programmed stimulation (as opposed to termination several cycles later). Triggered activity would be more likely to be induced by rapid pacing (rather than extrastimuli), would not be as consistent in mode of onset, and may have a more variable tachycardia rate dependent on mode of induction. In general, a faster initiating drive results in an earlier first beat of tachycardia and one expects a direct relationship between the first tachycardia cycle and prematurity of an extrastimulus initiating the tachycardia (Tables 5-2 and 5-3). It must again be emphasized that the characteristics of triggered activity vary considerably with different experimental preparations and conditions, and it is impossible to be definitive in ascribing any clinical arrhythmia to triggered activity using these generalizations.[3,4,13,14]

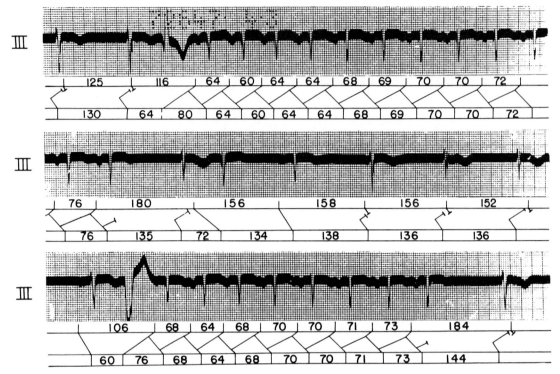

*Figure 5-11*   Determining mechanism by deductive analysis of surface ECG recordings. This early record from the collection of Pick and Langendorf illustrates analysis by picking the best hypothesis to fit the ECG data. The proposed mechanism of the observed tachycardia (as shown in the "laddergram") is AV junctional reentry utilizing a retrograde pathway with rate dependent conduction. The tachycardia is initiated by premature ventricular contractions that conduct retrogradely to the atrium with a prolonged conduction time. Self-termination occurs with a retrograde Wenckebach pattern. This analysis is remarkably insightful, although we currently know that the substrate for the observed tachycardia could be a retrogradely conducting accessory AV pathway with decremental properties. *(From Pick and Langendorf.*[29] *Reproduced by permission.)*

Even if mechanism cannot be definitively stated, the issue of "inducibility" is critical to the clinical electrophysiologist. Inducibility provides a means of studying the arrhythmia and assessing potential pharmacologic and nonpharmacologic therapies objectively.

ACTIVATION SEQUENCE MAPPING   Activation sequence for a tachycardia can be determined during electrophysiology studies, especially those done intraoperatively (Chap. 20). The demonstration of a zone of slow conduction and a plausible anatomic reentrant circuit support reentry. Interruption of a hypothesized

critical link in the circuit (for example, by "ice" mapping) adds considerable credibility to the demonstrated circuit.

MONOPHASIC ACTION POTENTIALS (MAPs)   Monophasic action potential recordings are extracellular recordings using contact (suction) electrodes and dc-coupled preamplifiers.[32] These can be used in standard electrophysiologic studies and provide an electrogram resembling an action potential with a detailed assessment of local repolarization. It may be possible to record after-depolarizations in the clinical setting with this technique[8] to study further the contribution of triggered activity to clinical arrhythmias.

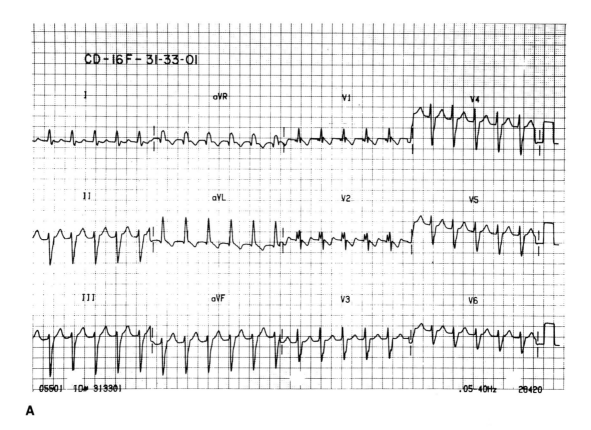

**A**

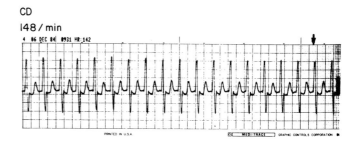

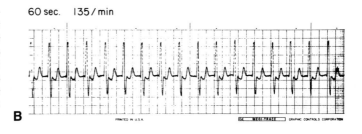

**B**

*Figure 5-12* "Verapamil-sensitive" ventricular tachycardia. This characteristic tachycardia has a uniform ECG appearance with right bundle branch block, left axis morphology (panel *A*). After verapamil, 5 mg, the cycle length gradually prolongs and the tachycardia stops (panel *B*). The tachycardia is frequently misdiagnosed as "supraventricular."

125 / min

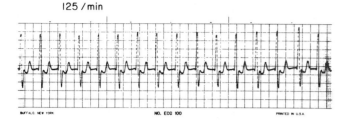

120 / min

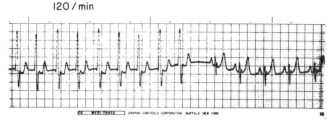

*Figure 5-12B* (*Continued*)

# References

1. Hoffman BF, Cranefield PF: The physiological basis for cardiac arrhythmias. *Am J Med* 37:670, 1964.

2. Hoffman BF, Cranefield PF: *Electrophysiology of the Heart*. Mount Kisco, New York, Futura, 1976.

3. Zipes DP: Genesis of cardiac arrhythmias: Electrophysiological considerations, in Braunwald, E (ed): *Heart Disease: A Textbook of Cardiovascular Medicine*. Philadelphia, Saunders, 1988, pp 581–620.

4. Wit AL, Rosen MR: Cellular electrophysiology of cardiac arrhythmias, in Josephson ME, Wellens HJJ (eds): *Tachycardias: Mechanisms, Diagnosis, Treatment*. Philadelphia, Lea & Febiger, 1984, pp 1–27.

5. Rosen MR et al: Electrophysiology and pharmacology of cardiac arrhythmias: Cardiac effects of verapamil. *Am Heart J* 89:665, 1975.

6. Vasalle M: The relationship among cardiac pacemakers: Overdrive suppression. *Circ Res* 41:268, 1977.

7. Cranefield PF: Action potentials, afterpotentials and arrhythmias. *Cir Res* 41:415, 1977.

8. Jackman WM et al: The long QR syndromes: A critical review, new clinical observations and a unifying hypothesis. *Prog Cardiovasc Dis* 31:115, 1988.

9. Roden DM et al: Clinical features and basic mechanisms of quinidine-induced arrhythmias: The proceedings of the 4th annual joint US-USSR Symposium on Sudden Cardiac Death. *J Am Coll Cardiol* 8:73A, 1986.

10. Schwartz P et al: The long QT syndrome, in Zipes DP, Jalife J (eds): *Cardiac Electrophysiology from Cell to Bedside*. Philadelphia, Saunders, 1990, pp 589–605.

11. Moak JP, Rosen MR: Induction and termination of triggered activity by pacing in isolated canine Purkinje fibers. *Circulation* 69:149, 1984.

12. Wit AL, Cranefield PF: Triggered and automatic activity in the canine coronary sinus. *Circ Res* 41:435, 1977.

13. Rosen MR et al: Mechanisms of digitalis toxicity: Effects of oubain on phase four of canine Purkinje fiber transmembrane potentials. *Circulation* 47:681, 1973.

14. Johnson NJ, Rosen MR: The distinction between triggered activity and other cardiac arrhythmias, in Brugada P, Wellens HJJ (eds): *Cardiac Arrhythmias: Where to Go from Here?* Mount Kisco, New York, Futura, 1987, pp 129–145.

15. Ferrier GR: Digitalis arrhythmias: Role of oscillatory afterpotentials. *Progr Cardiovasc Dis* 19:459, 1977.

16. Zipes DP et al: Atrial induction of ventricular tachycardia: Reentry versus triggered automaticity. *Am J Cardiol* 44:1, 1979.

17. Wu D et al: Exercise triggered paroxysmal ventricular tachycardia. *Ann Intern Med* 95:794, 1981.

18. Mines GR: On circulating excitations in heart muscle and their possible relations to tachycardia and fibrillation. *Trans R Soc Can Ser* 8:43, 1914.

19. Hoffman BF, Rosen MR: Cellular mechanisms for cardiac arrhythmia. *Circ Res* 49:1, 1981.

20. Allessie MA et al: Circus movement in rabbit atrial muscle as a mechanism of tachycardia. The "leading circle" concept: A new model of circus movement in cardiac tissue without the involvement of an anatomical obstacle. *Circ Res* 41:9, 1977.

21. Spach MS et al: Influence of the passive anisotropic properties on directional differences in propagation following modification of the sodium conductance in human atrial muscle: A model of reentry based on anisotropic discontinuous propagation. *Circ Res* 62:811, 1988.

22. El-Sherif N et al: Ventricular activation patterns of spontaneous and induced ventricular rhythms in canine one-day-old myocardial infarction: Evidence for focal and reentrant mechanisms. *Circ Res* 51:152, 1982.

23. Antzelevitch C et al: Characteristics of reflection as a mechanism of reentrant arrhythmias and its relationship to parasystole. *Circulation* 61:182, 1980.

24. Rosenthal ME et al: Resetting of ventricular tachycardia with electrocardiographic fusion: Incidence and significance. *Circulation* 77:581, 1988.

25. Gilliam FR et al: Characterization and differentiation of reset response curves in automaticity and reentry. *J Am Coll Cardiol* 2:115A, 1988.

26. Waldo AL et al: Transient entrainment and interruption of AV bypass pathway type paroxysmal atrial tachycardia: A model for understanding and identifying reentrant arrhythmias in man. *Circulation* 67:73, 1982.

27. Waldo AL et al: Demonstration of the mechanism of transient entrainment and interruption of ventricular tachycardia with rapid atrial pacing. *J Am Coll Cardiol* 3:451, 1984.

28. Brugada P, Wellens HJJ: Entrainment as an electrophysiologic phenomenon. *J Am Coll Cardiol* 3:451, 1984.

29. Pick A, Langendorf R: *Interpretation of Complex Arrhythmias*. Philadelphia, Lea & Febiger, 1979, pp 127–174.

30. Schwartz P, Priori SG: Sympathetic nervous system and cardiac arrhythmias, in Zipes DP, Jalife J (eds): *Cardiac Electrophysiology from Cell to Bedside*. Philadelphia, Saunders, 1990, pp 589–605.

31. Belhassen B et al: Response of recurrent sustained ventricular tachycardia to verapamil. *Br Heart J* 46:679, 1981.

32. Franz MR: Method and theory of monophasic action potential recording. *Prog Cardiovasc Dis* 33:347, 1991.

# Part II
## Arrhythmias

# Chapter 6

# Supraventricular Tachycardia

## Classification

Supraventricular tachycardia may be defined as tachycardia in which the atrium or atrioventricular (AV)
junction is the source or a vital link of the arrhythmia
mechanism. Specific tachycardia entities have been
traditionally cataloged descriptively using criteria

of
n,
ul
ar
y-
te
n
e
a
m
e
e,
r-
i-
g-
y

as

al

Atrial tachycardia              tachycardia
Atrial flutter
Atrial fibrillation

a brief period of AV block in these cases. The AV
reentrant tachycardias are considered in detail elsewhere (Chap. 7).

## Sinus Tachycardia

Sinus tachycardia is associated with a variety of
physiologic and pathologic states resulting in increased sympathetic and decreased vagal stimulation
of the sinus node. These are numerous and include
exercise, anxiety, hypovolemia, hypoxia, fever, hyperthyroidism, and anemia. Agents such as alcohol
and nicotine and many drugs with atropinic or
sympathomimetic effects cause sinus tachycardia.
The heart rate is greater than 100/min (by definition)
and can be 200/min or greater, although the maximal
rate decreases with age. Sinus tachycardia is "nonparoxysmal," with a graduated onset and offset. It may
be slowed transiently by carotid massage or other
vagotonic maneuvers. A shift in the site of the
dominant pacemaker within the node may cause
slight changes in rate and P-wave morphology. Sinus
tachycardia is managed by dealing with the primary
cause. Occasionally, if it is not related to cardiac or
respiratory failure, sinus tachycardia may be treated
with beta blockers for symptomatic relief. Sinus
node reentry and "chronic" sinus tachycardia are not
related to the usual physiologic stimuli causing sinus
tachycardia but are considered here because the site
of impulse formation is in the sinus node region and
they resemble sinus tachycardia electrocardiographically.

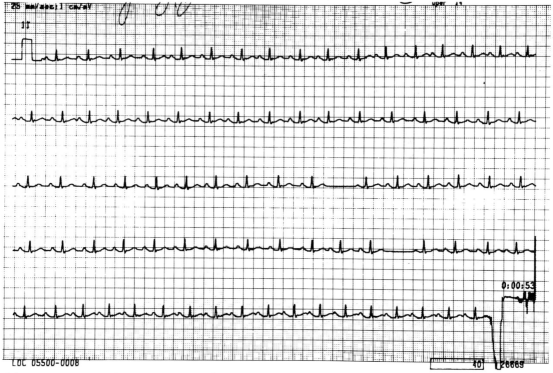

*Figure 6-1*    Sinus-node reentrant tachycardia. This patient had paroxysmal tachycardia at a rate of approximately 100/min with sudden onset and offset. It could be induced and terminated by atrial extrastimuli. The rhythm strip is continuous. Spontaneous termination is observed in the third and fourth lines followed by a sinus beat and subsequent resumption of tachycardia.

### Sinus Node Reentry

The sinus node consists of a central zone with densely packed cells and a transitional zone merging into atrial tissue. Conduction in this region can be sufficiently slow to allow reentry, and sinus node reentrance has been demonstrated in isolated rabbit preparations of atrium.[2] A clinical diagnosis of sinus node reentry is less precise and cannot entirely exclude reentry in atrial tissue very near the sinus node.[3]

Sinus node reentry is more prevalent in older patients of either sex with organic heart disease. It is an uncommon cause of problematic supraventricular tachycardia referred for electrophysiologic testing, although its prevalence as an asymptomatic arrhythmia is probably higher. In contrast to physiologic tachycardia, the onset and offset are paroxysmal. The

tachycardia rate is often less than 130/min and the P waves during tachycardia are identical or nearly so to those seen in sinus rhythm (Fig. 6-1). At electrophysiologic testing, tachycardia can be induced and terminated with single atrial extrastimuli. Intra-atrial conduction delay is not necessary for initiation. Earliest atrial activation during tachycardia is in the sinus node region, and the activation sequence is "high to low." Carotid sinus massage and other vagal maneuvers typically slow and terminate tachycardia, since increased vagal tone prolongs sinus nodal refractoriness but shortens atrial refractoriness. This observation supports the involvement of sinus node tissue as part of the reentrant circuit.

Treatment, when necessary, is empirical, and beta blockers or calcium antagonists are generally successful. Other antiarrhythmics, including class 1 and class 3 agents, can be equally efficacious.

### "Chronic" Sinus Tachycardia

An ill-defined "syndrome" of chronic, nonparoxysmal, apparently inappropriate sinus tachycardia has been described in the literature.[7,8] The heart rate is variable but consistently greater than 100/min. The tachycardia is indistinguishable from sinus tachycardia electrocardiographically and electrophysiologically except that the "resting" rate seems to be reset higher than normal. It has been suggested that the fundamental abnormality is altered autonomic modulation,[7] although this is not well established. Treatment with beta blockers has been recommended, although occasionally sinus node ablative therapy has been suggested for refractory patients.[8] In the experience of the authors, such patients are generally younger women, not infrequently health care workers. Abuse of adrenergic or atropinic compounds may be suspected in some patients, but others appear psychologically stable and no evidence of substance abuse is found. At this point, it is unclear whether this is a homogeneous pathologic entity or if some of these patients have a primary cause of sinus tachycardia that remains elusive.

## Atrial Tachycardia

Atrial tachycardia may be defined as tachycardia originating in atrial muscle at a site or sites other than the sinus node or AV node. Atrial flutter and fibrillation are "atrial" by this definition but are sufficiently unique to be described separately. The nomenclature for this tachycardia is not uniform. We have used the term *atrial tachycardia* in lieu of *ectopic atrial tachycardia* and consider the descriptor *ectopic* to be redundant.

Atrial tachycardia affects fewer than 10 percent of patients presenting with supraventricular tachycardia.[3] The resting electrocardiogram during sinus rhythm is not distinctive. During tachycardia, P waves dissimilar from sinus P waves are usually discernible, with rates between 100 and 240/min. The essence of diagnosis is observing that atrial tachycardia continues during AV node block occurring spontaneously or induced by vagal maneuvers or adenosine (Fig. 6-2). The absence of retrograde conduction at electrophysiologic study even after the administration of atropine or isoproterenol strongly points to a diagnosis of atrial tachycardia if the arrhythmia is not inducible even though AV block during spontaneous tachycardia has not been observed.

Atrial tachycardia is usually associated with cardiac or pulmonary disease, although it can occur in isolation, especially in the pediatric population.[9,10] Patients usually present with paroxysmal or nonparoxysmal tachycardia but can present with dyspnea and heart failure secondary to incessant tachycardia. The latter is dependent on the duration and rate of tachycardia. In one series, 94 percent of patients with a rate greater than 130/min on routine electrocardiogram presented with impaired left ventricular function.[10] Left ventricular dysfunction secondary to tachycardia-induced myopathy is generally reversible to some extent after the tachycardia is suppressed.[11,12]

The mechanism of atrial tachycardia may be difficult to establish unequivocally even with electrophysiologic testing.[9] The essential feature of intraatrial reentrant tachycardia is induction (and termination) by atrial extrastimuli within a consistently defined range of prematurity (Fig. 6-3). Induction occurs with closely coupled extrastimuli and onset of tachycardia is dependent on intraatrial conduction delay. Entrainment and reset may be demonstrated if the tachycardia rate is not excessive. Resting abnormalities of atrial conduction and refractoriness may be observed. Intraatrial reentrant tachycardia is usually seen in patients with heart disease and enlarged atria,[10,13,14] especially after atrial surgery for congenital heart disease. It frequently coexists with atrial flutter or fibrillation. The atrial rate is not affected by adenosine.[13] The mechanism is postulated to be abnormal automaticity when the tachycardia is not induced or terminated by pacing techniques. Triggered activity may be suggested when atrial tachycardia is induced by rapid atrial

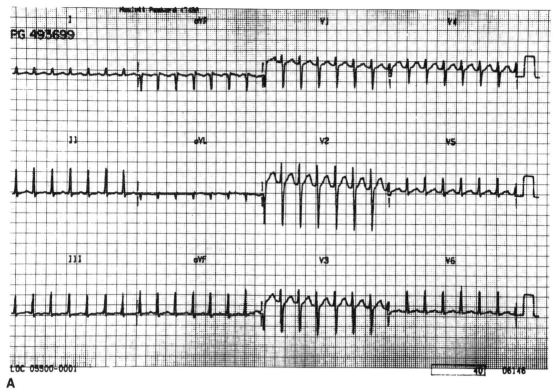

**A**

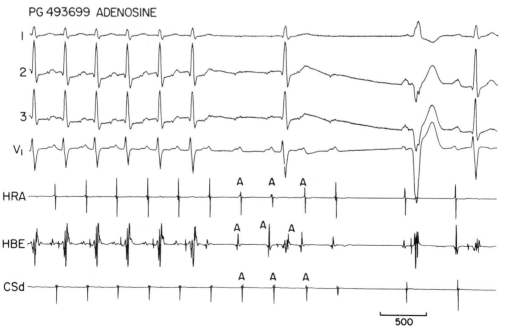

PG 493699  ADENOSINE

**B**

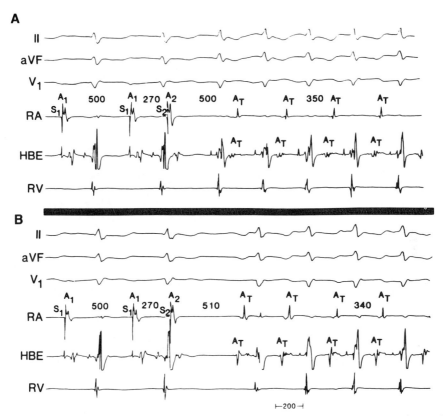

*Figure 6-3*  Induction of atrial tachycardia by programmed atrial extrastimuli. In panel *A*, onset of tachycardia appears to be related to prolongation of the AH interval, suggesting AV or AV-node reentry. In panel *B*, atrial tachycardia is initiated by an identical atrial extrastimulus which does *not* conduct to the AV node but initiates atrial tachycardia (AT) after a similar delay. (Key: II, AVF and $V_1$ = surface ECG leads; HBE = His bundle electrogram; RA = right atrial electrogram; RV = right ventricular electrogram; $S_1$ = atrial drive stimulus; $S_2$ = atrial extrastimulus; $A_1$ and $A_2$ = atrial activation as a result of $S_1$ and $S_2$, respectively.)

pacing without the other features associated with intraatrial reentry and is terminated by verapamil or adenosine (Fig. 6-2). The latter mechanisms (abnormal automaticity, triggered activity) are more

◀ *Figure 6-2*  Atrial tachycardia. Panel *A* shows supraventricular tachycardia at cycle length 380 ms without clearly discernible P waves. The administration of adenosine, 6 mg intravenously, during electrophysiologic testing (panel *B*) clarifies the diagnosis. Adenosine results in a brief period of AV block before terminating atrial tachycardia. (Key: 1, 2, 3, $V_1$ = surface ECG leads; CSd = distal coronary sinus; HBE = His bundle electrogram; HRA = high right atrium.)

frequent in children without other heart disease.[10,15] They may also be implicated in atrial tachycardia associated with pulmonary disease and digitalis toxicity, although the latter patients rarely undergo electrophysiologic testing.

Medical therapy for atrial tachycardia generally requires a drug to prolong AV node refractoriness and limit the ventricular response (verapamil, digitalis, beta blocker) and a second membrane-active drug (class 1a, 1c, or 3) to maintain sinus rhythm. Drugs such as sotalol and amiodarone may be used more frequently as monotherapy, since they prolong AV node refractoriness in addition to providing

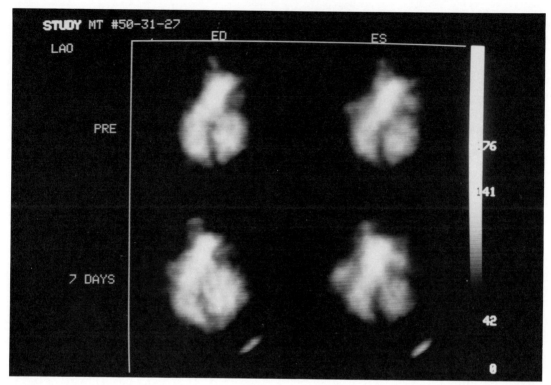

*Figure 6-4*   Radionuclide ventriculogram in a patient with incessant atrial tachycardia. The left anterior oblique (LAO) projections are shown. The *top panel* shows poor ventricular function with little difference between the end-diastolic (ED) and end-systolic (ES) frames. The ejection fraction was approximately 25 percent. Seven days after catheter ablation of a left atrial ectopic focus, ventricular function has improved considerably (*lower panel*), and the ejection fraction is now approximately 50 percent.

membrane stabilization. Operative ablation of the focus as determined by myocardial mapping has been successful in drug-refractory instances.[10,12] Multiple foci of tachycardia may emerge after successful elimination of the dominant focus, especially when this is localized to the right atrium.[10] Initial experience with catheter-ablative techniques for ectopic foci is encouraging but limited[10,16] (Fig. 6-4); AV-node ablation with implantation of a pacemaker may be useful.

## Multifocal Atrial Tachycardia

This atrial tachycardia is defined electrocardiographically by a heart rate greater than 100/min, three or more different ectopic P-wave morphologies, and an irregular ventricular response[17,18] (Fig. 6-5). It is usually seen in critically ill patients with diabetes mellitus, hypoxia, respiratory failure, acidosis, and electrolyte imbalance as concomitant features but may occasionally be found in ambulatory patients with no apparent heart disease. The tachycardia usually resolves with improvement of the patient's general condition. Beta-blocking agents may be useful but often are relatively contraindicated because of accompanying problems. Verapamil has been shown to be effective in providing symptomatic relief while other measures are being taken. Slowing of the atrial rate after verapamil suggests that the mechanism may be triggered activity.[19]

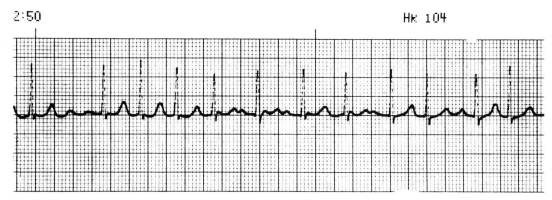

2:50                                                        HR 104

*Figure 6-5*   Rhythm strip with multifocal atrial tachycardia. The rate is "irregularly irregular," and multiple P-wave morphologies are noted.

## Atrial Fibrillation

Atrial fibrillation was observed in humans as a clinical entity as early as 1909.[20] It is the most common sustained arrhythmia in clinical practice and is present in approximately 0.4 percent of the population.[21] Its prevalence increases with age and heart disease to over 5 percent of the population aged 65 or above.[22] Atrial fibrillation is characterized electrocardiographically by low-amplitude, variable, and irregular baseline undulations corresponding to atrial rates in excess of 300/min. This "fibrillatory" activity has been described as fine or coarse, depending on amplitude but this distinction has not been useful clinically. Atrial fibrillatory activity is not associated with effective atrial contraction. The ventricular rate is totally irregular and has been described as "irregularly irregular." This irregularity may be more difficult to appreciate at rapid rates. The ventricular irregularity is related to both the atrial irregularity and repetitive concealed conduction of variable degree into the AV node by the atrial fibrillatory impulses. The mean ventricular rate is usually between 100 to 150/min in the absence of preexcitation and is markedly susceptible to acceleration by vagolysis and catecholamines (i.e., standing, exercise).

### Mechanisms

The mechanism of atrial fibrillation has been extensively investigated since initial observations of this arrhythmia. Two general mechanistic hypotheses have been proposed. The "focal" hypothesis suggests that atrial fibrillation is due to one or more areas of ectopic automaticity that account for the electrocardiographic appearance. Experimentally, aconitine produces rapid focal firing when applied to the atrium directly, and this produces an experimental type of atrial fibrillation electrocardiographically similar to clinical atrial fibrillation.[23] The rate of focal firing in this model is sufficiently rapid that the surrounding atrial tissue is not able to follow in a 1:1 fashion. Functional blocks and "fibrillatory" type of conduction then result. Fibrillation stops when the ectopic focus is abolished. An alternate "multiple wavelet" hypothesis was advanced by Moe,[24] in which atrial fibrillation is a result of multiple tiny reentrant wavelets all present simultaneously, constantly changing their paths in search of nonrefractory atrial muscle. Experimental support for this model was provided by Allessie and coworkers[25] in an animal model using programmed atrial stimulation and multichannel recording techniques. This type of reentry was called *leading circle* reentry by these authors, since it did not depend on a classic anatomic obstacle but rather a functional one based on refractoriness (see Fig. 5-10 in Chap. 5). Atrial fibrillation would stop if the reentrant circuits would randomly coalesce, and this probability is enhanced by the presence of fewer and larger wavelets. Multiple small wavelets are possible with very slow conduction velocity and short refractory periods of atrial tissue.

The "minimum" wavelet size is described by the product of conduction velocity and refractory period (wavelength = CV × RP) and can be thought of as the minimum route length that an impulse can travel within its refractory period.[25] Antiarrhythmic drugs that prolong refractoriness and/or accelerate conduction velocity would thus increase wavelet size and be "antifibrillatory." Conversely, vagal tone shortens atrial refractory period and is known to perpetuate atrial fibrillation experimentally[26] and clinically.[27,28] It has long been known that fibrillation requires a critical mass,[29] and this observation is compatible with the multiple wavelet hypothesis. Clinical atrial fibrillation is uncommon in small animals (rodents, cats) and relatively common in large mammals such as horses. Clinically, atrial fibrillation is uncommon in infants and young children. The multiple wavelet hypothesis is currently considered to explain the mechanism of atrial fibrillation by most observers. This does not, however, rule out focal, rapid firing as a provocative factor in clinical atrial fibrillation. Atrial fibrillation in the Wolff-Parkinson-White syndrome is known to be elicited by rapid reciprocating tachycardia.[30,31] Indeed, electrogram patterns in atrial fibrillation unassociated with the preexcitation syndromes sometimes suggest a more focal rapid firing which could conceivably be the trigger for atrial fibrillation and the rest of the atria (Fig. 6-6).

### Clinical Presentation

The disorders associated with atrial fibrillation are too numerous to provide a meaningful and useful catalog. It can be associated with virtually any cardiopulmonary or systemic disease, although the most common associated disorders are hypertension and ischemic heart disease. Atrial fibrillation may be related to hyperthyroidism, alcohol consumption, occult mitral valve disease, pulmonary embolism, and many other conditions (Fig. 6-7). In some instances, other supraventricular tachycardias may initiate atrial fibrillation, with the presentation simulating primary atrial fibrillation. This has best been demonstrated with reciprocating AV tachycardia but

can also occur with AV node reentrant tachycardia (Fig. 6-8) and probably other supraventricular tachycardias.[32] This is a potentially "curable" cause of atrial fibrillation and should be sought, especially in younger patients without any obvious associated factors. A loop event recorder may be useful for this if the tachycardia occurs frequently. Atrial fibrillation in the absence of apparent heart disease has been named "lone" atrial fibrillation[33] and may account for up to 25 to 35 percent of all cases. Lone atrial fibrillation is frequently attributed to occult degenerative atrial fibrosis and conduction disease. Atrial fibrillation has been an independent predictor of mortality in all groups of patients, although this excess in mortality is chiefly attributed to the associated cardiovascular or other disease. There is minimal if any excess mortality in lone atrial fibrillation[34] or atrial fibrillation associated with a reversible cause such as hyperthyroidism.

The clinical presentation with atrial fibrillation is also variable but includes the following:

1. Incidental finding in an asymptomatic individual
2. Palpitations
3. Systemic embolism
4. Miscellaneous factors such as syncope, angina, effort intolerance, and heart failure

Patients with severe organic heart disease such as obstructive hypertropic cardiomyopathy may decompensate rapidly with the onset of atrial fibrillation, due to both the uncontrolled ventricular rate and the loss of effective atrial contraction with its contribution to cardiac output. Patients may also present with paroxysmal or chronic atrial fibrillation. The natural history of paroxysmal atrial fibrillation can be variable. Paroxysms can be infrequent or progress to chronic atrial fibrillation in up to two-thirds of individuals if followed for a sufficient time period, especially those with organic heart disease.[33] The classic clinical signs of atrial fibrillation are well known and include an "irregularly irregular" heart rate, frequently associated with pulse deficit (heart rate by palpation less than by auscultation) and a

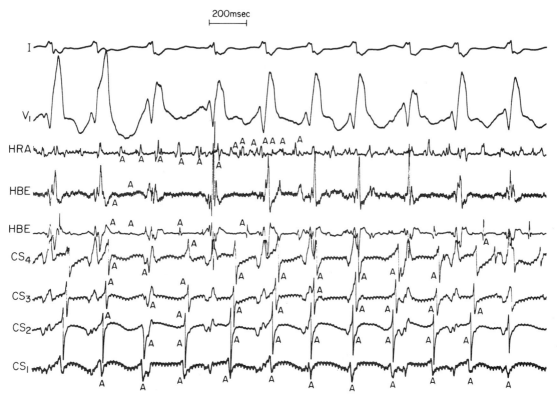

*Figure 6-6*   Intracardiac records in atrial fibrillation. The atrial fibrillatory pattern is clearly dissimilar in different parts of the atrium. This is most evident when examining the high right atrium, which shows rapid fibrillatory activity, and comparing it to the coronary sinus, which shows a slower, more organized atrial rhythm. This raises the possibility that focal atrial firing in the left atrium is responsible for atrial fibrillation, which is more desynchronized in the right atrium. Conversely, the higher frequency of responses in the high right atrium might suggest that the primary source of fibrillatory activity is in the right atrium, with the left atrium being activated secondarily. (Key: I, $V_1$ = surface ECG leads; $CS_4$, $CS_3$, $CS_2$, $CS_1$ = unipolar coronary sinus leads from proximal (4) to distal (1); HBE = His bundle electrogram; HRA = high right atrium.)

variable first heart sound. Fibrillatory waves may also be appreciated in the jugular venous pulse, and the pulse amplitude is variable.

## Management

The acute management of atrial fibrillation is not controversial. Associated correctable precipitating factors are corrected or minimized. Cardioversion is indicated early if there is severe hemodynamic decompensation. Otherwise, antiarrhythmic drug strategy is twofold, with initial attempts to control the ventricular rate using AV node blocking agents

such as digitalis, beta blockers, and calcium antagonists. Membrane-active agents are then added in an attempt to restore sinus rhythm. The latter agents include the class 1a drugs (quinidine, procainamide, disopyramide), 1c drugs (propafenone, flecainide), and class 3 drugs (sotalol, amiodarone). Cardioversion may be considered if atrial fibrillation persists after the above measures have been instituted. Management of the patient with recurrent or chronic atrial fibrillation initially involves a broad-based laboratory investigation focused by the results of history and physical examination. In the patient with no overt clinical findings, screening for thyroid abnormalities, pulmo-

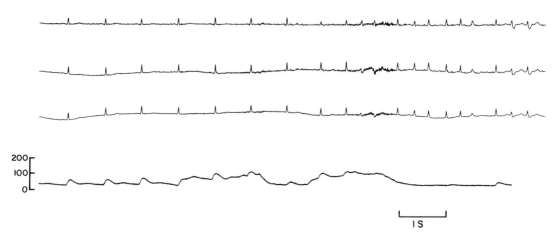

*Figure 6-7*    "Vagal" atrial fibrillation. This patient presented with syncope and was found to be in atrial fibrillation after the episode. Tilt testing revealed a positive vasodepressor response with atrial fibrillation occurring only after the onset of hypotension. In this figure, the blood pressure has already fallen to 50 mmHg (onset of record) and atrial fibrillation is evident after the ninth QRS complex. Atrial fibrillation in this instance may well be due to vagal stimulation, as has been observed in animal models.

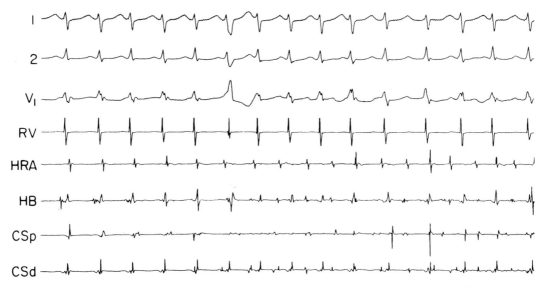

*Figure 6-8*    Atrial fibrillation secondary to AV node reentry. This patient presented with atrial fibrillation in the absence of other heart disease. AV node reentry was induced at electrophysiologic study (first five complexes) which quickly degenerated into atrial fibrillation (sixth and subsequent complexes). (Key: 1, 2, $V_1$ = surface ECG leads; CSp and CSd = proximal and distal coronary sinuses, respectively; HB = His bundle; HRA = high right atrium; RV = right ventricle.)

nary emboli, and occult heart disease is appropriate. Chronic antiarrhythmic drug management is largely by trial and error, based on the principles of rate control and maintenance of sinus rhythm with membrane-active drugs.[35] Electrophysiologic testing has a very limited role but may occasionally be useful as when a "primary" supraventricular tachycardia is suspected to be the trigger for atrial fibrillation. The clinician must choose one of two fundamental antiarrhythmic drug strategies, namely the acceptance of atrial fibrillation with rate control or the preservation of sinus rhythm with membrane-active antiarrhythmic drugs. The maintenance of normal sinus rhythm and prevention of atrial fibrillation is intuitively the preferred strategy, with many theoretical benefits, including

1.  Improved hemodynamics and cardiac output
2.  Prevention of systemic embolism
3.  Improved exercise tolerance
4.  Prevention of left atrial dilatation[36]

Aggressive attempts at maintaining sinus rhythm are indicated in severely symptomatic patients, especially those who are hemodynamically compromised during atrial fibrillation. Dual therapy is required in such patients, with an agent to control the ventricular response (in the event of breakthrough) in addition to a membrane-active drug to prevent atrial fibrillation. On the other hand, prevention of recurrent atrial fibrillation may be difficult or impossible even after aggressive drug trials. Concerns have been raised about increased mortality due to proarrhythmia with class 1a[37] and class 1c[38] agents even if sinus rhythm is maintained. The latter concerns may account for the increasing use of "low-dose" amiodarone (in the range of 200 mg daily) for the prevention of atrial fibrillation.[39] An alternate strategy is the acceptance of chronic atrial fibrillation, with the major end point of drug therapy being rate control. This is an especially viable strategy in patients in whom maintenance of sinus rhythm has not been successful, the latter frequently including patients with organic heart disease, enlarged left atria, and long-standing (more than 1 year) atrial fibrillation.[33] The preferred

drugs for rate control include the calcium antagonists and beta blockers. Although digitalis is a time-honored agent in atrial fibrillation, controlled trials have not verified efficacy in converting atrial fibrillation to sinus rhythm. In addition, rate control with digitalis is essentially lost with upright posture, especially during exercise.[40–42]

### Anticoagulation

Systemic emboli have been reported in 1 to 2 percent of patients undergoing cardioversion for atrial fibrillation.[43] Pharmacologic cardioversion can also result in emboli. Emboli occur immediately or up to 4 weeks after cardioversion. Although the efficacy of anticoagulation in preventing such emboli has not been demonstrated, anticoagulation with warfarin is currently recommended prior to cardioversion of atrial fibrillation of at least 3 to 4 days' duration. Generally, anticoagulation for 2 or 3 weeks prior to and after cardioversion is suggested.[43] Transesophageal echocardiography may identify patients with clot at risk for systemic emboli after cardioversion.[44]

The high incidence of systemic embolization in rheumatic mitral stenosis has long been appreciated. Routine anticoagulation with warfarin has been standard therapy in patients with atrial fibrillation and rheumatic valve disease who would otherwise face a 17-fold increase in the incidence of stroke.[45] In nonrheumatic atrial fibrillation, a fourfold increase in embolic stroke has been demonstrated for both chronic and paroxysmal atrial fibrillation.[46,47] This amounts to an incidence of approximately 5 percent per year in this condition, although a much smaller incidence of 0.5 percent has been reported in lone atrial fibrillation.[34] The results of four large, randomized, placebo-controlled trials have verified the efficacy of anticoagulation with warfarin in the prevention of stroke in patients with nonrheumatic atrial fibrillation. The risk reduction varied from 42 to 82 percent in these trials.[48,49] The incidence of major bleeding was generally less than 1 percent, largely due to the use of more modest doses of warfarin that were found to be effective (prothrombin time generally in the range of 1.5 times control or INR in the range of 2.7). It is probably not necessary to anticoagulate all patients. Risk factors have been identified that can be helpful in clinical decision making,[50,51] including the following:

1. Presence of hypertension
2. Recent (3 months) congestive heart failure
3. A history of previous systemic emboli
4. Age above 60
5. Left ventricular dysfunction
6. Enlarged left atrium

Conversely, patients who are not diabetic, below 60 years of age, and have lone atrial fibrillation are probably at very low risk of embolization. Aspirin, 325 mg/day, showed efficacy over placebo in one large trial,[52] with a 44 percent risk reduction. The ultimate role of aspirin remains to be clarified.

In spite of the results of these trials, individualization in patient management remains appropriate. For example, only 23 percent of the eligible 18,376 patients were randomized in one trial,[52] raising questions about the general applicability of the results to all patients. Certainly, considerations of compliance, occupation, lifestyle, and history of bleeding may lead a physician to choose to not anticoagulate. Aspirin may be a reasonable alternative in such individuals until further data regarding its role are available.

### Nonpharmacologic Therapy

Although there is no "curative" therapy for atrial fibrillation, several very useful nonpharmacologic options have emerged in the last decade. Catheter ablation of the AV node with implantation of a rate-responsive pacemaker is highly effective in the more severely symptomatic patients who have failed drug therapy.[53] Unfortunately, this therapy does not obviate the need for anticoagulation and requires a lifelong committment to pacing. Many patients achieve great symptomatic improvement, and the threshold to use this type of therapy is lessening among clinicians. Indeed, it has been suggested that good rate control after catheter ablation of the AV node results in long-term improvement in cardiac size and function.[54]

There have been two operative approaches to the prevention of atrial fibrillation. The "corridor" procedure described by Guiraudon.[55] isolates the atria into three electrically distinct fragments including the left atrium, right atrium, and a "corridor" between the sinus node and the AV node. Normal sinus node function can be maintained with a normal chronotropic response and the mass of the corridor is sufficiently small to prevent atrial fibrillation within it. Atrial fibrillation may continue in the "excluded" atrial segments, although this would not be appreciated by the patient. The need for anticoagulation is not obviated and atrial contractility is not maintained in a synchronized fashion. Cox et al.[56] have described an atrial procedure that they have termed the *maze*. This consists of a series of incisions in the atrium meant to prevent the perpetuation of multiple wavelets of reentry that are responsible for atrial fibrillation. Initial reports of this procedure ar encouraging. Unfortunately, both operative procedures involve major open-heart surgery and probably are not feasible for the majority of patients with atrial fibrillation who are frequently elderly with significant comorbid conditions.

## *Atrial Flutter*

Atrial flutter was recognized as a clinical arrhythmia as early as 1910.[57] It is characterized electrocardiographically as a supraventricular tachycardia with atrial rate between 250 and 350/min and with atrial rates as low as 200/min in the presence of membrane-active drugs.[1] There is typically a "saw-tooth" pattern of flutter waves with a continuously undulating baseline usually best appreciated in the inferior leads 2, 3, and AVF. The ventricular response is usually one-half of the flutter rate (150/min), but higher degrees of atrioventricular block are also seen, usually in even ratios (4:1, 6:1, and so on). There may be variable Wenckebach patterns, producing an "irregularly irregular" ventricular rate. Flutter waves may not be readily apparent with 2:1 AV conduction

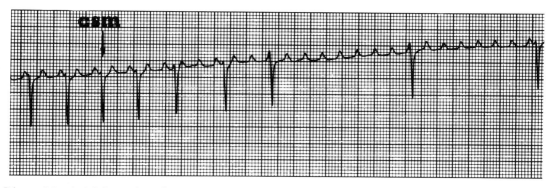

*Figure 6-9*   Atrial flutter. The flutter waves are not readily apparent until carotid sinus massage (CSM) is applied resulting in temporary increase in AV block and exposure of the flutter waves.

but can be readily exposed by carotid sinus massage, which causes transient AV block (Fig. 6-9). The flutter rate can be increased by maneuvers which decrease atrial size (i.e., standing), presumably by shortening the tachycardia circuit length.[58]

Two types of atrial flutter are recognized.[59] The "common," or type 1, flutter is characterized by atrial rates of 250 to 350/min and predominantly negative flutter waves recorded in the inferior limb leads (Fig. 6-10). This tachycardia can be terminated by atrial pacing. The "uncommon," or type 2, flutter is characterized by more rapid atrial rates, 350 to 450/min. The flutter waves have a predominantly positive deflection as recorded in the inferior leads. This flutter cannot be terminated by atrial pacing, although it may be converted to atrial fibrillation.

## Mechanisms

The mechanism of atrial flutter was debated for a long time with proponents of both focal abnormal automaticity[60] and reentry.[61] A great deal of evidence now supports the view that clinical atrial flutter is due to macroreentry in the right atrium.[62–67] Type 1 or common flutter has been most extensively studied and conforms to classic reentry with an excitable gap. The excitable gap can be demonstrated using single atrial extrastimuli (see Fig. 5-7 in Chap. 5) or entrainment by incremental atrial pacing (Fig. 6-11). Mapping of the circuit demonstrates a low to

high sequence up the anterior and septal walls, with a high to low sequence down the lateral and posterior walls (Fig. 6-12). A corridor of block characterized by "double spike" potentials can be demonstrated during endocardial mapping and probably corresponds to the crista terminalis.[65,67,68] The slow conduction zone of the circuit is near the isthmus between the inferior vena cava orifice and the inferior tricuspid ring, with the impulse emerging from this zone near the orifice of the coronary sinus. The latter zone is the "target" for operative or catheter ablation of the arrhythmia.

Type 2 flutter has not been as extensively studied. Evidence from endocardial mapping suggests that it is due to right atrial reentry, with the circuit described above reversed.[67] This arrhythmia cannot be entrained or reset. It is probable that the circuit does not have an excitable gap but is circulating at the maximal velocity allowed by the atrial functional refractory period.

## Clinical Presentation

Atrial flutter is observed in patients of any age but usually in those with organic heart disease.[1,69] The clinical setting overlaps considerably with that of atrial fibrillation, and both arrhythmias may be observed in the same individual. Generally, patients with both are treated as if they had atrial fibrillation. Factors predisposing to atrial fibrillation—including

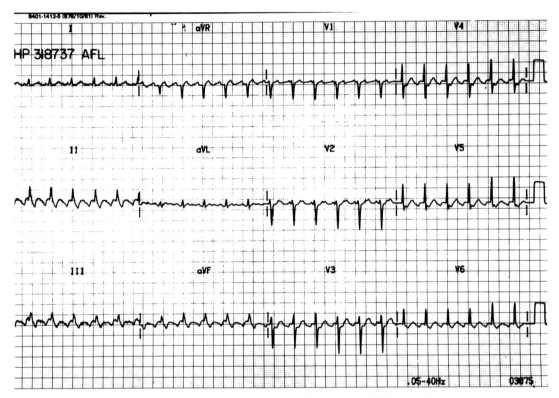

*Figure 6-10* 12 lead ECG during "common" atrial flutter. There is 2:1 AV block with predominately negative flutter waves in the inferior leads.

hyperthyroidism, pulmonary embolism, alcohol, and cardiac surgery—also predispose to atrial flutter. Atrial flutter may be paroxysmal or chronic. It usually presents as palpitations but can present with syncope, hypotension, and even cardiac arrest in individuals capable of one-to-one AV conduction during flutter.[70] Patients may also present with effort intolerance, dyspnea, or congestive heart failure.

### Acute Therapy

The basic principles of drug therapy are identical for all atrial tachycardias.[1,71] The first goal is control of the ventricular rate using AV node blocking drugs; the second goal is reversion to sinus rhythm using membrane-active agents, as outlined previously. Elective cardioversion is considered after adequate AV node blockade is achieved and a therapeutic level of the selected membrane-active drug is attained.

Cardioversion is always indicated at any point in the presence of hemodynamic compromise. This "classic" approach is frequently difficult to apply in atrial

*Figure 6-11* Entrainment during atrial flutter. Panel *A* illustrates atrial pacing at progressively more rapid rates, with acceleration of the flutter cycle length to the paced rate. A is the control strip and the paced rate is progressively increased from strip B to strip D. The pacing has not altered the flutter-wave morphology, and the arrhythmia resumes at its former rate after cessation of pacing in each strip. Panel *B* illustrates the effect of further acceleration of the pacing rate. At the first asterisk in strip A, there is a sudden change in the flutter-wave morphology, signifying the transition from entrainment of the circuit to cessation of reentry. Sinus rhythm ensues after discontinuation of pacing in strip B and continues in strip C. S denotes stimulus artifact. *(From Waldo AL et al: The role of transient entrainment in atrial flutter, in Touboul P, Waldo AL (eds): Atrial Arrhythmias: Current Concepts and Management. St. Louis, Mosby Year Book, 1990. Reproduced by permission.)* ⟶

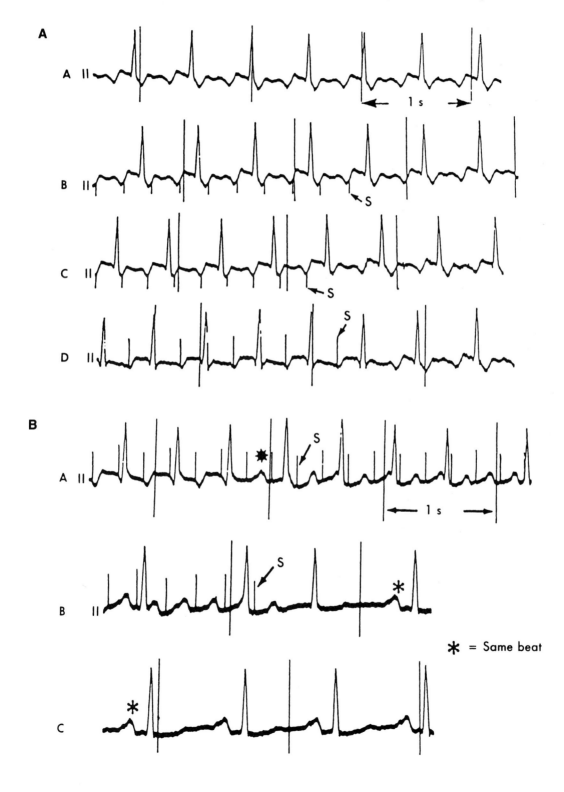

* = Same beat

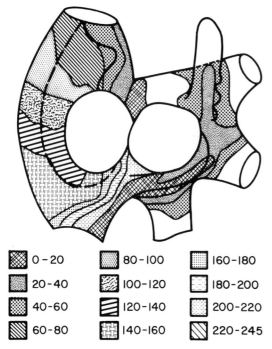

| ▨ | 0 - 20 | ▨ | 80 - 100 | ▦ | 160 - 180 |
|---|--------|---|----------|---|-----------|
| ▨ | 20 - 40 | ▧ | 100 - 120 | ▤ | 180 - 200 |
| ▨ | 40 - 60 | ▨ | 120 - 140 | ▦ | 200 - 220 |
| ▨ | 60 - 80 | ▤ | 140 - 160 | ◨ | 220 - 245 |

*Figure 6-12* Epicardial mapping during common atrial flutter. The heart is displayed as if the atria were removed from the ventricles and viewed from below, with the tricuspid valve orifice to the left and the mitral valve orifice to the right. Atrial activation proceeds from the posteroseptal region counterclockwise around the tricuspid valve orifice to return to the posteroseptal region via the atrial septum. The left atrium is activated passively. Numbers indicate isochrone lines (lines of equal activation time) which are 20 ms apart.

flutter. Control of the ventricular rate is difficult to achieve and abrupt transitions from "too fast" to "too slow" can occur. Membrane-active drugs, especially the 1c agents propafenone and flecainide, are very effective at prolonging the flutter cycle length but less effective at terminating flutter. For these reasons, it is not inappropriate to consider early cardioversion or the use of atrial pacing techniques, the latter being very effective for type 1 flutter.[72] Atrial pacing can be achieved by transvenous catheterization, by the esophageal route, or by epicardial wires in the postoperative patient. Atrial pacing is begun at 10 cycles/min faster than the spontaneous flutter rate and periodically incremented by 10/min. An abrupt change in flutter-wave morphology

indicates termination of flutter (Fig. 6-11). The critical rate required to terminate type 1 flutter is usually between 115 and 125 percent of the flutter rate. Attempts at pace termination of atrial flutter may result in induction of atrial fibrillation, which is frequently self-terminating in the patient without a history of atrial fibrillation.

### Chronic Management

Electrophysiologic testing in the patient with recurrent flutter will frequently demonstrate atrial conduction defects, including intraatrial conduction delays.[73] Flutter can be induced by atrial extrastimuli or atrial pacing resulting in atrial conduction delay and can be terminated as described. Generally, however, pharmacologic prophylactic therapy for atrial flutter is empirical with efficacy determined by trial and error. Dual therapy with both an AV node blocking drug and a membrane-active drug is recommended except for drugs such as sotalol and amiodarone, which have both properties. The use of membrane-active drugs alone may slow the atrial rate sufficiently to allow one-to-one AV conduction in some patients and are thus potentially "proarrhythmic" when used alone (Fig. 6-13).

Nonpharmacologic options are available for drug-refractory patients. Catheter ablation of the AV node (with implantation of a rate-responsive pacemaker) is useful, especially for patients with coexistent atrial fibrillation. More recently, catheter ablation in the region near the isthmus between the inferior tricuspid ring and the orifice of the inferior vena cava has been applied to common atrial flutter, using both DC energy[74] and radiofrequency energy.[75] This will probably become the nonpharmacologic therapy of choice for problematic atrial flutter.

Operative therapy has been described for type 1 flutter.[64] Intraoperative mapping during flutter verified the mechanism of flutter and provided the rationale for cryosurgery of the narrowest part of the right atrial reentrant circuit, the region bounded by the orifice of the inferior vena cava, the inferior tricuspid valve margin, and the orifice of the coronary sinus. This procedure has been largely supplanted by catheter ablation.

Finally, indications for anticoagulation in atrial flutter, either chronically or prior to cardioversion, are not clearly established. Theoretically, atrial flutter is associated with more synchronized atrial contraction than atrial fibrillation and might not be associated with thrombus formation in the atrium. There is currently no clear evidence of increased risk of systemic embolism in atrial flutter, and anticoagulation is not generally recommended.

## AV Node Reentry

Moe and coworkers[76] originally demonstrated AV node reentry in the dog and introduced the concept

of *dual pathways* in the AV junctional region as the substrate for this arrhythmia. This concept was supported in human studies by Kisten,[77] who observed two populations of PR intervals in selected patients during electrocardiographic recording, with short PR intervals postulated to be over the "fast pathway" and long PR intervals postulated to be over the "slow pathway" (see Figs. 17-14 and 17-15 in Chap. 17). Schuilenburg and Durrer[78] first demonstrated dual-pathway curves in humans utilizing the extrastimulus technique, relating interatrial interval ($A_1$-$A_2$) to prematurity of a ventricular extrastimulus. Finally, Rosen,[79] Denes et al.,[80] Wu,[81] and others proposed the connection between paroxysmal supraventricular tachycardia in humans and dual-pathway physiology demonstrated by the extrastimulus technique.

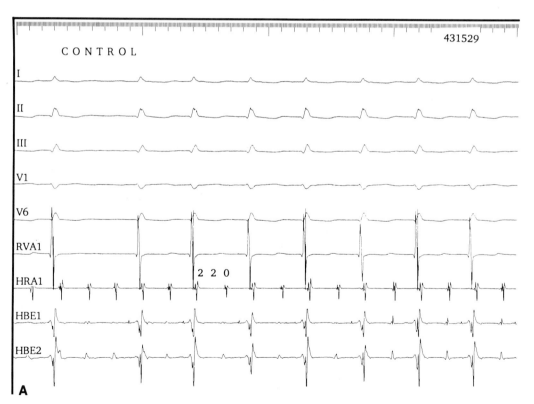

*Figure 6-13*  Propafenone in atrial flutter. The records are from a patient treated with propafenone as monotherapy for prophylaxis of atrial flutter. The patient returned with wide QRS tachycardia necessitating cardioversion. Electrophysiological testing in the absence of drug revealed inducible atrial flutter (panel *A*) at an atrial cycle length of 220 ms. The addition of propafenone (panel *B*) 140 mg intravenously resulted in   *(continues overleaf)*

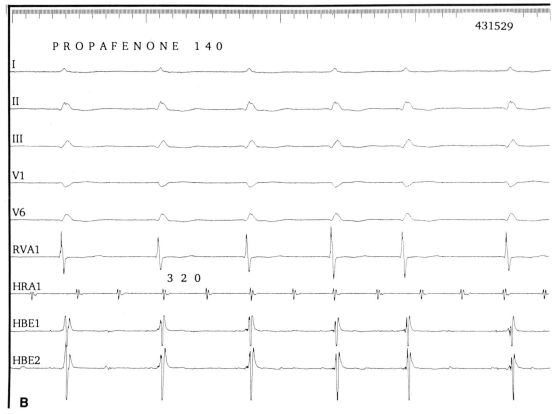

*Figure 6-13 (Continued)*   prolongation of the flutter cycle length considerably, to 320 ms. At this point, upright tilt (panel *C*) resulted in a slight shortening of cycle length to 285 ms with the occurrence of 1:1 AV conduction with aberrancy and reproduction of the patient's clinical tachycardia. One-to-one AV-node conduction during tilt was related to tilt induced autonomic changes, namely, vagolysis and enhanced sympathetic tone. This "pro-arrhythmia" would have been prevented by addition of an agent to provide AV node blockade.

### Clinical Presentation and Electrocardiographic Recognition

AV-node reentry accounts for approximately 60 percent of cases of paroxysmal supraventricular tachycardia referred to an electrophysiology laboratory.[81–85] It can occur in any age group but most frequently presents in young to middle-aged adults, being slightly more prevalent in women than in men. After presentation, further episodes will vary in frequency and duration but will usually persist for years. Once tachycardia has established a pattern, recurrence is the rule. There are generally no precipitating factors,

although some patients will report a consistent relationship of exercise, posture, or gastrointestinal symptoms to initiation of tachycardia. The onset is typically sudden and paroxysmal, and termination occurs abruptly. However, spontaneous termination is frequently perceived as gradual, possibly related to the occurrence of sinus tachycardia after abrupt termination of AV node reentry tachycardia in some patients. Symptoms are not specific, the most common being palpitation or the sensation of a rapid heartbeat. This may be accompanied by light-headedness, dyspnea, or chest pain. A sensation of throbbing in the neck is common. Syncope may

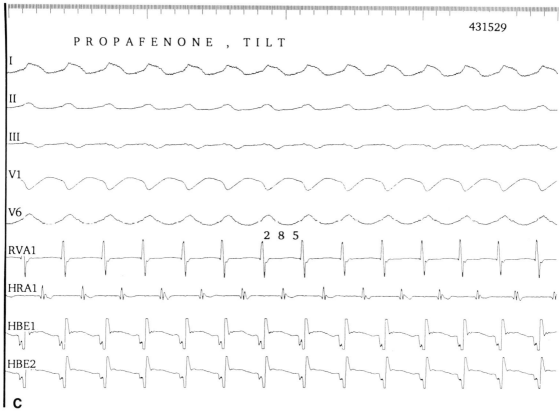

431529

PROPAFENONE , TILT

I

II

III

V1

V6

2 8 5

RVA1

HRA1

HBE1

HBE2

C

*Figure 6-13 (Continued)*

occur and usually does so either at the onset of tachycardia or well into the tachycardia episode. Syncope is usually related more to impaired vasomotor adaptation to tachycardia than to a prohibitively rapid rate.[86] Occasionally, syncope may be the presenting symptom, with the patient not having any awareness of a rapid heartbeat. The signs are similarly nonspecific, with most patients presenting with a diminished, regular pulse. The prognosis is generally excellent in the absence of concomitant heart disease.

Electrocardiographically, a regular supraventricular tachycardia is observed with rates ranging from 120 to 220/min (Fig. 6-14). Minor oscillations in cycle length may be observed and QRS alternans of QRS amplitude may be present with more rapid tachycardia. Functional bundle branch block does not affect the rate of tachycardia, since the bundle branches are not part of the reentrant circuit. The P wave is invariably simultaneous with a QRS complex or may be seen slightly before or after the QRS complex (Fig. 6-15). The uncommon type of AV node reentry has a long ventriculoatrial interval (RP > PR) (Fig. 6-16). P-wave locations intermediate between the two described are distinctly uncommon. If the P wave cannot be identified, it may be impossible to distinguish AV node reentry from AV reentry electrocardiographically.[87] ST depression of considerable magnitude is frequently observed and is a nonspecific phenomenon generally not related to coronary artery disease. The onset of tachycardia, when observed electrocardiographically, is frequently heralded by a premature atrial depolarization which results in a sudden prolongation of the PR interval, marking the onset of tachycardia. When spontaneous

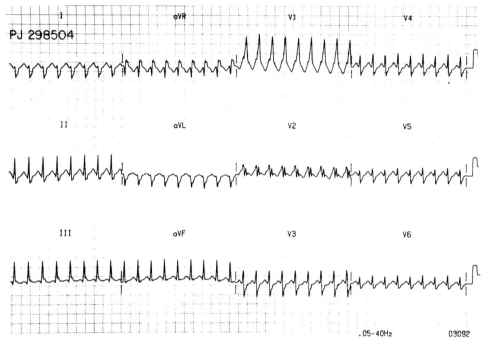

*Figure 6-14*  Typical AV node reentry. Right bundle branch block aberration is observed and P waves are not visible.

termination is observed and the P wave can be identified, the last QRS of the tachycardia is associated with a P wave, since reentry usually stops by block in the anterograde limb (PR) of the circuit. In fact, consistent termination of tachycardia with a P wave not followed by a QRS invariably represents an AV node-dependent tachycardia, either AV or AV node reentry (Chap. 12).

### Electrophysiologic Features

The fundamental concept for the substrate of AV node reentry is dual AV nodal pathways with disparate electrophysiologic properties. One pathway has a shorter conduction time and a longer refractory period (the fast pathway), while the other has a longer conduction time and a shorter refractory period (slow pathway). Unidirectional block in one of the pathways allows conduction over the alternate route, with retrograde conduction over the previously blocked pathway allowing for reentrance. This basic concept

is well established and no longer a subject of debate, although the specific anatomic correlates underlying the physiologic phenomena are less clear.[81,83,88–92] Typical AV node reentry is by far the most prevalent and is associated with "slow" anterograde conduction and "fast" retrograde conduction. The RP interval is short (< 90 ms) and the retrograde activation sequence as measured by intracardiac recordings usually demonstrates earliest atrial activity at the standard His catheter recording site. The atypical or uncommon variety is observed in fewer than 5 percent of patients presenting with supraventricular tachycardia.[93,94] It is characterized by a long RP interval (RP > PR) with retrograde conduction occurring over a "slow" pathway. Earliest retrograde atrial activation as assessed by electrophysiologic testing occurs near or at the orifice of the coronary sinus, at some distance from the recorded His electrogram. Very rarely, patients will experience a rare type of tachycardia related to "two for one" conduction, in which each sinus impulse produces

**A**

**B**

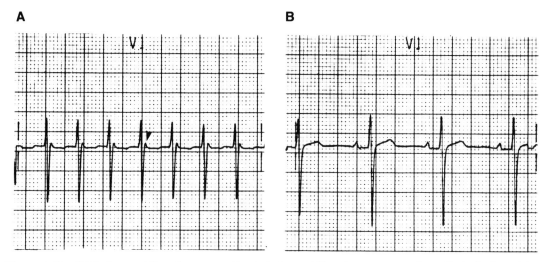

*Figure 6-15*   ECG clue to AV node reentry. Panel *A* shows AV node reentrant tachycardia in lead V₁. The P wave is observed as a tiny hump (r prime) at the end of the QRS complex (*arrowhead*); this is best appreciated by comparing the QRS complex to that in sinus rhythm (panel *B*).

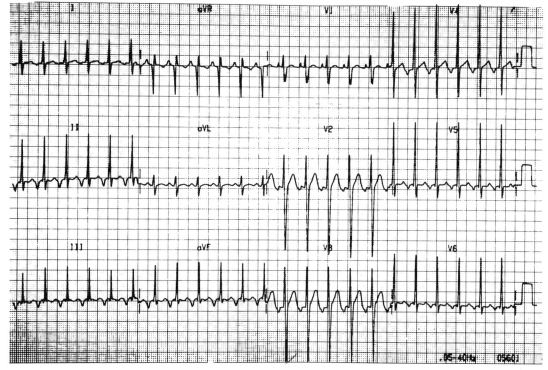

*Figure 6-16*   ECG during the uncommon type of AV node reentry. The RP interval is longer than the PR interval and the P wave is characteristically negative in leads 2, 3, and AVF.

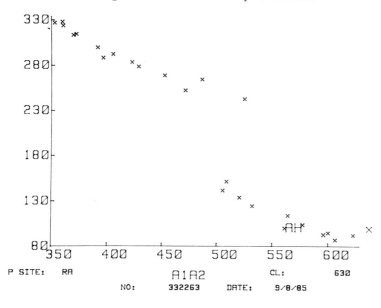

**Antegrade Refractory Period**

*Figure 6-18* Dual-pathway physiology. The curve relates prematurity of an atrial extrastimulus ($A_1$, $A_2$) on the x axis to the AH interval on the y axis in a patient with AV node reentrant tachycardia. At an $A_1$, $A_2$ interval of approximately 500 ms, there is an abrupt increase in the AH interval coinciding with the onset of tachycardia. There is frequently some minor variability of the coupling interval producing this transition.

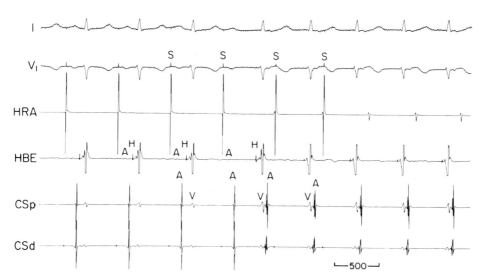

*Figure 6-19* Atrioventricular reentry with dual-pathway physiology. The figure demonstrates atrial pacing at a constant cycle length with a sudden prolongation of the AH interval (fourth cycle), initiating supraventricular tachycardia. The mechanism of tachycardia is, however, AV reentry utilizing a left lateral accessory pathway as the retrograde limb, as is evident by the fact that earliest retrograde atrial activation is at the distal coronary sinus (CSd). In this particular patient, atrioventricular reentry was dependent upon slow-pathway conduction. Either ablation of the slow pathway or ablation of the concealed left lateral pathway would be curative.

### Chronic Management

Patients with relatively infrequent and better-tolerated episodes may choose to deal with them on an "as required" basis, seeking medical help when needed. Some patients may also be successful at learning vagotonic maneuvers that may terminate tachycardia, such as the Valsalva maneuver, carotid sinus massage, facial ice-water immersion, or assuming a supine position. The mainstay of chronic prophylactic therapy in the past has been pharmacologic. Drug therapy may be electrophysiologically guided in patients with severe symptoms during tachycardia or it may be done on a trial-and-error (empirical) basis. Drug therapy may be directed at the anterograde limb of the circuit (verapamil, beta blocker, digoxin) or the retrograde limb (class 1a, class 1c; see Chap. 19). Combination therapy or drugs that combine more than one mode of action (for example, sotalol with class 3 and beta-blocking effect) may be used in difficult cases. The success of AV-node modification with radiofrequency current (see Chap. 17) directed at either the "fast" pathway or the "slow" pathway has had a great impact on the chronic management of patients with AV node reentrant tachycardia.[101–103] The slow-pathway approach, in particular, is associated with success rates in excess of 90 percent and a risk of inadvertent AV block in the range of 1 percent. This has had the effect of relegating radiofrequency modification of the node to a primary status in the management of this disorder and it is more frequently being offered as a reasonable alternative to a lifelong commitment to antiarrhythmic drugs. Operative therapy is very successful for AV node reentrance (see Chap. 20) but has been made virtually obsolete by the success of radiofrequency ablation. In a similar vein, antitachycardia pacemakers are also essentially obsolete for this particular arrhythmia.

### Anatomic Considerations

There remains very little dispute about the functional validity of the dual-pathway physiology concept to explain AV node reentrance. The anatomic correlates

of the constituents of the circuit are not as well established. Electrophysiologic data support the view that the entire circuit in AV node reentry is in the AV "junctional" area. This is most evident from the following observations during tachycardia:

1.  The ventricles are not required for maintenance of tachycardia. Block below the recorded His electrogram does not affect tachycardia[104–106] (Fig. 6-20).
2.  The His bundle is not essential to perpetuation of tachycardia. Tachycardia can continue with block above the recorded His,[105] and AV node reentry is inducible in the face of ventricular atrial block at the AV node level.[107]
3.  Atrial activity as measured by electrode catheters is not necessary for perpetuation of tachycardia.[91,108]

Observations after operative and ablative therapy of AV node reentry have also provided insights into AV node function. It is clear that either the "fast" pathway or the "slow" pathway can be ablated rather selectively, the fast pathway being posterior and inferior to the recorded His bundle site and the slow pathway at the "base" of Koch's triangle between the orifice of the coronary sinus and the tricuspid leaflet. In addition, there may be multiple slow pathways. The anterograde fast pathway and retrograde fast pathway are usually but not necessarily ablated together, suggesting that they may be anatomically distinct.[109]

Whether or not fast and slow pathways are "extranodal" or "intranodal" may be a moot issue. The AV junctional area in its entirety is situated at the base of the atrial septum on the right atrial aspect of the central fibrous body. The boundary between atrium and AV node is indistinct and irregular, both anatomically[89] and physiologically.[90] It is probable that the slow and fast pathways are in the "transitional zone" as described by Becker and Anderson (Fig. 6-21), with the slow pathway corresponding to the crista terminalis "extension" of the AV node. Transitional cells at the "boundary" of the AV node and atrium have rapid upstroke action

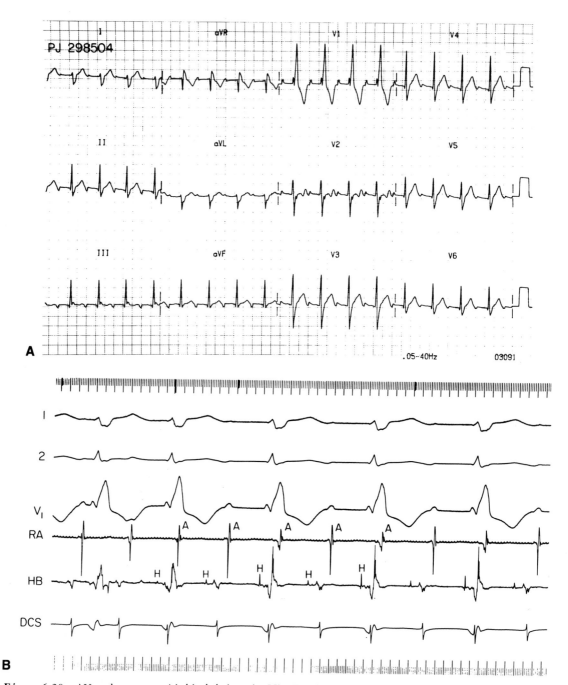

*Figure 6-20*   AV node reentry with block below the His. Panel *A* shows supraventricular tachycardia with a P wave discernible precisely at mid-diastole. Electrophysiologic testing demonstrated typical AV nodal reentry with dual-pathway physiology. Intermittently, 2:1 block below the recorded His-bundle electrogram was observed (panel *B*). Abbreviations as in previous figures.

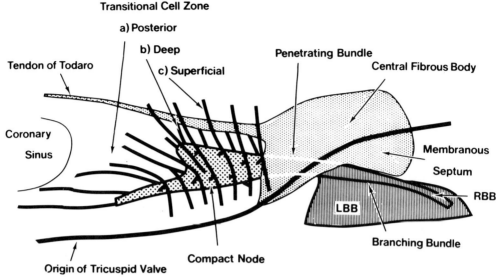

*Figure 6-21*   Schematic representation of the anatomy of the AV node. The AV node is seen as an irregular structure with multiple atrial imputs. It is tempting to hypothesize that the so-called slow pathway is the posterior protuberance of the AV node toward the coronary sinus as depicted in this diagram. *(From Becker and Anderson.*[89] *Reproduced by permission.)*

potentials but transitional morphology when examined histologically. The transitional zone is thought to account for the normal delay in AV nodal conduction, whereas the compact AV node is thought to account for most of the delay during Wenckebach periodicity. Because the transition between AV node and atrium is not a clear boundary, this issue may never be resolved for the purist.

## Junctional Tachycardia

Junctional tachycardia not related to reentry is relatively uncommon.[110] In addition, patients do not usually undergo electrophysiologic testing for this arrhythmia and the mechanism remains less clearly defined. Junctional tachycardia is observed in infants less than 6 months old and as a perioperative arrhythmia in children. It generally occurs within 12 h of cardiac surgery and gradually dissipates over the subsequent hours to days if the patients survives

the perioperative period.[111] Pediatric patients may present with congestive heart failure and tachycardia-induced myopathy. The QRS during tachycardia has supraventricular morphology and a widely variable rate. The tachycardia rate and regularity is much more variable within a patient than that seen in AV node reentry. Although the mechanism of junctional tachycardia is frequently quoted as "automatic," large, systematic studies using intracardiac recording techniques are not available.

Pick and Dominquez[112] coined the term *nonparoxysmal AV nodal tachycardia* (nonparoxysmal junctional tachycardia) to describe the type of junctional tachycardia generally seen in adults. The descriptor *nonparoxysmal* refers to the onset, which more typically shows acceleration rather than an abrupt onset with immediate reversion to the tachycardia rate. The major clinical settings include the acute phase of myocardial infarction, the postoperative phase of cardiac surgery (especially valve surgery), digitalis intoxication, and acute myocarditis.[113] Electrocardiographically, the QRS morphology is supraventricular and the rate is generally between 70 and 130/min, although it can be as high as 200/min or greater. The rate is frequently variable and the tachycardia may be irregular. AV dissociation is frequently observed, potentially creating an impression of ventricular tachycardia, especially if bundle branch block aberration is present. When spontaneous onset is observed, tachycardia begins with a premature atrial or ventricular depolarization. The tachycardia rate increases with exercise and isoproterenol and decreases with beta blockers. Evidence supporting a mechanism is sparse but nonparoxysmal junctional tachycardia in adults is generally thought to be a triggered rhythm due to delayed after-depolarizations.[114,115]

Therapy for nonparoxysmal junctional tachycardia in adults is rarely needed but is done by trial and error when necessary. Beta blockers will slow the rate and systematic drug studies with other agents are not available. Tachycardia generally resolves with resolution of the primary associated problem. Atrial pacing greater than the spontaneous tachycardia rate may be helpful in instances where tachycardia is hemodynamically problematic. In automatic junctional tachycardia in children, digitalis and verapamil are usually not helpful and beta blockers may decrease the tachycardia rate. Experience with other antiarrhythmic agents is largely anecdotal, but a number of class 1 agents and amiodarone have had reported success. Tachycardia may be incessant and require nonpharmacologic measures such as AV node ablation.

## References

1. Zipes DP: Specific arrhythmias: Diagnosis and treatment, in Braunwald E (ed): *Heart Disease: A Textbook of Cardiovascular Medicine.* Philadelphia, Saunders, 1988, pp 658–716.

2. Bonke FIM et al: Effect of an early atrial premature beat on activity of the sinoatrial node and atrial rhythm in the rabbit. *Circ Res* 29:704, 1971.

3. Josephson MW, Seides SF: Supraventricular tachycardias, in Josephson ME, Seides SF (eds): *Clinical Cardiac Electrophysiology: Techniques and Interpretations.* Philadelphia, Lea & Febiger, 1979, pp 147–190.

4. Curry PVL et al: Paroxysmal reciprocating sinus tachycardia. *Br Heart J* 38:311, 1976.

5. Prystowsky EN et al: An analysis of the effects of acetylcholine on conduction and refractoriness in the rabbit sinus node and atrium. *Circ Res* 44:112, 1979.

6. Prystowsky EN et al: Enhanced parasympathetic tone shortens atrial refractoriness in man. *Am J Cardiol* 51:96, 1983.

7. Bauernfeind RA et al: Chronic paroxysmal sinus tachycardia in otherwise healthy persons. *Ann Intern Med* 91:702, 1979.

8. Yee R et al: Refractory paroxysmal sinus tachycardia: Management by subtotal right atrial exclusion. *J Am Coll Cardiol* 3:400, 1984.

9. Akhtar M: Mechanisms of supraventricular tachycardia originating in the atria, in Touboul P, Waldo A (eds): *Atrial Arrhythmias: Current Concepts and Management.* St. Louis, Mosby Year Book, 1990, pp 270–281.

10. Garson A Jr et al: Atrial automatic ectopic tachycardia in children, in Touboul P, Waldo A (eds): *Atrial Arrhythmias: Current Concepts and Management.* St. Louis, Mosby Year Book, 1990, pp 282–287.

11. O'Neill BJ et al: Results of operative therapy in the permanent form of junctional reciprocating tachycardia. *Am J Cardiol* 63:1074, 1989.

12. Packer DL et al: Tachycardia induced cardiomyopathy: A reversible form of left ventricular dysfunction. *Am J Cardiol* 57:563, 1986.

13. Haines DE, DiMarco J: Sustained intraatrial reentrant tachycardia: Clinical, electrocardiographic and electrophysiologic characteristics and long-term follow up. *J Am Coll Cardiol* 15:1345, 1990.

14. Coumel P et al: Sustained Intra-atrial reentrant tachycardia: Electrophysiologic study of 20 cases. *Clin Cardiol* 2:167, 1979.

15. Gillette PC et al: Mechanisms of atrial tachycardias, in Zipes DP, Jalife J (eds): *Cardiac Electrophysiology: from Cell to Bedside.* Philadelphia, Saunders, 1990, pp 559–563.

16. Walsh EP et al: Transcatheter ablation of ectopic

atrial tachycardia in young patients using radiofrequency current. *Circulation* 86:1138, 1992.

17. Habibzadeh MA: Multifocal atrial tachycardia: A 66 month follow-up of 50 patients. *Heart Lung* 9:328, 1980.

18. Bisset GS et al: Chaotic atrial tachycardia in childhood. *Am Heart J* 101:268, 1981.

19. Levine JH et al: Treatment of multifocal atrial tachycardia with verapamil. *N Engl J Med* 312:21, 1981.

20. Lewis T: Auricular fibrillation: A common clinical condition. *Br Med J* 2:1529, 1909.

21. Ostrander LD et al: Electrocardiographic findings among the adult population of a total natural community, Tecumseh, Michigan. *Circulation* 31:888, 1965.

22. Kannel WB et al: Epidemiologic features of chronic atrial fibrillation: The Framingham Study. *New Engl J Med* 306:1018, 1982.

23. Moe GK, Abildskov JA: Atrial fibrillation as a self sustaining arrhythmia independent of focal discharge. *Am Heart J* 58:59, 1959.

24. Moe GK: On the multiple wavelet hypothesis of atrial fibrillation. *Arch Int Pharmacodyn Ther* 140:183, 1962.

25. Allessie MA et al: Circus movement in rabbit atrial muscle as a mechanism of tachycardia: III. The "leading circle" concept: A new model of circus movement in cardiac tissue without the involvement of an anatomic obstacle. *Circ Res* 41:9, 1977.

26. Burn JH et al: Effects of acetylcholine in the heart-lung preparation including production of auricular fibrillation. *J Physiol* 128:277, 1955.

27. Coumel P et al: Syndrome of d'arythmie auriculaire d'origine vagale. *Arch Mal Coeur* 71:645, 1978.

28. Leitch JW et al: Neurally mediated atrial fibrillation and syncope. *N Engl J Med* 324:495, 1991.

29. Garrey WE: The nature of fibrillatory contraction of the heart. Its relation to tissue mass and form. *Am J Physiol* 33:397, 1914.

30. Fujimura O et al: The mode of onset of atrial fibrillation in the Wolff-Parkinson-White syndrome: how important is the accessory pathway? *J Am Coll Cardiol* 15(5):1082, 1990.

31. Chen PS et al: New observations on atrial fibrillation before and after surgery in patients with Wolff-Parkinson-White syndrome. *J Am Coll Cardiol* 19:974, 1992.

32. Hurwitz JL et al: Occurrence of atrial fibrillation in paients with paroxysmal supraventricular tachycardia due to atrioventricular nodal reentry. *PACE* 13:705, 1990.

33. Nunain SO et al: Determinants of the course and prognosis of atrial fibrillation, in Touboul P, Waldo A (eds): *Atrial Arrhythmias: Current Concepts and Management.* St. Louis, Mosby Year Book, 1990, pp 350–358.

34. Kopecky SL et al: The natural history of lone atrial fibrillation: A population based study over three decades. *N Engl J Med* 317:669, 1987.

35. Antman EM et al: Therapy of refractory symptomatic atrial fibrillation and atrial flutter: A staged care approach with new antiarrhythmic drugs. *J Am Coll Cardiol* 60:572, 1987.

36. Sanfilippo AJ et al: Atrial enlargement as a consequence of atrial fibrillation: A prospective, echocardiographic study. *Circulation* 82:792, 1990.

37. Coplen SE et al: Efficacy and safety of quinidine therapy for maintenance of sinus rhythm after cardioversion: A meta analysis of randomized controlled trials. *Circulation* 82:1106, 1990.

38. The cardiac arrhythmia suppression trial (CAST) investigators: Preliminary report: Effect of encainide and flecainide on mortality in a randomized trial of arrhythmia suppression after myocardial infarction. *N Engl J Med* 321:406, 1989.

39. Gosselink ATM et al: Low-dose amiodarone for maintenance of sinus rhythm after cardioversion of atrial fibrillation or flutter. *JAMA* 267:3289, 1992.

40. Falk RH, Leavitt JI: Digoxin for atrial fibrillation: A Drug whose time has gone? *Ann Intern Med* 114:573, 1991.

41. Rawles JM et al: Time of occurrence, duration and ventricular rate of paroxysmal atrial fibrillation: The effect of digoxin. *Br Heart J* 639:225, 1990.

42. Galun E et al: Failure of long term digitalization to prevent rapid ventricular response in patients with paroxysmal atrial fibrillation. *Chest* 99:1038, 1991.

43. Mancini GBJ, Goldberger AL: Cardioversion of atrial fibrillation: Consideration of embolization, anticoagulation, prophylactic pacemaker and long-term success. *Am Heart J* 104:617, 1982.

44. Manning WJ et al: Cardioversion from atrial fibrillation without prolonged anticoagulation with use of transesophageal echocardiography to exclude the presence of atrial thrombi. *N Engl J Med* 328:750, 1993.

45. Wolf PA et al: Epidemiological assessment of chronic atrial fibrillation and the risk of stroke. *Neurology* 28:973, 1978.

46. Flegel KM et al: Risk of stroke in nonrheumatic atrial fibrillation. *Lancet* 526, 1987.

47. Petersen P, Godtfredsen J: Embolic complications in paroxysmal atrial fibrillation. *Stroke* 17:622, 1986.

48. Albus GW et al: Stroke prevention in nonvalvular atrial fibrillation. *Ann Intern Med* 115:727, 1991.

49. Cairns JA, Connolly SJ: Nonrheumatic atrial fibrillation: Risk of stroke and role of antithrombotic therapy. *Circulation* 84:469, 1991.

50. The stroke prevention in atrial fibrillation investigators: Predictors of thromboembolism in atrial fibrillation: I. Clinical features of patients at risk. *Ann Intern Med* 116:1, 1992.

51. The stroke prevention in atrial fibrillation investigators: Predictors of thromboembolism in atrial fibrillation: II. Echocardiographic features of patients at risk. *Ann Intern Med* 116:6, 1992.

52. Stroke prevention in atrial fibrillation study group investigators: Preliminary report of stroke prevention in atrial fibrillation study. *N Engl J Med* 322:863, 1990.

53. Langberg JJ et al: Catheter ablation of the atrioventricular junction with radiofrequency energy. *Circulation* 80:1527, 1989.

54. Xie B et al: Does left ventricular ejection fraction change after ablation of AV nodal conduction in patients with atrial fibrillation? *J Am Coll Cardiol* 19:228A, 1992.

55. Leitch JW et al: Sinus node atrioventricular node isolation: long-term results with the "corridor operation" for atrial fibrillation. *J Am Coll Cardiol* 17:970, 1991.

56. Cox JL et al: The surgical treatment of atrial fibrillation: III. Development of a definitive surgical procedure. *J Thorac Cardiovasc Surg* 101:569, 1991.

57. Jolly WA, Ritchie WJ: Auricular flutter and fibrillation. *Heart* 2:177, 1910–1911.

58. Waxman MB et al: Effects of posture, Valsalva maneuver and respiration on atrial flutter rate: An effect mediated through cardiac volume. *J Am Coll Cardiol* 17:1545, 1991.

59. Waldo AL: Some observations concerning atrial flutter in man. *PACE* 6:1181, 1983.

60. Scherf D: Studies on auricular tachycardia caused by aconitine administration. *Proc Soc Exp Biol Med* 64:233, 1947.

61. Lewis T: Theory and circus movement and its application to atrial flutter, in *The Mechanism and Graphic Registration of the Heart Beat*, 3d ed. London, Shaw, 1925, pp 319–327.

62. Disertori M et al: Evidence of a reentry circuit in the common type of atrial flutter in man. *Circulation* 67:434, 1983.

63. Frame LH et al: Circus movement in the canine atrium around the tricuspid ring during experimental atrial flutter and during reentry in vitro. *Circulation* 76:1155, 1987.

64. Klein GJ et al: Demonstration of macroreentry and feasibility of operative therapy in the common type of atrial flutter. *Am J Cardiol* 57:587, 1986.

65. Olshansky B et al: Characterization of double potentials in human atrial flutter: Studies during transient entrainment. *J Am Coll Cardiol* 15:833, 1990.

66. Olshansky B et al: Demonstration of an area of slow conduction in human atrial flutter. *J Am Coll Cardiol* 16:1639, 1990.

67. Cosio FG et al: Atrial endocardial mapping in the rare for of atrial flutter. *Am J Cardiol* 66:715, 1990.

68. Tanoiri T et al: Study on the genesis of the double potential recorded in the high right atrium in atrial flutter and its role in the reentry circuit of atrial flutter. *Am Heart J* 121:57, 1991.

69. Garson A Jr et al: Atrial flutter in the young: A collaborative study of 380 cases. *J Am Coll Cardiol* 6:871, 1985.

70. Kennelly BM et al: Electrophysiological studies in four patients with atrial flutter with 1:1 atrioventricular conduction. *Am Heart J* 96:723, 1978.

71. Waldo AL et al: Clinical evaluation in therapy of patients with atrial fibrillation or flutter. *Cardiol Clin* 8:479, 1990.

72. Waldo AL et al: Atrial flutter: Transient entrainment and related phenomena, in Zipes DP, Jalife J (eds): *Cardiac Electrophysiology from Cell to Bedside*. Philadelphia, Saunders, 1990, pp 530–537.

73. Watson RM et al: Atrial flutter: I. Electrophysiological substrates and modes of initiation and termination. *Am J Cardiol* 45:732:741, 1980.

74. Saoudi N et al: Catheter ablation of the atrial myocardium in human type I atrial flutter. *Circulation* 81:762, 1990.

75. Feld GF et al: Radiofrequency catheter ablation of human type 1 atrial flutter: Identification of a critical zone in the reentrant circuit by endocardial mapping techniques. *Circulation* 86:1233, 1992.

76. Moe GK et al: Physiologic evidence for a dual AV transmission system. *Circ Res* 4:357, 1956.

77. Kisten AD: Multiple pathways of conduction and reciprocal rhythm with interpolated ventricular premature systoles. *Am Heart J* 65:162, 1963.

78. Schuilenburg RM, Durrer D: Atrial echo beats in the human heart elicited by induced atrial premature beats. *Circulation* 37:680, 1968.

79. Rosen KM et al: Demonstration of dual atrioventricular nodal pathways in man. *Am J Cardiol* 33:291, 1974.

80. Denes P et al: Demonstration of dual AV nodal pathways in patients with paroxysmal supraventricular tachycardia. *Circulation* 48:549, 1973.

81. Wu D: Dual atrioventricular nodal pathways: A reappraisal. *PACE* 5:72, 1982.

82. Josephson MW, Seides SF: Supraventricular tachycardias, in Josephson ME, Seides SF (eds): *Clinical Cardiac Electrophysiology: Techniques and Interpretations.* Philadelphia, Lea & Febiger, 1979, pp 147–163.

83. Sung RJ et al: Atrioventricular node reentry: Evidence of reentry and functional properties of fast and slow pahways, in Zipes DP, Jalife J (eds): *Cardiac Electrophysiology from Cell to Bedside.* Philadelphia, Saunders, 1990, pp 513–525.

84. Sharma AD et al: AV nodal reentry—Current concepts and surgical treatment. *Prog Cardiol* 1:129, 1988.

85. Akhtar M: Supraventricular tachycardias electrophysiologic mechanisms, diagnosis and pharmacologic therapy, in Josephson ME, Wellens HJJ (eds): *Tachycardias: Mechanisms, Diagnosis, Treatment.* Philadelphia, Lea & Febiger, 1984, pp 137–169.

86. Leitch JW et al: Syncope associated with supraventricular tachycardia: An expression of tachycardia rate or vasomotor response? *Circulation* 85:1064, 1992.

87. Kay GN et al: Value of the 12 lead electrocardiogram in discriminating atrioventricular nodal reciprocating tachycardia from circus movement atrioventricular tachycardia utilizing a retrograde accessory pathway. *Am J Cardiol* 59:296, 1987.

88. Ilnuma H et al: Role of the perinodal region in atrioventricular nodal reentry: Evidence in an isolated rabbit preparation. *J Am Coll Cardiol* 2:465, 1983.

89. Becker AE, Anderson RH: Morphology of the human atrioventricular junctional area, in Wellens HJJ, Lie KI, Janse MJ (eds): *The Conduction System of the Heart: Structure, Function and Clinical Implications.* Philadelphia, Lea & Febiger, 1976, pp 263–286.

90. Janse MJ et al: Electrophysiology and structure of the atrioventricular node of the isolated rabbit heart, in Wellens HJJ, Lie KI, Janse MJ (eds): *The Conduction System of the Heart, Structure, Function and Clinical Implications.* Philadelphia, Lea & Febiger, 1976, pp 296–315.

91. Josephson ME, Miller JM: Atrioventricular node reentry tachycardias: Is the atrium a necessary link? In Touboul P, Waldo A (eds): *Atrial Arrhythmias: Current Concepts and Management.* St. Louis, Mosby Year Book, 1990, pp 311–329.

92. Schuger CD et al: The excitable gap in atrioventricular nodal reentrant tachycardia. Characterization with ventricular extrastimuli and pharmacologic intervention. *Circulation* 80:324, 1989.

93. Sung RJ et al: Initiation of two distinct forms of atrioventricular nodal reentrant tachycardia during programmed ventricular stimulation in man. *Am J Cardiol* 42:681, 1983.

94. Wu D et al: An unusual variety of atrioventricular nodal reentry due to retrograde dual atrioventricular nodal pathways. *Circulation* 56:50, 1977.

95. Casta A et al: Dual atrioventricular nodal pathways: A benign finding in arrhythmia-free children with heart disease. *Am J Cardiol* 46:1013, 1980.

96. Wu O et al: Effects of atropine on induction and maintenance of atrioventricular nodal reentrant tachycardia. *Circulation* 59:779, 1979.

97. Huycke EC et al: Role of intravenous isoproterenol in the electrophysiologic induction of atrioventricular node reentrant tachycardia in patients with dual atrioventricular node pathways. *Am J Cardiol* 64:1131, 1989.

98. Hariman RJ et al: Catecholamine dependent atrioventricular nodal reentrant tachycardia. *Circulation* 67:681, 1983.

99. Wu D et al: Effects of procainamide on atrioventricular nodal reentrant paroxysmal tachycardia. *Circulation* 27:1171, 1978.

100. Wu D et al: Effects of quinidine on atrioventricular nodal reentrant paroxysmal tachycardia. *Circulation* 64:823, 1981.

101. Lee MA et al: Catheter modification of the atrioventricular junction with radiofrequency energy for control of atrioventricular nodal reentry tachycardia. *Circulation* 83:827, 1991.

102. Jackman WM et al: Treatment of supraventricular tachycardia due to atrioventricular node reentry by radiofrequency catheter ablation of slow pathway conduction. *N Engl J Med* 327:313, 1992.

103. Jazayeri MR et al: Selective transcatheter ablation of the fast and slow pathways using radiofrequency energy in patients with atrioventricular nodal reentrant tachycardia. *Circulation* 85:1318, 1992.

104. Wellens HJJ et al: Second degree block during reciprocal atrioventricular nodal tachycardia. *Circulation* 53:595, 1976.

105. DiMarco JP et al: Paroxysmal supraventricular tachycardia with Wenckenbach block: Evidence for reentry within the upper portion of the atrioventricular node. *J Am Coll Cardiol* 3:1551, 1984.

106. Schmitt C et al: Atrioventricular nodal supraventricular tachycardia with 2:1 block above the bundle of His. *PACE* 11:1018, 1988.

107. Zayas MR et al: Atrioventricular node tachycardia in the absence of retrograde conduction. *Can J Cardiol* 5:143, 1989.

108. Bauernfeind RA et al: Retrograde block during dual pathway atrioventricular nodal reentrant paroxysmal tachycardia. *Am J Cardiol* 42:499, 1978.

109. Fujimura O et al: Operative therapy of atrioventricular node reentry: Results of an anatomically guided procedure. *Am J Cardiol* 64:1327, 1989.

110. Swerdlow CW, Liem LB: Atrial 'and junctional tachycardias: Clinical presentation, course and therapy, in Zipes DP, Jalife J (eds): *Cardiac Electrophysiology: From Cell to Bedside*. Philadelphia, Saunders, 1990, pp 742–755.

111. Garson A et al: Usefulness of intravenous propafenone for control of postoperative junctional ectopic tachycardia. *Am J Cardiol* 59:1422, 1987.

112. Pick A, Dominquez P: Nonparoxysmal AV nodal tachycardia. *Circulation* 16:1022, 1967.

113. Rosen KM: Junctional tachycardia: Mechanisms, diagnosis, differential diagnosis and management. *Circulation* 67:654, 1973.

114. Rosen MR et al: Can accelerated atrioventricular junctional escape rhythms be explained by delayed after depolarizations? *Am J Cardiol* 45:1272, 1980.

115. Tenczer J et al: Atrioventricular junctional rhythm induced by atrial stimulation: A suspected clinical manifestation of "triggered" activity. *Int Cardiol* 11:359, 1986.

# Chapter 7

# Preexcitation Syndromes

Under usual circumstances, an impulse originating in the atrium conducts over the normal atrioventricular (AV) node–His-Purkinje system to activate the ventricles. When an accessory pathway (AP) is present, the opportunity exists to bypass some or all of the normal conducting system. The term *ventricular preexcitation* denotes that an atrial impulse activates at least some part of the ventricular muscle earlier than anticipated, assuming conduction had occurred over the normal AV conduction system.[1] Several anatomic forms of accessory pathways have been identified (Fig. 7-1).[1,2] However, an accessory AV muscle connection is the cause of preexcitation in more than 90 percent of patients.

Recent data have clarified certain pathway characteristics. For example, a slowly conducting AV connection that is ordinarily only used for retrograde conduction in a specific type of tachycardia termed the *permanent form of junctional reciprocating tachycardia* (PJRT) can also be used for anterograde conduction.[3] In addition, a form of reentrant preexcited tachycardia previously thought to use a nodoventricular or nodofascicular fiber for anterograde conduction in most cases actually conducts over an atriofascicular tract (atrium to right bundle) (Fig. 7-1).[4–6]

The preexcitation syndrome commonly referred to as Wolff-Parkinson-White (WPW) syndrome has an interesting history.[1] The WPW syndrome more properly defines patients with accessory AV connections that have tachyarrhythmias.[7] Ventricular preexcitation should be used to identify the presence of a delta wave in an asymptomatic patient. These acces-

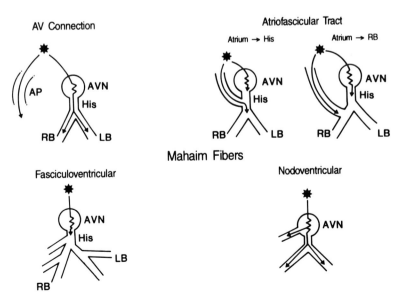

*Figure 7-1* Classification of the preexcitation syndromes. The European Study Group for Preexcitation suggested an anatomic classification for accessory pathways (APs) with use of tract to designate APs that insert into specialized conduction tissue and connection when they terminate into working myocardium. Four generalized types of preexcitation syndromes are demonstrated. Recent data suggest variations of some of these broad categories, as detailed in the text. AVN = atrioventricular node; RB = right bundle; LB = left bundle. (*Reproduced with permission from Prystowsky EN et al: Med Clin North. Am 68:831, 1984.*)

sory pathways are sometimes referred to as *bundles of Kent*, named after the investigator Stanley Kent, who suggested in a series of articles that impulses could conduct from atrium to ventricle over tissue other than the normal AV conduction system.[8] Kent actually described a nodelike structure, but the vast majority of patients with WPW syndrome likely conduct from atria to ventricles over a musclelike structure. Thus, although Kent's conclusion that accessory connections commonly occur in normal hearts appears to be incorrect and the term *Kent bundle* should probably not be used in describing accessory pathways, his observations enabled Mines,[9] in 1914, to postulate the mechanism of AV reentry correctly.

Electrophysiologic studies over the past two decades have enabled investigators from around the world to define more precisely mechanisms of preexcitation and the reentrant circuits involved in tachycar-

dia. The study of patients with this disorder involves the placement of several catheters in multiple areas of the heart (Chap. 17). Cardiac pacing and recording of electrograms from these various sites are done to identify pathway location and mechanisms of tachycardia.

In general, we perform electrophysiologic studies on almost all patients with WPW syndrome, typically followed by catheter ablation of the accessory pathway(s) during the same session (Chap. 17). The approach to the asymptomatic patient with ventricular preexcitation is more controversial.[10] Patients can have atrial fibrillation with a rapid preexcited ventricular response (Fig. 7-2) that can rarely degenerate into ventricular fibrillation and cause sudden cardiac death.[1,10–13] Since the risk for sudden death is exceedingly small in the asymptomatic patient, we do not favor routine testing of all these individuals. Some exceptions are (1) persons in high-

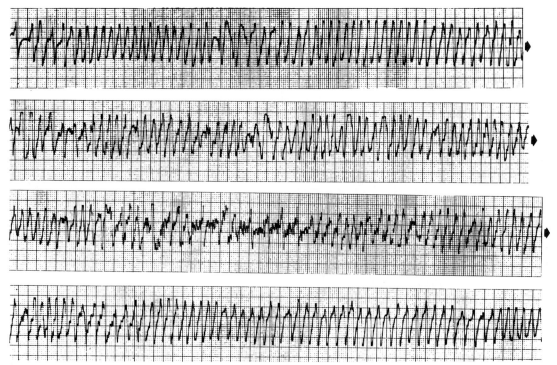

*Figure 7-2*   Atrial fibrillation with a rapid preexcited ventricular response.

risk employment, for example, airline pilots; (2) persons with a family history of sudden death or rapid tachycardia; and (3) individuals who want to engage in competitive athletics. To aid the clinician in decision making, we[10] have developed general risk categories determined from the preexcited ventricular rate during induced atrial fibrillation at electrophysiologic study. These are (1) definite-risk—shortest preexcited RR interval less than 220 ms; (2) probable risk—shortest preexcited RR interval less than 250 ms but more than 220 ms; (3) possible risk—shortest preexcited RR interval less than 300 ms but more than 250 ms; and (4) negligible risk—shortest preexcited RR interval more than 300 ms.

## Mechanisms of Preexcitation

A typical electrocardiographic (ECG) pattern from a patient with an AV connection is noted in Fig. 7-3. The PR interval is short (<0.12 s); the early portion of the QRS complex has a slurred upstroke (delta wave); and the QRS complex is prolonged (≥0.12 s). In most patients the preexcited complex is present constantly, but in some, intermittent preexcitation is present (Fig. 7-4). Intermittent preexcitation implies a poor margin of safety of conduction over the accessory pathway; rapid preexcited ventricular responses during atrial fibrillation rarely occur in this situation. Although relatively rare in our experience, preexcitation may become manifest only during situations resembling supernormal conduction over the accessory pathway (Fig. 7-5).[14,15]

The preexcited QRS complex represents fusion of a supraventricular impulse depolarizing ventricular myocardium over the normal AV conduction system and the accessory pathway (Fig. 7-6). In panel *A*, a QRS complex with a late premature atrial beat is recorded. The blackened portion of the ventricular myocardium represents that area of the ventricle that is activated over the accessory pathway and forms the delta wave, which is blackened in ECG lead I. Note that conduction over the AV node and His-Purkinje system occurs with similar timing to activa-

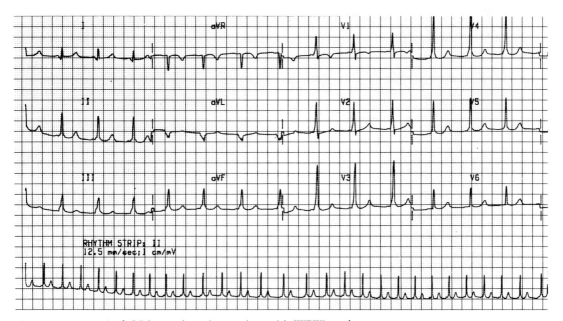

*Figure 7-3*  Preexcited QRS complexes in a patient with WPW syndrome.

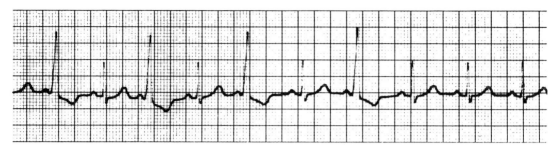

**Figure 7-4**   Intermittent preexcitation. During normal sinus rhythm, preexcitation occurs in complexes 1, 3, 5, and 7 and a narrow QRS morphology representing normal conduction from the atrium to ventricle is present in complexes 2, 4, 6, and 8 to 10.

tion of the ventricle over the accessory pathway; therefore minimal preexcitation is present. Panel *B* represents conduction of an early premature atrial complex. As expected, AV nodal delay occurs, as represented by increased conduction time through the AV node on the bottom schematic. However, conduction time over the accessory pathway usually remains the same even with premature atrial complexes; therefore more of the ventricle can be activated over the accessory pathway, which results in a widened QRS complex. The His bundle deflection is no longer identified. A premature atrial complex that occurs early enough when the accessory pathway is still refractory will block over the accessory pathway (panel *C* ). Then AV node conduction will be delayed

and the QRS complex will normalize, since ventricular activation results entirely by the normal AV conduction system. Thus, the PR interval prolongs but a delta wave is now absent.

Ventricular preexcitation is a classic case of fusion, and the resultant QRS complex depends on several factors. These include the relative conduction times over the accessory pathway and normal conduction system and the relationship of the origin of the atrial impulse to the location of the accessory pathway. For example, minimal preexcitation often occurs in a patient with a left lateral free-wall accessory pathway with relatively short AV nodal–His-Purkinje activation time (Fig. 7-7). This figure demonstrates ventricular preexcitation during normal sinus

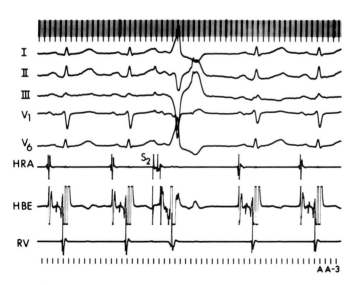

**Figure 7-5**   Supernormal conduction over an AP. Tracings from top to bottom are ECG leads I, II, III, V1, and $V_6$ and intracardiac electrograms from the high right atrium (HRA), His bundle area (HBE), and right ventricle (RV). A premature atrial stimulus ($S_2$) is initiated in the high right atrium and results in ventricular preexcitation. Note that the QRS complex widens and the His bundle electrogram moves into the ventricular electrogram. In this patient ventricular preexcitation was noted only during slow sinus rates and with very early atrial premature complexes. This suggests supernormal conduction over the accessory pathway.

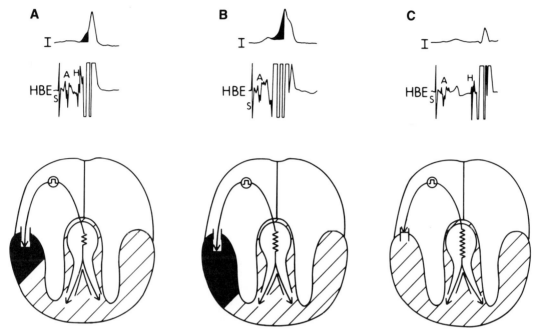

*Figure* 7-6   Mechanism of preexcitation with AV connection. From top to bottom, tracings are ECG lead I, His bundle electrogram, and a schematic of AV conduction that can occur over the AP identified on the left side of the figure or the normal AV node–His-Purkinje system seen in the center. (See text for details.)

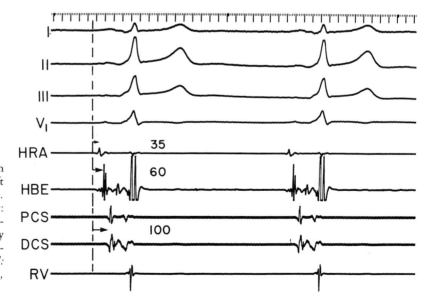

*Figure*     7-7   Activation times from the right and left atria during sinus rhythm. (See text for details.) (Key: PCS = proximal coronary sinus; DCS = distal coronary sinus.) *(Reproduced with permission from Prystowsky EN et al: Med Clin North Am 68:831, 1984.)*

rhythm. Note that atrial activation near the AV node occurs 60 ms after the onset of the P wave, whereas activation of the base of the lateral left atrium occurs at 100 ms. Preexcitation is minimal because the accessory pathway is located in the left atrium relatively far from the origin of the sinus impulse. If this patient had very short AV conduction times over the normal system, preexcitation might not be apparent on the standard ECG. This concept is explored further in Fig. 7-8. This patient has a left lateral accessory pathway, and minimal preexcitation is present during sinus rhythm (Fig. 7-8*A*); note the often observed characteristic feature of this location of the QS configuration in aVL with an R:S $\geq 1.0$ in $V_1$. Pacing from the right atrium produced AV nodal delay and ventricular preexcitation is more marked (Fig. 7-8*B*). However, pacing from the coronary sinus near the atrial origin of the accessory pathway at the same heart rate dramatically increases ventricular preexcitation, as is most evident in the precordial leads (Fig. 7-8*C* ). Since the pacing site is near the accessory pathway, conduction proceeds quickly from the atrium to the ventricle over this structure and the QRS complex is maximally preexcited. The differential effect of site of origin of the atrial impulse and activation time over the normal conduction system is useful in identifying pathway locations, and recent data suggest that in the presence of preexcitation a left free-wall accessory pathway is almost always present if the PR interval is $>0.12$ s.[16]

---

## *Mechanism of Atrioventricular Reentrant Tachycardia*

Atrioventricular reentrant tachycardia (AVRT) is the paradigm of reentry. Reentrant excitation can occur when at least two functionally distinct pathways

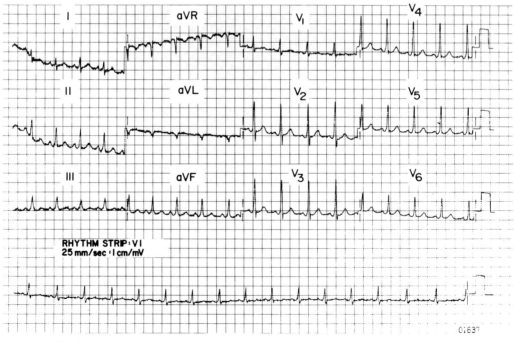

**A**

*Figure 7-8*   Variable degrees of ventricular preexcitation. (See text for details.)

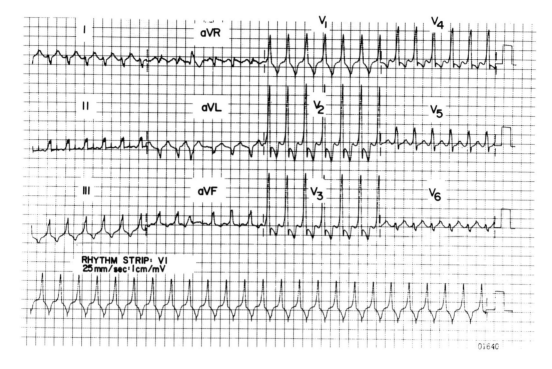

**B**

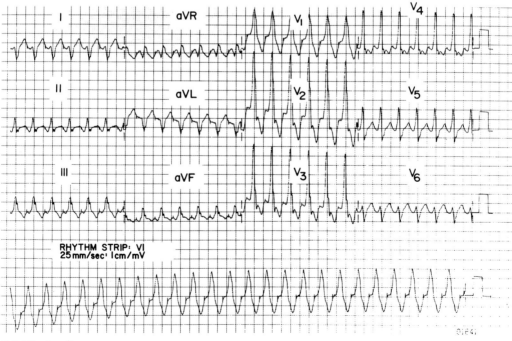

**C**

*Figure 7-8 (Continued)*

of conduction are present. Unidirectional block is initiated in one pathway, and the ensuing conduction time is slow enough over the nonblocked pathway to allow recovery of excitability in the blocked pathway. This permits retrograde conduction over the previously blocked pathway and completion of the reentrant circuit (Fig. 7-9).

Reentrant AV tachycardia is defined as either orthodromic or antidromic. *Orthodromic* refers to propagation of an impulse in the normal direction. In AV reentry, this occurs when conduction proceeds in the anterograde direction from the atrium over the normal conduction system to the ventricle and retrogradely back to the atrium over the accessory pathway. *Antidromic* reentry designates retrograde conduction over the normal AV node–His-Purkinje system with anterograde conduction over an accessory pathway (see later). With orthodromic reentry, the QRS is narrow unless bundle branch block is present.

Premature atrial or ventricular complexes can initiate orthodromic AV reentry.[1,17] Figure 7-10 demonstrates induction of AV reentry with a premature atrial complex. In panel *A*, the high right atrium is paced at a cycle length of 600 ms and a premature atrial complex is introduced at an interval

of 300 ms. The premature complex blocks anterogradely over the accessory pathway and conducts through the AV node, as demonstrated by the His depolarization ($H_2$). However, tachycardia is not initiated because the impulse does not conduct to the ventricle, which is a requisite part of the AV reentrant tachycardia circuit. In fact, this is very important to remember, since this is the only form of supraventricular tachycardia in which ventricular activation is necessary for initiation and maintenance of the arrhythmia. Panel *B* demonstrates a premature atrial complex introduced with an earlier coupling interval of 280 ms. The accessory pathway is blocked again and conduction through the AV node is accomplished. In this instance, however, conduction proceeds slowly through the His-Purkinje system and reaches the ventricle with a His to ventricle ($H_2 - V_2$) interval of 70 ms. Note that the QRS complex is no longer preexcited, although right bundle branch block morphology is present. Conduction occurs retrogradely over the accessory pathway, which in this case is in the left atrium, as demonstrated by earliest retrograde activation at the distal coronary sinus electrogram (DCS and $CS_1$). Tachycardia starts as anterograde conduction occurs again

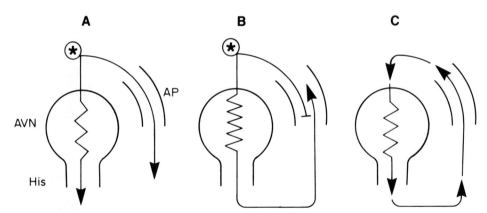

*Figure 7-9*   Schematic representation of induction of AV reentrant tachycardia. *A.* Conduction of an atrial impulse over the AV node (AVN) and His-Purkinje system (HIS) as well as over the accessory pathway (AP). *B.* A premature atrial complex blocks anterogradely over the accessory pathway and conducts slowly enough over the normal system to allow retrograde conduction over the AP. *C.* Retrograde conduction proceeds over the AP with ensuing anterograde conduction, thus completing the tachycardia circuit. *(Reproduced with permission from Prystowsky EN: Curr Probl Cardiology 13:225, 1988.)*

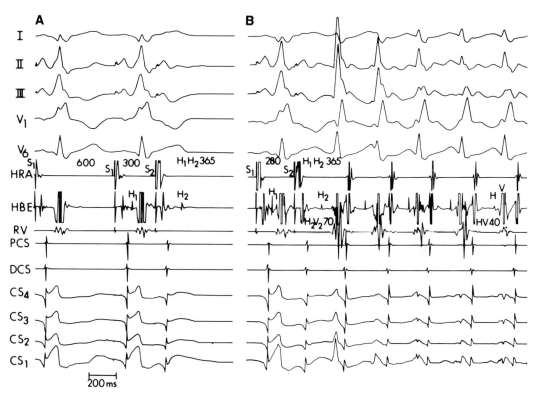

**Figure 7-10**   Initiation of AV reentry with a premature atrial complex. $CS_4$ through $CS_1$ are unipolar recordings from the proximal pole to the distal pole of a quadripolar catheter in the coronary sinus (CS). (See text for details.)

over the normal system. Note that the HV interval shortens after a few complexes—a common occurrence—and the HV interval is now 40 ms. If the interval from the His bundle electrogram to a constant atrial electrogram is measured, the His-to-atrial interval will be found to shorten as the HV interval shortens. This critical observation demonstrates that the His-Purkinje system is part of the tachycardia circuit, which is specific for AV reentry. In summary, initiation of orthodromic AV reentry with a premature atrial complex requires block over the accessory pathway, conduction to the ventricle over the normal system, and retrograde activation of the atrium over the accessory pathway, with subsequent conduction over the normal conducting system.

Atrioventricular reentry can also occur in a patient with a concealed accessory pathway. A con-cealed accessory pathway is one that is incapable of anterograde conduction but can conduct in the retrograde direction.[18-22] In this situation, tachycardia is initiated with a premature atrial complex that provides sufficient anterograde delay to allow retrograde conduction to occur over the accessory pathway (Fig. 7-11). Although manifest or overt preexcitation is not present in these patients, it is possible that total anterograde block in the accessory pathway is not always present and that, for induction of tachycardia, the premature atrial complex is required to provide this block in addition to AV nodal conduction delay. Some patients with left-sided accessory pathways capable of anterograde conduction have rapid conduction over the normal AV conduction system and demonstrate no ventricular preexcitation in sinus rhythm. These are *not* concealed accessory

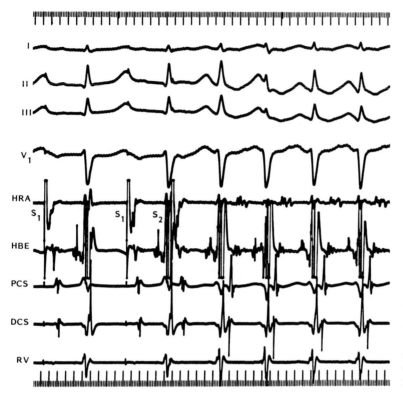

*Figure 7-11*  Induction of AV reentry with a concealed left-sided AP. Note that during high right atrial pacing (S$_1$), a premature atrial complex (S$_2$) increases AV nodal conduction time. This is followed by retrograde conduction over a left free-wall AP identified by earliest retrograde atrial activation in the distal coronary sinus lead. (See text for further details.)

pathways, since preexcitation can become manifest when AV nodal delay occurs—for example, with premature atrial complexes or during adenosine administration.

Premature ventricular complexes can also induce AV reentry (Fig. 7-12). The same concepts of reentry apply in this situation except that the PVC blocks retrogradely in the normal conducting system and progresses over the accessory pathway for tachycardia induction. Panel *A* of Fig. 7-12 shows a relatively late PVC conducting over both the accessory pathway and the normal ventriculoatrial conduction system. In panel *B*, an earlier PVC blocks retrogradely in the His-Purkinje system and progresses over the accessory pathway, with subsequent anterograde penetration into the normal conducting system. Panel *C* shows completion of the reentrant circuit. Initiation of AV reentry during programmed ventricular stimulation is shown in Fig. 7-13. In panel *A*, the right

ventricle is paced at 500 ms (120/min) and two PVCs are introduced. The first PVC (S$_2$) never initiated tachycardia; this is explained by the presence of a retrograde His bundle depolarization (H$_2$), indicating that retrograde conduction proceeded into the AV node.[23] Thus, unidirectional AV nodal block was never present. However, a second premature complex (S$_3$) demonstrates no retrograde His depolarization but still conducts over a left-sided accessory pathway, noted by earliest retrograde atrial activation recorded in the distal coronary sinus electrogram. Tachycardia occurs with anterograde AV node conduction, with left bundle branch block aberrancy yielding a wide QRS tachycardia. In panel B, the left bundle branch block aberrancy disappears and a narrow QRS complex tachycardia is now present. Note that the cycle length of the tachycardia shortens from 350 to 300 ms with disappearance of left bundle branch block. This important observation is

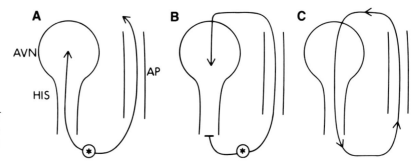

**Figure** *7-12* Initiation of AV reentry with a premature ventricular complex. (See text for details.)

diagnostic of AV reentry and identifies the site of the accessory pathway to the ipsilateral site of bundle branch block. The primary reason for a shortening in tachycardia cycle length is a decrease of ventriculoatrial conduction time from 160 to 70 ms as measured on the distal coronary sinus lead.[24–26] The reentrant tachycardia circuit is represented schematically for this situation in Fig. 7-14.

The length of the AV reentry cycle depends on the total time through all tissues involved in the tachycardia circuit. In reality, variation among patients in conduction characteristics of the accessory pathway, His-Purkinje system, and atria and ventricles are usually minimal and the major difference occurs because of AV nodal conduction properties. This is also the reason that patients may sometimes have faster tachycardia rates during exercise than at rest. Figure 7-15 shows the effects, demonstrated at the time of electrophysiologic study, of intravenous isoproterenol and atropine on the rate of AV reentry in one patient. The heart rate is approximately 150/min during control; but the tachycardia rate increased to 230/min with isoproterenol at a dose of 1 μg/min (middle panel). Adequate time was allowed for washout of isoproterenol; then atropine 0.4 mg was given and tachycardia reinitiated. The tachycardia rate again increased to approximately 230/min (right-hand panel). In both instances the acceleration of the tachycardia rate resulted directly from a shortening of AV nodal conduction time. Please note also that during the more rapid rates with either isoproterenol or atropine, QRS amplitude alternans is present and

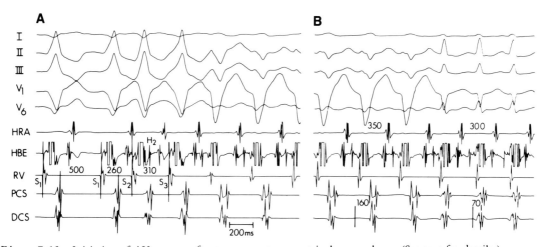

**Figure** *7-13* Initiation of AV reentry after two premature ventricular complexes. (See text for details.)

wave changes commonly appears during tachycardia and has no prognostic significance. Whether these events are due to a relative ischemic state is not known, but these patients typically have rapid AVRT induced at electrophysiologic study. Patients with AVRT can also have atrial fibrillation with a rapid preexcited ventricular response; if this arrhythmia degenerates to ventricular fibrillation, cardiac arrest can occur. Although this is a relatively rare presentation of this syndrome, it has been well documented.[1,11-13] In our experience, most patients do not give a history of onset of tachycardia with a consistent initiating event—for example, exercise. The usual situation is a tachyarrhythmia that can occur with rest or exercise, and, uncommonly, can even awaken the patient from sleep. If an etiologic factor is predominant, this is important in the therapeutic approach to the patient (e.g., beta-adrenergic blockade to prevent episodes of exercise-induced AVRT).

## Laboratory Data

### Electrocardiographic Observations

Atrioventricular reciprocating tachycardia is usually a narrow QRS tachycardia unless bundle branch block is present (Chap. 12). In many patients, a retrograde P wave is evident in the early ST segment, but this is often not discernible, especially when tachycardia rates are >180/min. If a retrograde P wave is present and the RP interval is less than half of the RR interval, AVRT is a likely diagnosis. If a P wave is not evident on the surface ECG during tachycardia, an esophageal lead may be inserted through the nares. If the resulting VA interval is <95 ms, it is against the diagnosis of AVRT; whereas a VA interval of >95 ms suggests but does not prove this diagnosis.[31] Electrical QRS alternans (Fig. 7-15) was discussed earlier and suggests the presence of an accessory pathway in the tachycardia circuit.[27] The most helpful clue is the transition from bundle branch block to narrow QRS tachycardia with a change in the tachycardia cycle length[24-26] (Fig. 7-13). Acceleration of tachycardia with loss of

bundle branch block conduction identifies an accessory pathway as part of the retrograde limb of the tachycardia circuit, and the accessory pathway is anatomically ipsilateral to the blocked bundle branch; the relatively rare situation of two separate tachycardias in this situation must always be considered. In our opinion, this is the only absolute ECG observation that identifies an accessory pathway as part of the retrograde tachycardia circuit. Practically, if the 12-lead ECG in sinus rhythm demonstrates preexcitation, the most likely diagnosis of tachycardia is AVRT, even though other forms of tachycardia can occur in such a patient with an accessory pathway.

### Electrophysiologic Study

In a patient with AVRT, electrophysiologic investigation is undertaken for several reasons and can identify the presence and location of the accessory pathways (APs) as well as document the participation of the AP in multiple types of arrhythmias.[32] The location of the AP can be identified by several methods that are listed in Table 7-1. A complete description of all of these electrophysiologic methods is discussed in detail elsewhere.[1] Regarding electrocardiographic criteria for accessory pathway location, the following general rules are helpful.[1,7,16,33] During maximal preexcitation, a positive initial (first 40 ms) delta wave in ECG lead $V_1$ identifies a left-sided AP; negative delta waves in ECG leads II, III, and aVF locate pathways on the posterior portion of the ventricles; a positive delta wave in $V_2$ through $V_6$

**Table 7-1    Anatomic Location of Accessory Pathway**

Delta wave morphology
Differential atrial pacing
Retrograde atrial activation sequence
Ventriculoatrial prolongation with ipsilateral bundle branch block
Preexcitation index
Number of PVCs needed for preexcitation
Earliest ventricular contraction

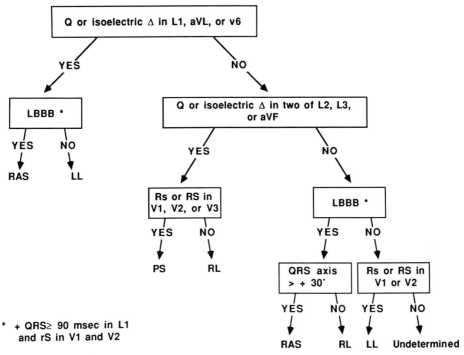

*Figure* 7-17    Algorithm to localize accessory pathway. Δ = delta wave; + = positive. RAS = right anteroseptal; LL = left lateral; PS = posteroseptal; RL = right lateral. *(Reproduced with permission from Milstein et al.[33])*

with a negative or isoelectric delta wave in $V_1$ strongly suggests a posteroseptal location; positive delta waves in leads II, III, and aVF suggests that the pathway is located on the anterior portion of the heart; the presence of isoelectric to negative delta waves in $V_1$ through $V_4$ represents an anteroseptal or anterior location. As $V_2$ through $V_4$ become positive, the AP on the right side of the heart is located in a progressively more posterior direction around the tricuspid ring. Figure 7-17 is an ECG algorithm to provide a first approximation to AP locations.

Differential atrial pacing consists of stimulating different areas of the right and left atria to determine the shortest stimulus to delta-wave interval, which occurs when the pacing site is near the atrial insertion of the accessory pathway. An example of differential pacing is noted in Fig. 7-8B and C, taken from a patient with a left-sided AP in which a shorter

stimulus to delta wave occurs during coronary sinus pacing (Fig. 7-8C). The retrograde atrial activation sequence is a very important method for locating the AP. Analysis of Figs. 7-13 and 7-16 demonstrates the earliest retrograde atrial activation during AVRT to be in the left atrium, defined by an early coronary sinus atrial electrogram, and in the right atrium, noted by an early right atrial electrogram, respectively, in these two patients with a left sided and right sided AP.

The concept of introducing PVCs during AVRT to cause retrograde preexcitation is represented in Figs. 7-18 and 7-19. Figure 7-18 shows the AVRT tachycardia circuit schematically. During AVRT, retrograde atrial activation occurs over the AP and anterograde conduction is over the normal AV conduction system. In this figure, the tachycardia cycle length is identified as $X$ and a premature ventricular stimulus (St) is introduced during tachycardia. This

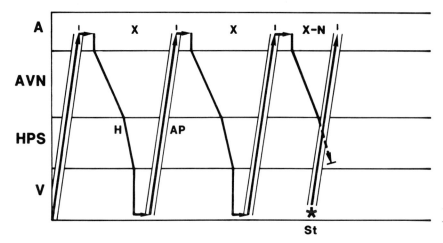

*Figure   7-18* Schematic representation of atrial preexcitation. A = atrium, AVN = AV node; HPS = His-Purkinje system; V = ventricle; H = His; AP = accessory pathway; St(*) = stimulus. (See text for details.) *(Reproduced with permission from Prystowsky EN: Heart Lung 10:465, 1981.)*

PVC conducts retrogradely over the AP to the atrium at a time when anterograde conduction from the previous tachycardia beat has activated the His bundle. This results in shortening of the tachycardia cycle length and is represented by X minus N (X − N). Since the His bundle has been anterogradely activated from the prior tachycardia beat, conduction can proceed to the atrium only by an alternative route, that is, over an AP. Although this confirms the existence of an AP that functions in a retrograde direction, it does not confirm that the AP is involved in the tachycardia. It is also important that the

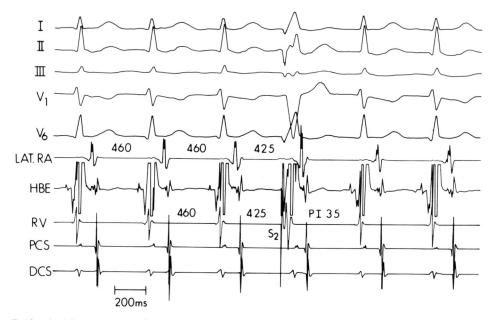

*Figure 7-19*   Atrial preexcitation during AVRT. A PVC (S₂) initiated late in diastole preexcites the atrium with an identical retrograde atrial activation sequence as that which first activated the lateral right atrium (Lat. RA). The preexcitation index (PI) is 35 ms. (See text for details.)

retrograde atrial activation sequence during tachycardia and following the PVC are identical.

Preexcitation of the atrium during AVRT can be used to locate the AP. One method, the preexcitation index, is based on the principle that during right ventricular pacing, a PVC introduced relatively late in diastole can preexcite the atrium in a patient with a right free-wall or septal AP location, whereas a much earlier PVC is necessary to do this for a left free-wall AP location.[34] In Fig. 7-19, AVRT is present and utilizes a right free-wall AP for retrograde conduction. Note that a relatively late PVC ($S_2$) preexcites the atrium (atrial cycle length shortens from 460 to 425 ms) and the preexcitation index equals 35 ms. This index is derived by subtracting the first premature ventricular interval that initiates preexcitation from the baseline tachycardia cycle length ($V_1V_1 - V_1V_2$).[34] In patients with left-sided APs, the ability of one PVC to preexcite the atrium suggests a more posterior AP location, compared with two PVCs required for atrial preexcitation. Two PVCs are more commonly needed if the AP is in a more lateral position.[35] Accessory pathways can also be localized by a variety of methods that identify ventricular excitation sequences. These techniques localize the earliest area of activation of the ventricle and represent the site of the AP's insertion into the ventricle.[36,37]

### Evidence for Accessory Pathway Participation in Tachycardia

Several methods that are discussed in detail elsewhere[1] can be used at electrophysiologic investigation to confirm the participation of the AP in AVRT. These are (1) ventriculoatrial (VA) prolongation with ipsilateral bundle branch block (Figs. 7-13 and 7-14); (2) His–atrial prolongation with increase in HV interval (Fig. 7-10); and (3) termination of tachycardia with a PVC that does not conduct to the atria and occurs when the His bundle is refractory. Two other methods strongly suggesting that the AP is involved in the tachycardia circuit but that do not absolutely prove this point are atrial preexcitation with a PVC introduced when the His bundle is

refractory (Fig. 7-19) and eccentric retrograde atrial activation during tachycardia (Figs. 7-13 and 7-19).

### Therapy

The approach to the patient with AVRT involves acute therapy to terminate the arrhythmia and an approach to chronic suppression of further recurrences. Chronic therapy for these individuals depends on several factors, including the frequency of arrhythmic episodes, the severity of symptoms associated with the arrhythmia, as well as the patient's age and state of myocardial function. No therapy may be necessary for an arrhythmia that occurs infrequently, is not sustained, and is associated with only minimal symptoms. In contrast, an arrhythmia that produces substantial hemodynamic compromise such as syncope needs aggressive suppressive therapy even if it occurs infrequently.

Chronic therapy can be pharmacologic or nonpharmacologic, such as surgery, an implantable antitachycardia pacemaker, or intracardiac catheter ablation.[1] Prior to catheter ablation, surgical therapy was often suggested to treat patients who (1) have a history of atrial fibrillation with rapid preexcited ventricular response; (2) are young and face decades of pharmacologic treatment; (3) have AVRT as the primary arrhythmia but associated with marked hemodynamic consequences such as syncope; and (4) are young women of childbearing age who may face the difficult decision of whether to continue pharmacologic therapy, with its potential danger to the developing fetus, during pregnancies or risk recurrent episodes of tachyarrhythmias that may also cause harm to mother or child. Data from Duke University demonstrated that the quality of life after surgery was excellent and supported nonpharmacologic treatment as first-line therapy in many instances.[38] A description of surgical techniques can be found in Chap. 20. However, endocardial catheter ablation has eliminated the need for surgery in most patients, and it is our usual treatment of choice if chronic therapy is needed[39–43] (Chap. 17).

Pharmacologic therapy is directed toward the AV nodal limb of the tachycardia circuit, the acces-

*Table 7-2    Site of Primary Antiarrhythmic Effect*

| AV Node | Accessory Pathway | AV Node and Accessory Pathway |
|---|---|---|
| Digitalis | Quinidine | |
| Beta-adrenergic blockers | Procainamide | Flecainide |
| | Disopyramide | Propafenone |
| Slow channel blockers | Lidocaine | Sotalol |
| | Mexiletine | Amiodarone |
| Purines | Moricizine | |

sory pathway, or both[1] (Table 7-2). A proposed schema for the acute therapy of WPW tachyarrhythmias is demonstrated in Fig. 7-20. In a patient in whom AVRT is hemodynamically unstable, DC cardioversion is the initial treatment of choice. This is a relatively rare situation; most patients can undergo acute drug therapy or maneuvers to increase vagal tone. If carotid sinus massage or the Valsalva maneuver do not terminate tachycardia, intravenous adenosine (6 to 12 mg), verapamil (5 to 10 mg), or diltiazem (15 to 20 mg) is recommended. If tachycardia still has not terminated, which would be rare, vagal maneuvers can be repeated. Persistent AVRT can be treated with additional intravenous adenosine, verapamil, or diltiazem. Alternatively, procainamide given as 50 mg/min intravenously to a total dosage of 10 mg/kg with constant recording of the blood pressure can be used. Maneuvers such as atrial pacing—using either a catheter inserted into the atrium or an esophageal lead—can also be employed, as can DC cardioversion. One may also opt for an observation period if the patient is stable and the tachycardia has slowed. With continued rest, it is not uncommon for the arrhythmia to terminate. If pharmacologic therapy is chosen for chronic suppression of the arrhythmia, drugs that affect the AV node or APs may be chosen. In our experience, efficacy can be achieved with many of these agents. It is recommended that digitalis not be used unless the electrophysiologic properties of the AP are known, since this agent can shorten AP refractoriness and might increase the chance for the development of

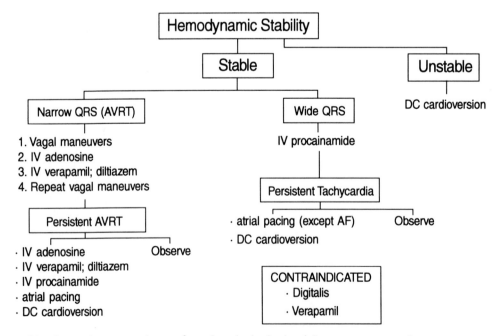

*Figure 7-20*    Approach to acute therapy for tachyarrhythmias involving an accessory pathway.

ventricular fibrillation.[44] If a rapid preexcited ventricular response is demonstrated during atrial fibrillation at electrophysiologic study, it is recommended that drugs that affect the AP be given either alone or in combination with agents that affect the AV node.

## Preexcited Tachycardia

### Clinical Diagnosis

Preexcited tachycardias present as a wide QRS complex arrhythmia. A differential diagnosis is supraventricular tachycardia with anterograde conduction over an accessory pathway, supraventricular tachycardia with bundle branch block aberrancy, and ventricular tachycardia (Chap. 13). In most instances, the patients have a history and physical examination similar to those of patients who present with AVRT, and the two arrhythmias often occur in the same patient. The one exception may be the marked hemodynamic compromise that can occur during atrial fibrillation with a rapid ventricular response due to conduction over an accessory pathway (Fig. 7-2).

### Laboratory Data

The ECG is a valuable tool in the diagnosis of these arrhythmias. Since anterograde conduction occurs over one or more accessory pathways during tachycardia, it is important to compare the 12-lead ECG morphology of tachycardia with the ECG recorded during sinus rhythm. Electrophysiologic evaluation will be necessary to identify the mechanism of preexcited tachycardia in most instances.

### Electrophysiologic Evaluation

Preexcited tachycardias can be subdivided into those in which the AP is a requisite part of the tachycardia circuit and those in which it is used only as a bystander for conduction of anterograde impulses to the ventricle (Fig. 7-21). When the AP is a requisite

### I. ACCESSORY PATHWAY REQUISITE PART OF CIRCUIT

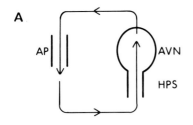
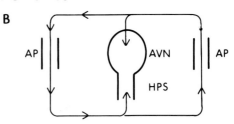

### II. ACCESSORY PATHWAY USED FOR BYSTANDER ANTEROGRADE CONDUCTION

**A. ATRIAL TACHYARRHYTHMIA**          **B. AVN REENTRY**

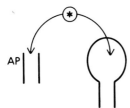
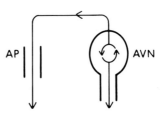

*Figure 7-21*  Preexcited tachycardias with anterograde conduction over an accessory atrioventricular connection. See text for details. AP = accessory pathway; AVN = atrioventricular node; HPS = His–Purkinje system *(Reproduced with permission from Prystowsky EN, Ref. 13.)*

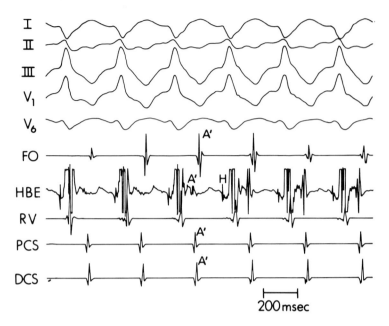

I

II

III

V₁

V₆

FO

HBE

RV

PCS

DCS

A'

A'

H

A'

A'

├──────┤
200 msec

*Figure 7-22* Antidromic reciprocating tachycardia. FO = foraman ovale. During tachycardia, earliest retrograde atrial activation occurs in the septum near the AV node, as identified on the HBE lead. The His bundle deflection occurs after the onset of the preexcited QRS complex. At electrophysiologic study as well as at surgery to ablate this patient's left free-wall AP, only one AP was identified and the diagnosis of antidromic reciprocating tachycardia was confirmed.

part of the tachycardia circuit, two basic types of reentrant wavefronts can occur. The most common form is antidromic tachycardia (Fig. 7-21, IA), demonstrated in Fig. 7-22.[45,46] Antidromic tachycardia utilizes an AP for anterograde conduction and the normal AV node and His-Purkinje system for retrograde conduction. In patients who have both AVRT and antidromic reciprocating tachycardia, the rate of tachycardia is almost always faster with the antidromic type.[46] Patients with multiple APs, especially those with Ebstein's anomaly, can have a variety of preexcited tachycardias that may utilize the normal conduction system as well as one or more APs in the tachycardia circuit (Fig. 7-21, IB). The tachycardia circuit depicted in this instance utilizes one AP for retrograde conduction and a second AP for anterograde conduction, with the normal AV node–His-Purkinje system a nonfunctioning part of the tachycardia. However, several variations on this theme may occur,[45] and these arrhythmic mechanisms can only be identified at electrophysiologic study.

Preexcited tachycardia can also utilize the AP for anterograde conduction without requiring AP conduction to maintain the tachyarrhythmia

(Fig. 7-21, II). A potentially lethal variety of these arrhythmias is atrial fibrillation or flutter with rapid preexcited ventricular rates (Figs. 7-2 and 7-21, IIA). A relatively rare clinical occurrence but a diagnosis that must be entertained is AV nodal reentry with bystander AP participation (Fig. 7-21, IIB). Points to differentiate these arrhythmias are discussed in detail elsewhere.[13]

An unusual type of preexcited tachycardia may involve a nodoventricular pathway for anterograde conduction.[47] However, recent data suggest that most patients thought to have a nodoventricular pathway actually have a right free-wall AP that enters into the right bundle (atriofascicular) and acts as the anterograde limb of the tachycardia circuit.[5,6] If ventriculoatrial conduction is intermittent during persistence of tachycardia, the tachycardia circuit cannot involve an AV pathway—a helpful although uncommonly identified finding. The usual situation is demonstrated in Fig. 7-23. On the left-hand portion of the figure is a left bundle branch block QRS morphology tachycardia with 1:1 retrograde conduction. Mapping during tachycardia demonstrated earliest retrograde atrial activation to be in

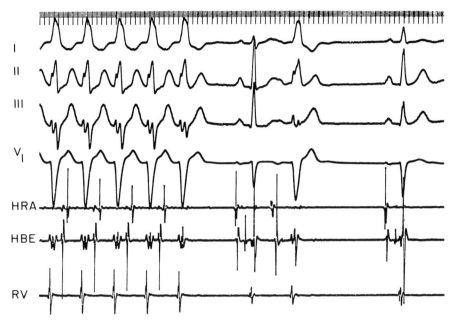

*Figure 7-23*   Preexcited tachycardia utilizing an accessory pathway for anterograde conduction. This patient did not undergo surgery, and it is unclear whether the anterograde limb is a nodoventricular pathway or a free-wall right-sided AP way. (See text for details.)

the His bundle area. Note that the fifth QRS tachycardia complex is not followed by retrograde atrial activation and tachycardia terminates. The subsequent sinus complex demonstrates a normal QRS morphology and a normal HV interval. This beat is followed by a premature atrial complex that conducts to the ventricle with a left bundle branch block QRS morphology, and the onset of the QRS complex occurs just prior to His bundle activation. This patient has an atriofascicular tract. The important clinical message is to consider atriofascicular reentry in the differential diagnosis of a "typical" left bundle branch block tachycardia, especially in a patient with a normal ventricle (Chaps. 9 and 13). These pathways are amenable to catheter ablation and surgery.

### Treatment

Consideration for chronic therapy in these individuals is similar to that in patients with AVRT. However, it is more common for these patients to present with a rapid tachycardia with significant symptoms; therefore chronic suppressive therapy is usually the rule. In patients without heart disease who present with atrial fibrillation and conduction over an AP, it is highly likely that atrial fibrillation is initiated by AVRT, as demonstrated at electrophysiologic study,[1,48] or possibly by involvement of the AP itself.[49] In more than 95 percent of such patients, surgical ablation of the AP will eliminate recurrent episodes of atrial fibrillation.[49,50] Similar results occur after catheter ablation of the accessory pathway. If there is adequate evidence that the atrial tachyarrhythmia is unrelated to AVRT—for example, onset of the arrhythmia during long-term event recordings—ablation of the AP will prevent the rapid preexcited ventricular response. However, the patient may still require antiarrhythmic therapy to suppress the atrial arrhythmia. In this instance, the patient should know that nonpharmacologic treatment may not eliminate the need to take drugs. Nonpharmacologic therapy still removes the potential threat to life that can arise for some of these patients (Fig. 7-2).

Acute treatment for a preexcited tachycardia is demonstrated in Fig. 7-20. As with AVRT, DC cardioversion is the treatment of choice if the arrhythmia is unstable. Intravenous procainamide is the preferred treatment in a stable hemodynamic situation; intravenous verapamil and especially digitalis should always be avoided. Beta blockers are usually ineffective in these situations. Although these agents could theoretically terminate tachycardia in a given individual by blocking retrograde conduction in the AV node, the exact mechanism of the wide QRS tachycardia often cannot be determined from the ECG, and other forms of preexcited tachycardia or ventricular tachycardia can be markedly worsened with these agents. If intravenous procainamide does not terminate the arrhythmia or substantially slow the rate, DC cardioversion is a reasonable option, although an observation period may be acceptable in some patients. Atrial pacing may be effective in arrhythmias other than atrial fibrillation.

## Commentary

The WPW syndrome is a common cause of paroxysmal, regular, narrow QRS complex supraventricular tachycardia. It often presents in the first few decades of life, and arrhythmias tend to worsen over time. Rarely, sudden death can occur due to atrial fibrillation, with rapid preexcited ventricular rates degenerating into ventricular fibrillation. Intravenous adenosine, verapamil, and diltiazem have made acute therapy of AVRT easy. Likewise, radiofrequency catheter ablation has enabled thousands of patients to undergo a nonpharmacologic cure without surgery and with minimal morbidity. At present, the risk of sudden death in asymptomatic people with ventricular preexcitation is too low to warrant wide-scale electrophysiologic evaluation for most of these individuals. Risk stratification is recommended in certain situations, as for individuals in high-risk occupations and for competitive athletes.

## References

1. Prystowsky EN: Diagnosis and management of the preexcitation syndromes. *Curr Probl Cardiol* 13:225, 1988.

2. Anderson RH et al: Ventricular preexcitation: A proposed nomenclature for its substrates. *Eur J Cardiol* 3:27, 1975.

3. Critelli G et al: The permanent form of junctional reciprocating tachycardia, in Benditt DG, Benson DW (eds): *Cardiac Preexcitation Syndromes*. Boston, Martinus Nijhoff, 1986, pp 233–253.

4. Gallagher JJ et al: Variants of preexcitation: Update 1989, in Zipes DP, Jalife J (eds): *Cardiac Electrophysiology: From cell to bedside*. Philadelphia, WB Saunders, 1990, pp 480–490.

5. Klein GJ et al: "Nodoventricular" accessory pathway: Evidence for a distinct accessory atrioventricular pathway with atrioventricular node-like properties. *J Am Coll Cardiol* 11:1035, 1988.

6. Tchou P et al: Atriofascicular connection or a nodoventricular Mahaim fiber? Electrophysiologic elucidation of the pathway and associated reentrant circuit. *Circulation* 77:837, 1988.

7. Gallagher JJ et al: The preexcitation syndromes. *Prog Cardiovasc Dis* 20:285, 1978.

8. Kent AFS: Observations on the auriculoventricular junction of the mammalian heart. *Q J Exp Physiol* 7:192, 1913.

9. Mines GR: On circulating excitations in heart muscles and their possible relation to tachycardia and fibrillation. *Trans R Soc Can* 8(IV):43, 1914.

10. Klein GJ et al: Asymptomatic Wolff-Parkinson-White: Should we intervene? *Circulation* 80:1902, 1989.

11. Dreifus LS et al: Ventricular fibrillation: A possible mechanism of sudden death in patients with Wolff-Parkinson-White syndrome. *Circulation* 43:520, 1971.

12. Klein GJ et al: Ventricular fibrillation in the Wolff-Parkinson-White syndrome. *N Engl J Med* 301:1080, 1979.

13. Prystowsky EN, Packer DL: Preexcited tachycardias, in Zipes DP, Jalife J (eds): *Cardiac Electrophysiology: From Cell to Bedside*. Philadelphia, Saunders, 1989, pp 472–479.

14. Chang MS et al: Supernormal conduction in accessory atrioventricular connections: An electrophysiologic study. *Am J Cardiol* 59:852, 1987.

15. Przbylski J et al: Supernormal conduction in the accessory pathway of patients with overt or concealed ventricular preexcitation. *J Am Coll Cardiol* 9:1269, 1987.

16. Fananapazier LK et al: Importance of preexcited QRS morphology during induced atrial fibrillation to the diagnosis and localization of multiple accessory pathways. *Circulation* 81:578, 1990.

17. Wellens JHH, et al: Electrical stimulation of the heart in patients with Wolff-Parkinson-White syndrome, type A. *Circulation* 43:99, 1971.

18. Barold SS, Coumel P: Mechanisms of atrioventricular junctional tachycardia: Role of reentry and concealed accessory bypass tracts. *Am J Cardiol* 39:97, 1977.

19. Coumel P, Attuel P: Reciprocating tachycardia in overt and latent preexcitation: Influence of bundle branch block on the rate of the tachycardia. *Eur J Cardiol* 1:423, 1974.

20. Neuss H et al: Analysis of reentry mechanisms in three patients with concealed Wolff-Parkinson-White syndrome. *Circulation* 51:75, 1975.

21. Pritchett ELC et al: Supraventricular tachycardia dependent upon accessory pathways in the absence of ventricular preexcitation. *Am J Med* 64:214, 1978.

22. Prystowsky EN et al: Postmyocardial infarction incessant supraventricular tachycardia due to concealed accessory pathway. *Am Heart J* 103:426, 1982.

23. Akhtar M et al: Role of retrograde His Purkinje block in the initiation of supraventricular tachycardia by ventricular premature stimulation in the Wolff-Parkinson-White syndrome. *J Clin Invest* 64:1047, 1981.

24. Pritchett ELC et al: Ventriculoatrial conduction time during reciprocating tachycardia with intermittent bundle branch block in the Wolff-Parkinson-White syndrome. *Br Heart J* 38:1058, 1976.

25. Kerr CR et al: Changes in ventriculoatrial intervals with bundle branch block aberration during reciprocating tachycardia in patients with accessory atrioventricular pathways. *Circulation* 66:196, 1982.

26. Motte G et al: Disappearance of a bundle branch block with acceleration of reciprocal tachycardia in Wolff-Parkinson-White syndrome. *Ann Cardiol Angeiol* 22:343, 1973.

27. Green M et al: Value of QRS alternation in determining the site of origin of narrow QRS supraventricular tachycardia. *Circulation* 68:368, 1983.

28. Kay GN et al: Value of the 12-lead electrocardiogram in discriminating atrioventricular nodal reciprocating tachycardia from circus movement atrioventricular tachycardia utilizing a retrograde accessory pathway. *Am J Cardiol* 59:296, 1987.

29. Morady F et al: Determinants of QRS alternans during narrow QRS tachycardia. *J Am Coll Cardiol* 9:489, 1987.

30. Pritchett ELC et al: "Dual atrioventricular nodal pathways" in patients with Wolff-Parkinson-White syndrome. *Br Heart J* 43:7, 1980.

31. Pressley JC et al: The effect of Ebstein's anomaly on the short and long-term outcome of surgically treated patients with Wolff-Parkinson-White syndrome. *Circulation* 86:1147, 1992.

32. Prystowsky EN: Indications for intracardiac electrophysiologic studies in patients with supraventricular tachycardia. *Circulation* 75:111, 1987.

33. Milstein S et al: An algorithm for the electrocardiographic localization of accessory pathways in the Wolff-Parkinson-White syndrome. *PACE* 10:555, 1987.

34. Miles WM et al: The preexcitation index: An aid in determining the mechanism of supraventricular tachycardia and localizing accessory pathways. *Circulation* 74:493, 1986.

35. Packer DL et al: Effect of left free wall accessory pathway location and left bundle branch aberrancy on the response to ventricular premature complexes during reciprocating tachycardia. *PACE* 10:408, 1987.

36. Windle JR et al: Determination of the earliest site of ventricular activation in Wolff-Parkinson-White syndrome: Application of digital continuous loop two dimensional echocardiography. *J Am Coll Cardiol* 7:1286, 1986.

37. Nakajima K et al: Phase analysis in the Wolff-Parkinson-White syndrome with surgically proven accessory conduction pathways: Concise communication. *J Nucl Med* 25:7, 1984.

38. Prystowsky EN et al: The quality of life and arrhythmia status after surgery for Wolff-Parkinson-White syndrome: An 18 year perspective. *J Am Coll Cardiol* 9:100A, 1987.

39. Warin JF et al: Catheter ablation of accessory pathways with a direct approach. *Circulation* 78:800, 1988.

40. Jackman WM et al: Catheter ablation of accessory atrioventricular pathways (Wolff-Parkinson-White syndrome) by radiofrequency current. *N Engl J Med* 324:1605, 1991.

41. Calkins H et al: Diagnosis and cure of the Wolff-Parkinson-White syndrome or paroxysmal supraventricular tachycardias during a single electrophysiologic test. *N Engl J Med* 324:1612, 1991.

42. Kuck KH et al: Radiofrequency current catheter ablation of accessory atrioventricular pathways. *Lancet* 337:1557, 1991.

43. Leather RA et al: Radiofrequency catheter ablation of accessory pathways: A learning experience. *Am J Cardiol* 68:1651, 1991.

44. Sellers RD, et al: Digitalis in the preexcitation syndrome: Analysis during atrial fibrillation. *Circulation* 56:260, 1977.

45. Bardy GH et al: Preexcited reciprocating tachycardia in patients with Wolff-Parkinson-White syndrome: Incidence and mechanisms. *Circulation* 70:377, 1984.

46. Packer DL et al: Physiologic substrate for antidromic reciprocating tachycardia: Prerequisite characteristics of the accessory pathway and AV conduction system. *Circulation* 85:574, 1992.

47. Gallagher JJ et al: Role of Mahaim fibers in cardiac arrhythmias in man. *Circulation* 64:176, 1981.

48. Campbell RWF et al: Atrial fibrillation in the preexcitation syndrome. *Am J Cardiol* 40:514, 1977.

49. Chen PS et al: New observations on atrial fibrillation before and after surgery in patients with Wolff-Parkinson-White syndrome. *J Am Coll Cardiol* 19:974, 1992.

50. Sharma AD et al: Atrial fibrillation in patients with Wolff-Parkinson-White syndrome: Incidence after surgical ablation of the accessory pathway. *Circulation* 72:161, 1985.

# Chapter 8

# Ventricular Tachycardia

Ventricular tachycardia (VT) is protean in form, duration, clinical setting, and prognosis. There is no uniformly accepted classification of VT, and this arrhythmia may be subdivided using many factors, as noted in Table 8-1. Unfortunately, no single subcategory provides enough information for correct classification of all patients with VT, and in many instances there is substantial crossover. For example, in many patients the mechanism of tachycardia is not certain. Whereas reentry is the presumptive mechanism for sustained VT in patients who have coronary artery disease with a previous myocardial infarction and ventricular scar, the mechanism of exercise-induced VT may include enhanced automaticity, triggered activity, and probably reentry. Thus, our present state of knowledge regarding mechanism of VT precludes use of this sole criterion for classification. The other potential classification variables listed in Table 8-1 also have deficiencies. It is often more useful to define a set of variables for a particular type of tachycardia so as to provide the clinician with a meaningful approach to the patient who has that arrhythmia. For example, patients with no definable structural heart disease who have right bundle branch block, left axis morphology sustained VT are a select subgroup for whom the location of this tachycardia is known and response to therapy—for example, endocardial radiofrequency catheter ablation or oral verapamil—has been well documented.[1-3] We will approach the classification of VT by clinical presentation in order to aid the clinician taking care of these patients. Sustained monomorphic VT and ventricular fibrillation are covered in more detail in Chaps. 9 and 15, respectively.

## Table 8-1 Classification of Ventricular Tachycardia

Mechanism
Location
Morphology
Duration
Cardiac pathology
Exercise-related
Drug responsiveness
Isoproterenol inducibility
Electrophysiologic inducibility

## Accelerated Idioventricular Rhythm

Accelerated idioventricular rhythm (AIVR) is a form of VT that is probably due to automaticity. The rate of tachycardia is usually between 50 and 110/min, and it becomes manifest in most instances as sinus slowing occurs. Thus, the sinus node competes with the idioventricular focus for capture of the ventricles. Although this arrhythmia usually occurs in the presence of heart disease, we have noted it in patients with no definable structural heart disease. The arrhythmia is self-terminating and rarely requires any therapeutic intervention. In some prolonged episodes of AIVR with sinus nodal dysfunction, there may be a decrease in blood pressure because of the

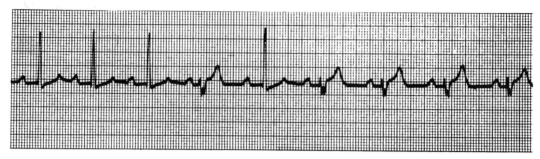

***Figure 8-1***   Accelerated idioventricular rhythm. (See text for details.)

ventricular origin of the arrhythmia and lack of atrioventricular synchrony, and enhancement of the sinus rate or suppression of the ventricular focus may be necessary. The former can be accomplished with drugs such as atropine or isoproterenol if not contraindicated, or by atrial pacing. Examples of AIVR are noted in Figs. 8-1 and 8-2. Note that in Fig. 8-1 the fourth QRS complex is slightly premature, 120 ms in duration, and ventricular in origin. The PR interval is suddenly shortened, consistent with the ventricular origin of the QRS complex. The last four QRS complexes represent AIVR, with a rate of approximately 65/min, a rate only slightly faster than that of the underlying sinus rhythm. There also appears to be some slight variability in the QRS morphology during AIVR (Fig. 8-1). The QRS complexes with the longer PR intervals during AIVR most likely have slight degrees of fusion due to partial depolarization of the ventricles from the supraventricular impulse. Figure 8-2 demonstrates AIVR at a faster rate of approximately 107/min and, as expected, the underlying sinus rate is also faster than that noted in Fig. 8-1.

## Nonsustained Ventricular Tachycardia

The definition of nonsustained VT differs among investigators in the field of clinical electrophysiology.

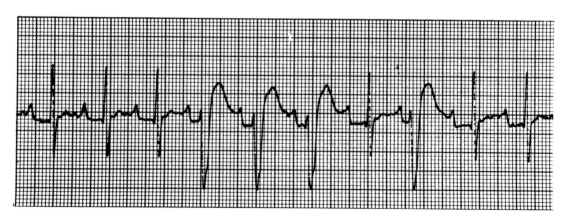

***Figure 8-2***   Electrocardiographic tracing of accelerated idioventricular rhythm for the fourth through sixth complexes. The P-P intervals are relatively constant throughout.

We currently define nonsustained VT as a tachycardia lasting from three consecutive ventricular complexes to <30 s in duration with a rate ≥110/min. In contrast, VT induced with programmed electrical stimulation techniques (see Chap. 9) is defined as *sustained* if it lasts ≥30 s or needs to be terminated sooner because of hemodynamic compromise. In most instances nonsustained VT is relatively brief in duration, usually less than 10 complexes. As noted below, nonsustained VT can be monomorphic or polymorphic, and patients can have both forms of tachycardia at different times.

### Repetitive Monomorphic Ventricular Tachycardia

Repetitive monomorphic VT (RMVT) is an arrhythmia characterized by runs of monomorphic VT or single or paired ventricular QRS complexes, all with the same QRS morphology, which occur in a patient with no definable structural heart disease. The intervening supraventricular QRS complexes are normal. An example of this arrhythmia is noted in Fig. 8-3 in a patient who had recurrent presyncope that was replicated during a tilt-table evaluation. The syndrome of RMVT has been well documented in the medical literature for many years.[4–9] Froment et al.[6] recognized the benign course of patients with RMVT and labeled it "curable and mild monomorphic ventricular extrasystoles with paroxysms of tachycardia." Rahilly and colleagues[7] reported on 18 patients with RMVT. Of these, 10 were men and 8 women; the mean age was 37 years. Only 2 patients had syncope, and there were 8 without any symptoms. The QRS morphology during ventricular tachycardia was left bundle branch block in 10 patients, 9 with a normal axis. Tachycardia rates were quite variable but in 16 patients ranged from 100 to 150/min. Exercise testing increased episodes of tachycardia in

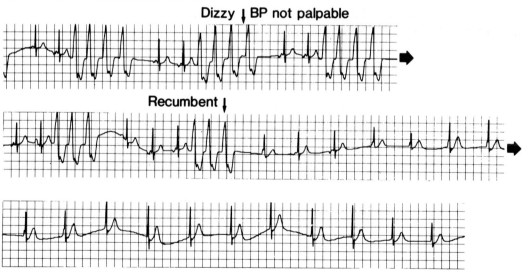

*Figure 8-3* Repetitive monomorphic VT in a patient who has neurally mediated syncope. The arrhythmia noted in the top and middle ECG strips is repetitive monomorphic VT that the patient had throughout the day and was never associated with any symptoms. The patient had repeated episodes of presyncope and underwent held-up tilt evaluation. In the absence of isoproterenol, no symptoms occurred. During head-up tilt at 70° with isoproterenol at 3 μg/min infusion, the patient's clinical symptoms of presyncope were reproduced and the blood pressure was not palpable. The repetitive monomorphic VT was unchanged throughout the pretilt evaluation and during tilt testing. Thus, the patient's symptoms were unrelated to VT. Of note, this patient had normal cardiac function.

5 patients, decreased episodes in 5 patients, and there was no change in 3. Of note, during Holter monitoring, there were frequently large variations in number of episodes of tachycardia throughout the day, and clustering of episodes was not uncommon. Programmed electrical stimulation initiated VT in 2 of 9 patients. During a 2-year mean follow-up evaluation there were no deaths, although many patients were treated because of initial symptoms. In 5 of 6 patients who were not treated, no VT was identified during Holter evaluation several years later. Thus, this arrhythmia can resolve spontaneously in some patients.

In another series of patients with RMVT, all 22 had left bundle branch block, inferior axis morphology.[8] This suggests a right ventricular outflow tract site, which has been successfully approached using endocardial catheter ablation techniques.[10–11] Of the 22 patients reported by Buxton et al.,[8] 7 were induced during electrophysiologic testing, 9 with isoproterenol infusion and 11 of 18 during exercise testing. This series of patients clearly differs from those reported by Rahilly et al.,[7] and it is quite possible that RMVT can be caused by various mechanisms, highlighting the difficulty of attempting to subclassify even a relatively narrow clinical syndrome. Coumel et al.[9] discussed 70 patients with RMVT who had a mean age of 40 years. Left bundle branch block with normal or right axis morphology occurred in 51 percent. These authors suggested that the arrhythmia was related to sympathetic tone and there were sinus rates below which repetitive beating did not occur.

Episodes of VT that are repetitive and monomorphic can occur in patients who have underlying structural heart disease, and the arrhythmia does not presage as good a clinical outcome in these patients as it does in patients with no structural heart disease. Two examples are demonstrated in Figs. 8-4 and 8-5. The arrhythmia noted in Fig. 8-4 demonstrates single premature ventricular complexes with a fixed coupling interval to the preceding sinus QRS complex and one run (three complexes) of nonsustained VT. In this single-lead tracing, all QRS ventricular complexes appear similar. This patient had underlying structural heart disease, and this arrhythmia should not be characterized as RMVT. In Fig. 8-5, the patient has runs of rapid monomorphic VT with only infrequent sinus complexes. This patient with heart disease was highly symptomatic and required urgent therapy to suppress the VT. Thus, runs of nonsustained monomorphic VT can occur in patients with and without structural heart disease, but the syndrome of repetitive monomorphic VT requires the absence of underlying structural heart disease.

It is always important to consider the diagnosis of supraventricular tachycardia (SVT) with fixed or functional bundle branch block aberrancy or a preexcited QRS morphology in patients with a wide QRS complex tachycardia. Figure 8-6 shows a patient with no structural heart disease who was referred with a diagnosis of RMVT. The recurrent episodes of wide QRS complex tachycardia are due to supraventricular complexes conducted over a left lateral accessory pathway in this patient, who had no previous electrocardiogram (ECG) for comparison.

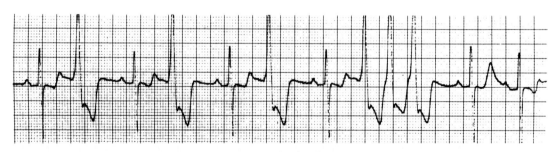

*Figure 8-4*   Nonsustained monomorphic VT. (See text for details.)

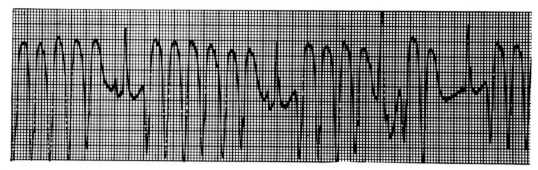

*Figure 8-5*   Runs of rapid monomorphic nonsustained VT.

This diagnosis was confirmed at electrophysiologic study. Thus, although one should always consider VT as the initial diagnosis in such a patient, one must also realize that alternative mechanisms can be present.

Treatment of patients with repetitive monomorphic VT should be directed primarily at relief of symptoms, since the occurrence of sudden cardiac death in an otherwise asymptomatic patient with RMVT is rare. Drug therapy in symptomatic individuals is usually first-line treatment, but endocardial radiofrequency catheter ablation is also appropriate in some of these patients. The necessity for long-term therapy should be reevaluated after 1 to 2 years of treatment, since the arrhythmia can resolve over time.

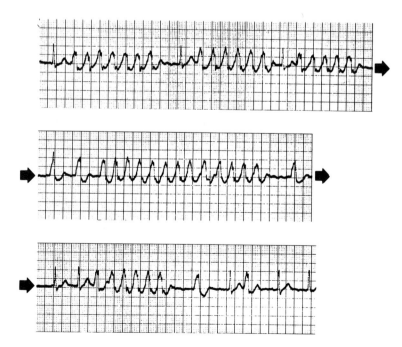

*Figure 8-6*   Repetitive episodes of a wide QRS complex tachycardia diagnosed as a preexcited tachycardia at electrophysiologic study. (See text for details.)

### Paroxysmal Nonsustained Ventricular Tachycardia

Isolated episodes of nonsustained VT are common in patients with structural heart disease but infrequently occur in patients who have normal ventricular function. Ventricular tachycardia can be monomorphic, polymorphic, or monomorphic with each episode but with more than one morphology being noted in a given patient. Typically patients have only a few episodes a day, often merely one, and the duration is less than 10 complexes with a rate <160/min. However, nonsustained VT is highly variable and may be much more rapid and longer in duration. Patients are often asymptomatic and the arrhythmia is discovered incidentally. When symptoms occur, they are most commonly palpitations, but presyncope and dizziness are occasionally noted. The significance of nonsustained VT in asymptomatic individuals depends on the presence and severity of underlying heart disease.

Patients with structural heart disease, especially those with substantial decrease in left ventricular function, frequently have episodes of asymptomatic nonsustained VT recorded during 24-h ambulatory ECG monitoring.[12-20] Some investigators have documented an independent association of nonsustained VT with subsequent sudden cardiac death in patients with dilated cardiomyopathy.[14-16] Figure 8-7 is a common example of nonsustained VT. The rate of tachycardia is somewhat variable, ±150/min, and the duration is short, 8 complexes. Figure 8-8

represents a run of rapid polymorphic VT that occurs less commonly but is not rare. Analysis of the VT in Figs. 8-7 and 8-8 might suggest a greater risk for the patient with tachycardia represented in Fig. 8-8. The supposition would be that if this tachycardia sustained, it would undoubtedly lead to hemodynamic compromise and possibly sudden cardiac death. In contrast, sustained VT of 150/min, as noted in Fig. 8-7, would be more likely to be associated with hemodynamic stability and probably would not lead to cardiac arrest. In fact, a poor correlation has been noted between characteristics of nonsustained VT and mortality or sudden cardiac death. For example, Meinertz et al.[15] reported that ≥20 episodes of ventricular pairs or nonsustained VT in a 24-h ECG recording correlated with sudden cardiac death in patients with idiopathic dilated cardiomyopathy. However, the authors did not suggest that any characteristics of VT—such as rate, duration, or morphology—were prognostically useful. In a retrospective analysis of the outcome of patients who had nonsustained VT during 24-h ambulatory monitoring,[12] 10 of 37 patients died suddenly. All 10 had structural heart disease and 9 of 10 had congestive heart failure, compared with only 10 of 27 patients with nonsustained VT who did not experience sudden death. Patients who died suddenly had 2.4 episodes of VT per day and 3.8 complexes per episode; the rate was 160 ± 36/min. Importantly, these characteristics were similar to those noted in patients who did not die suddenly. Nonsustained VT is also an independent risk factor for arrhythmic mortality

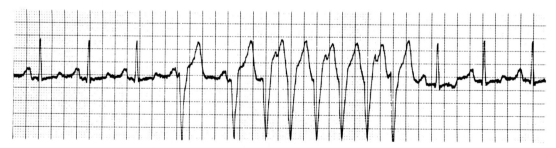

*Figure 8-7*  Example of nonsustained VT that starts with the fourth QRS complex and is eight complexes in duration. Ventriculoatrial dissociation is present and the first complex of tachycardia merges with the end of the sinus P-wave. Emergence of VT late in diastole (R-on-P wave) is not unusual.

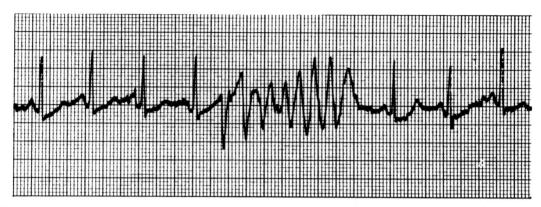

*Figure 8-8*   Rapid polymorphic nonsustained VT.

in patients in whom it was identified a mean of 11 days after acute myocardial infarction, but individual parameters of the nonsustained VT episodes were not predictive of sudden death.[18] Nonsustained VT also occurs commonly in patients with hypertrophic cardiomyopathy, but recent data suggest its significance is minimal in asymptomatic individuals.[20]

There are several potential explanations for the poor predictive capability of individual parameters of nonsustained VT—such as rate, duration, and morphology—in patients who are asymptomatic from this arrhythmia. The assumption that patients have only one type of nonsustained VT is incorrect.[21] Quite frequently patients have multiple types of VT with variable duration and rate, and the more episodes per day of tachycardia the greater is the variability in rate.[21] Figure 8-9 is taken from a patient with atrial fibrillation and multiple runs of VT recorded during continuous in-hospital ECG telemetry. All three episodes of nonsustained VT differ from each other in morphology, duration, and rate. It would be impossible to predict which one of these arrhythmias, if any, would correlate with a future episode of sustained VT. Further, if this patient were included in an epidemiologic study, it would be very difficult to characterize the various tachycardias and risks for future occurrence of sudden cardiac death.

The assumption that the nonsustained VT will resemble sustained VT is also incorrect,[21] as noted in Figs. 8-10 and 8-11. In Fig. 8-10, panel A, two runs of nonsustained VT that are polymorphic but with similar appearance are followed at the end of the tracing with the initiation of sustained monomorphic VT, which is also demonstrated in panel B. The rate of sustained VT is approximately 167/min, whereas some portions of the nonsustained VT are as rapid as 250/min. In Fig. 8-11 three panels of simultaneously recorded 12-lead ECGs are demonstrated. In panel A, single and paired ventricular premature complexes have a similar morphology. In panel B, a nonsustained VT run begins with a QRS complex that has a similar morphology to the premature QRS complexes noted in panel A, but the subsequent two QRS complexes of tachycardia are clearly different. Sustained VT in this patient (panel C) closely resembles the 12-lead ECG morphology noted in panel A. Thus, one premature ventricular complex morphology presaged the morphology noted during VT, whereas the other was markedly different. In summary, except for the observations noted by Meinertz et al.[15] regarding frequency of runs of nonsustained VT, our own experience and that documented by other investigators suggests that the presence of nonsustained VT in patients with heart disease, especially those with significant left ventricular dysfunction, is a risk factor for the future occurrence of sudden cardiac death. Individual characteristics of VT are of no prognostic significance in patients with asymptomatic nonsustained VT.

Apparently healthy individuals with asymptom-

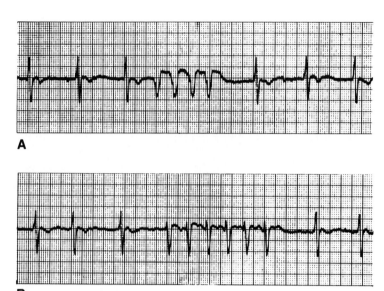

A

B

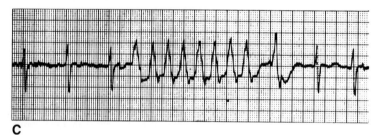

C

*Figure 8-9*  Multiple episodes of VT in a patient with underlying atrial fibrillation. The three episodes noted in panels *A, B,* and *C* differ in rate, duration, and morphology.

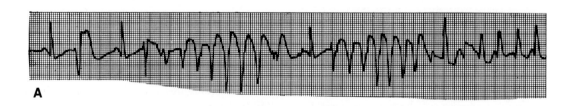

A

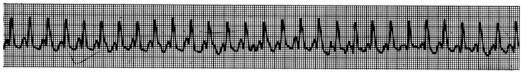

B

*Figure 8-10*  Nonsustained (panel *A*) and sustained (panel *B*) VT. (See text for details.)

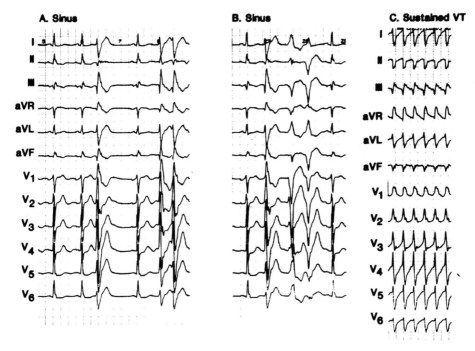

**A. Sinus**   **B. Sinus**   **C. Sustained VT**

*Figure 8-11*   Single and repetitive ventricular complexes of different morphology (panels *A* and *B*) and sustained VT that resembles one of the ectopic morphologies (panel *C*).

atic nonsustained VT are at minimal risk for sudden cardiac death.[22] Kennedy and colleagues[22] evaluated 73 such patients with a mean age of $46 \pm 13$ years, and the mean follow-up was 6.5 years. One patient had a cardiac arrest, survived, and was documented to have disease of the right coronary artery. Another patient died suddenly approximately 7 years after entry into the study and was known to have normal coronary angiography when initially evaluated. The incidence of sudden death during follow-up was therefore very low. Since the risk of sudden cardiac death is minimal in patients with no structural heart disease, therapy should be given only to those individuals who have substantial symptoms associated with nonsustained VT. In general, we recommend reassurance for those patients who have palpitations, but symptoms such as presyncope or syncope need to be evaluated in more detail. Noninvasive and invasive electrophysiologic testing may be needed to define the problem, and therapy is warranted to

suppress ventricular arrhythmias if they are documented to be the cause of the symptoms. Therapy should be individualized to the patient; some may require only beta blockers, whereas others may need more potent antiarrhythmic agents, for example, disopyramide or propafenone.

Treatment to suppress symptoms may also be warranted in patients who have structural heart disease. Such therapy should be individualized. For example, we would avoid the use of disopyramide in patients with a history of congestive heart failure and, as a general rule, do not recommend flecainide for patients with structural heart disease. As noted previously, patients with left ventricular dysfunction, for example, ejection fraction $\leq 40$ percent, who have asymptomatic nonsustained VT are at risk for sudden cardiac death, but no study to date has demonstrated that any form of therapy will decrease mortality in these patients. Several prospective studies are evaluating this question (see Chap. 15).

## *Exercise-Induced Ventricular Tachycardia*

Exercise is associated with many physiologic changes, including an increase in systolic blood pressure, heart rate, contractility, sympathetic tone, secretion of catecholamines, and decreased parasympathetic tone. The role of decreased parasympathetic tone in arrhythmogenesis has been evaluated in many models. For example, atropine can facilitate initiation of AV nodal reentrant tachycardia at electrophysiologic study in some patients in whom heightened vagal tone has prolonged AV nodal refractoriness and depressed conduction.[23] In canine models as well as humans, data are available to suggest that a decrease in parasympathetic tone after myocardial infarction increases the risk of mortality.[24,25] The relative contribution of parasympathetic withdrawal or heightened sympathetic tone to initiation of ventricular arrhythmias during exercise is unclear. The changes in autonomic tone can facilitate initiation of VT by a variety of mechanisms including reentry, automaticity, and triggered automaticity.[26] Further, patients with or without structural heart disease can have exercise-induced ventricular arrhythmias by one of several mechanisms. Thus, the appearance of VT, whether sustained or nonsustained, during exercise requires further investigation to determine, if possible, the electrophysiologic mechanism and to define whether cardiac structural abnormalities are present. Exercise can also induce ischemia, and it is critically important to identify patients with ischemia-initiated VT. In our experience such VT is often polymorphic, not infrequently degenerating to ventricular fibrillation. The approach to patients with ischemia-provoked malignant arrhythmias is quite different, as noted below.

Sung et al.[26,27] have devised a useful method to try to classify mechanisms of exercise-induced VT. This classification is based on the method of induction of VT at electrophysiologic testing as well as the responsiveness of the arrhythmia to intravenous verapamil.[26] In the group of patients with sustained VT not responsive to verapamil, tachycardia was subcategorized into initiation using programmed electrical stimulation or induction with isoproterenol infusion but not using atrial or ventricular stimulation techniques. Ten patients, all with heart disease, had VT induced by programmed electrical stimulation and reentry was the postulated mechanism. Automaticity was thought to be the cause of VT initiated during isoproterenol infusion but not with programmed stimulation of the heart. There were an additional 12 patients, 11 without any apparent heart disease, in whom verapamil could completely suppress the VT. Programmed electrical stimulation characteristically initiated VT in this group of patients, and propranolol could slow VT but did not prevent inducibility as a rule. Triggered automaticity was considered a potential mechanism.

The use of verapamil to treat patients with VT is not advisable except in very specific circumstances such as verapamil-sensitive tachycardia originating from the right ventricular outflow tract or left ventricle (see Chap. 9). Of note, Lerman et al.[28] reported that some patients with verapamil-sensitive VT are also responsive to intravenous adenosine, propranolol, and heightened vagal tone. These authors suggested that VT was due to cyclic AMP–mediated triggered activity. Table 8-2 lists several studies of patients with exercise-induced VT and demonstrates the diversity of findings in these patients.[29-36]

### *Therapy*

In most cases, patients with sustained VT, regardless of mechanism, should be treated, and the method of treatment will depend upon the mechanism of the arrhythmia and the type of heart disease present. For example, patients with ischemia-initiated polymorphic VT or ventricular fibrillation[37] require anti-ischemic therapy, pharmacologic or nonpharmacologic, as primary treatment and reevaluation afterward for the need for specific antiarrhythmic drugs. The arrhythmia of patients with no obvious structural heart disease may be suppressed with beta blockers, verapamil, or one of several membrane-active antiarrhythmic drugs. Therapy will have to be individual-

*Table 8-2 Exercise-Induced Ventricular Tachycardia*

| Author | Number of Patients | Heart Disease | VT Morphology | VT Duration | Therapy Effective | |
|---|---|---|---|---|---|---|
| | | | | | Beta Blockers | Verapamil |
| Woelfel[29] | 14 | NHD—6 CAD—6 NCAD—2 | RBBB—6 LBBB—5 Pleo—3 | VT-S—5 VT-NS—9 | 10/11 (IV) | — |
| Woelfel[30] | 16 | NHD—5 CAD—7 NCAD—4 | RBBB—5 LBBB—7 Pleo—4 | VT-S—6 VT-NS—10 | — | 12/16 (IV) 8/12 (O) |
| Sung[31] | 12 | NHD—3 CAD—6 NCAD—3 | RBBB—7 LBBB—5 | VT-S—12 | 3/6 (IV) | — |
| Wu[32] | 3 | NHD—3 | LBBB—3 | VT-S—3 | 3/3 (O) | 3/3 (IV) |
| Palileo[33] | 6 | NHD—2 RVCM—3 MVP—1 | LBBB—6 | 6/6 > 10 s but self-terminating | 6/6 (O) | — |
| O'Hara[34] | 17 | CAD—17 | RBBB—16 Other—1 | VT-S—17 | — | — |
| Mont[35] | 37 | NHD—37 | RBBB—22 LBBB—9 | VT-S—19 VT-NS—18 | 2/8 | — |
| Sokoloff[36] | 10 | NHD—3 CAD—4 NCAD—3 | LBBB—10 | VT-NS—10 | 9/10 (IV) | — |
| Lerman[28] | 4 | NHD—4 | LBBB—3 LBBB/RBBB—1 | VT-S—4 | 3/3 (IV) | 3/3 (IV) |

*Abbreviations:* CAD = coronary artery disease; NCAD = no CAD; NHD = no obvious heart disease; RVCM = right ventricular cardiomyopathy; MVP = mitral valve prolapse; VT-S = sustained VT; VT-NS = nonsustained VT; pleo = pleomorphic; RBBB = right bundle branch block; LBBB = left bundle branch block.

ized to the patient. In some of these patients, radiofrequency endocardial catheter ablation can be used to cure VT; this will be discussed in more detail in Chap. 9. Patients with structural heart disease and inducible VT at electrophysiologic study will almost always require therapy with specific antiarrhythmic drugs or nonpharmacologic treatment, although beta blockers may be useful adjunctive therapy.

The need for therapy of patients who have asymptomatic nonsustained VT detected during treadmill evaluation is uncertain and controversial. The incidence of sudden cardiac death during exercise is rare—for example, one death in 396,000 person-hours of activity during jogging—but it appears to be more prevalent in patients who have underlying structural heart disease.[38] Cardiac arrest due to ventricular fibrillation during exercise in a patient with no obvious structural heart disease appears to occur rarely.[39] One must always remember that atrial fibrillation with a very rapid preexcited ventricular response in patients with Wolff-Parkinson-White syndrome can lead to sudden cardiac death, and in these individuals cardiac function is usually normal (Chap. 7).

The incidence and predictability for survival of patients with exercise-induced VT during routine treadmill testing has been extensively investigated[40–48]

*Table 8-3    Incidence and Characteristics of VT during Treadmill Evaluation*

| Author | Frequency | Heart Disease | VT Occurrence | VT Duration | Prognosis of VT-NS for SCD |
|---|---|---|---|---|---|
| Yang[41] | 55/3351 (1.6%) | NHD—5 CAD—45 NCAD—5 | During ex—28 Recovery—27 | VT-S—50 VT-NS—5 | None |
| Milanes[42] | 48/2600 (1.9%) | NHD—5 CAD—36 NCAD—7 | During ex—76% Recovery—53% | VT-S—1 VT-NS—47 | — |
| Codini[43] | 47/5730 (0.8%) | NHD—7 CAD—30 NCAD—10 | During ex—17 Recovery—23 Both—7 | VT-S—5 VT-NS—42 | — |
| Busby[45] | 18/1160 (1.6%) | NHD—18 | — | VT-S—1 VT-NS—17 | None |
| Mokotoff[48] | 26 | NHD—8 CAD—16 NCAD—2 | During ex—13 Recovery—13 | — | None |

*Abbreviations:* NHD = no obvious heart disease; CAD = coronary artery disease; NCAD = no CAD; Ex = exercise; VT-S = sustained ventricular tachycardia; VT-NS = nonsustained VT; SCD = sudden cardiac death.

(Table 8-3). In essence, these studies demonstrate that asymptomatic nonsustained VT occurring during exercise is much more common in patients with underlying structural heart disease, especially coronary artery disease; has an incidence of approximately 1 to 2 percent; is usually of short duration; frequently presents in the early recovery period; and is not predictive of subsequent sudden cardiac death. Since asymptomatic exercise-provoked nonsustained VT is not associated with a higher incidence of sudden death, a compelling argument can be made to withhold therapy in these patients.

## Sustained Monomorphic Ventricular Tachycardia

We define sustained VT as tachycardia that lasts at least 30 s or has to be terminated prior to 30 s because of hemodynamic compromise.[49] Although this definition was proposed to classify VT induced at electrophysiologic testing, we also use it to define spontaneous sustained VT, since there is no alternative, universally accepted definition. Sustained VT can be monomorphic, polymorphic, or combinations of the two. An episode of sustained monomorphic VT is noted in Fig. 8-12 and is characterized by a similar QRS morphology throughout the episode of tachycardia and usually minimal variability in cycle length between QRS complexes. Sustained polymorphic VT displays changes in QRS morphology throughout the episode of tachycardia, sometimes as frequently as every few QRS complexes, and frequently degenerates into ventricular fibrillation; alterations in cycle length throughout the episode of tachycardia are also frequent (Fig. 8-13). In one sense, ventricular fibrillation is the ultimate polymorphic VT. In some patients, polymorphic nonsustained VT can organize into monomorphic sustained VT (Fig. 8-14). In this patient with a history of monomorphic sustained VT, nonsustained polymorphic VT was initiated at electrophysiologic testing with two extrastimuli ($S_2S_3$) introduced during right ven-

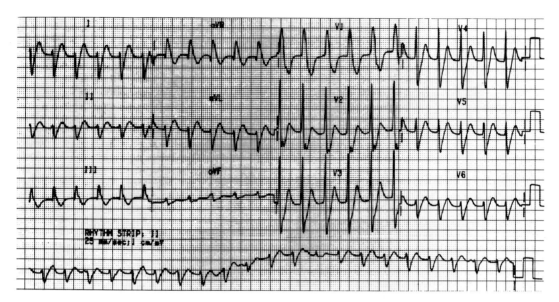

***Figure 8-12***   Sustained monomorphic VT with a right bundle branch block morphology.

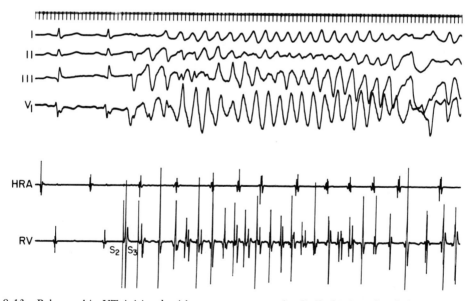

***Figure 8-13***   Polymorphic VT initiated with two premature stimuli ($S_2$-$S_3$) introduced during sinus rhythm. Simultaneous ECG leads I, II, III, and VI are recorded with intracardiac leads from the high right atrium (HRA) and right ventricle (RV). Note the frequent alterations in QRS morphology and cycle length between QRS complexes. *(Reprinted with permission from Prystowsky EN, PACE 11:225, 1988.)*

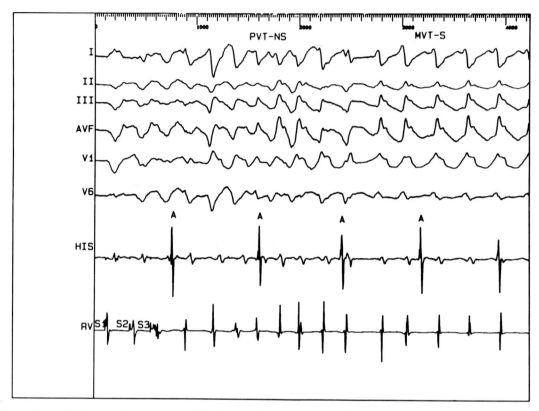

*Figure 8-14*    Polymorphic nonsustained VT that organizes into sustained monomorphic VT. (See text for details.)

tricular pacing (S₁). There was ventriculoatrial disso-ciation, as noted in the His bundle electrogram. This same phenomenon can occur during spontaneous initiation of monomorphic VT. Some patients will demonstrate long runs of monomorphic VT that spontaneously change into a different monomorphic QRS morphology lasting for some time. In these individuals, it is difficult to characterize this arrhythmia as either monomorphic sustained VT or polymorphic sustained VT. In our opinion, these arrhythmias are often stable and more closely fit the clinical characteristics of a monomorphic sustained VT.

There are many causes for sustained monomorphic VT and several clinical entities exist with specific therapeutic approaches. The evaluation and approach to patients with sustained monomorphic VT is discussed in detail in Chap. 9.

## Ventricular Flutter/Ventricular Fibrillation

Ventricular flutter and ventricular fibrillation are two forms of tachycardia that are very rapid and result in cardiac arrest if not promptly terminated. Cardiac arrest is discussed in detail in Chap. 15. Ventricular flutter is often very difficult to distinguish from a very rapid monomorphic sustained VT. The QRS

## Control EP

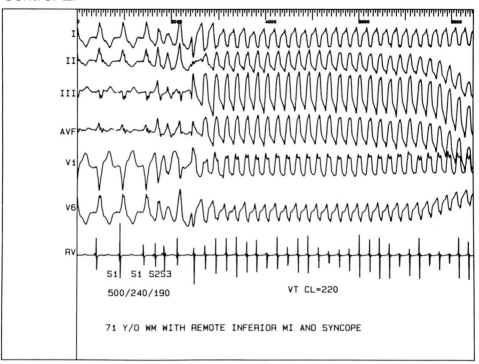

*Figure 8-15*  Initiation of ventricular flutter with a ventricular pacing cycle length of 500 ms (S₁) and two extrastimuli (S₂S₃).

complexes have a sine wave appearance, as noted in Fig. 8-15. In this 71-year-old man with a history of syncope and an inferior wall myocardial infarction, two ventricular premature extrastimuli introduced during pacing cycle length 500 ms, initiated ventricular flutter that caused rapid loss of consciousness. One could argue that this is a very rapid sustained monomorphic VT, but the distinction is of no real clinical significance since the consequences are the same and it is often very difficult to differentiate these two arrhythmias. Ventricular fibrillation (Fig. 8-16) is a rapid VT with grossly disorganized QRS complexes that will lead to cardiac arrest and sudden death if not promptly terminated. Patients with ventricular flutter or ventricular fibrillation will usually present with cardiac arrest or, if the arrhyth-

mia terminates spontaneously, syncope; these individuals require aggressive workup and therapy, as noted in Chap. 15.

## Long QT Syndromes (LQTS) and Torsade de Pointes

Torsade de pointes is a serious type of VT initially described by Dessertenne.[50] It is characterized by a prolonged QT interval during baseline rhythm and a rapid VT with a phasic continuous alteration of QRS morphology (Fig. 8-17). It is also important to realize that artifacts of recording techniques can

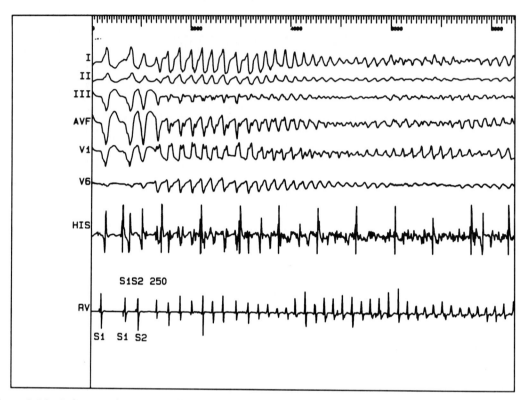

*Figure 8-16*    Induction of ventricular fibrillation with one extrastimulus ($S_2$) introduced during ventricular pacing ($S_1$). The patient had a low left ventricular ejection fraction and spontaneous nonsustained VT (VT-NS) 7 days after coronary artery bypass graft (CABG) surgery.

give the appearance of torsade de pointes (Fig. 8-18). We feel that it is very important to include a prolonged QT interval at baseline rhythm as part of this syndrome for diagnostic as well as therapeutic reasons. For example, patients with a normal QT interval at baseline rhythm can have polymorphic VT with a morphology that resembles torsade de pointes. These individuals may be treated successfully with intravenous agents, such as procainamide, that have a tendency to prolong the QT interval; one

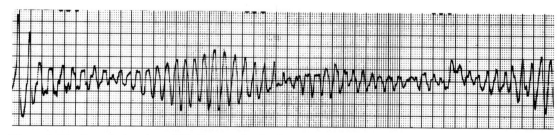

*Figure 8-17*    Torsade de pointes VT. (See text for details.)

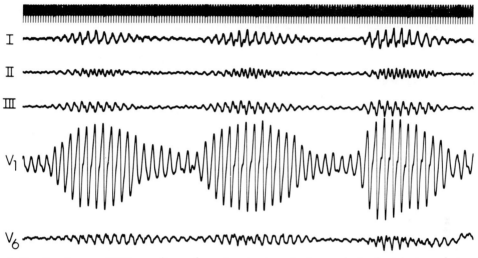

*Figure 8-18*   Simultaneous ECG recordings of a patient in sinus rhythm at electrophysiologic study in whom the recording wire connected to the patient was jiggled at regular intervals to give the artifactual appearance of torsade de pointes.

would not administer such a drug to a patient with torsade de pointes VT. The etiology for torsade de pointes is linked to the QT prolongation. If torsade de pointes is suspected, conditions or agents that prolong the QT interval should be sought. Accepting that there can be crossover in characteristics between the congenital and acquired form of LQTS[51] (Table 8-4), they will be discussed separately in this chapter. In this manner, diagnosis and therapy can be facilitated for a particular patient who presents with long QT syndrome. However, although drugs or other conditions that prolong ventricular repolarization

*Table 8-4   Long QT Syndromes with Torsade de Pointes*

| Features | Congenital | Acquired |
| --- | --- | --- |
| Initiating event for torsade de pointes/syncope | Intense emotions, vigorous physical activity, awakening | Pause-dependent; Short-long-short QRS sequence on ECG |
| Inheritance | Autosomal dominant (Romano-Ward); autosomal recessive with congenital deafness (Jervell and Lange-Nielsen) | — |
| Noninheritance causes (some) | — | Antiarrhythmic drugs, phenothiazines, tri and tetracyclic antidepressants, hypokalemia, hypomagnesemia, severe bradycardia |
| Therapy | Beta-adrenergic blockers, permanent pacemaker, left cervicothoracic sympathetic ganglionectomy, implantable defibrillator | Discontinue causative agent, IV magnesium, correct electrolyte abnormality, temporary pacing, IV isoproterenol |

may be the cause of acquired LQTS, they could also greatly exacerbate arrhythmias in a patient with congenital long QT syndrome.

### Congenital Long QT Syndrome (Table 8-4)

Jervell and Lange-Nielsen[52] reported a family with prolonged corrected QT($QT_c$) interval associated with congenital deafness and the occurrence of sudden death, which is thought to have an autosomal recessive inheritance. Another form of LQTS associated with autosomal dominant inheritance and lack of congenital deafness was described by both Romano et al.[53] and Ward.[54] Keating and colleagues[55] investigated a large family pedigree with LQTS and identified a DNA marker at the Harvey ras-1 locus on the short arm of chromosome 11 as the genetic basis for LQTS in these patients. In addition, Vincent et al.[56] evaluated the relationship of QTc intervals with carriers of the long-QT gene in 199 family members and reported that the QTc interval was longer in the gene carriers than noncarriers. Further, they had substantial overlap of the QTc interval between carriers and noncarriers and concluded that measurement of the QTc interval may not predict an accurate diagnosis in these families. These preliminary data are exciting and permit a glimpse of the future in our ability to unravel some of the pathophysiologic mechanisms associated with the LQTS. At present, we still rely on the family history as well as ECG QTc measurement to identify affected and nonaffected individuals.[57]

The pathogenesis of the idiopathic (congenital) LQTS has undergone intense investigation and several theories exist that are not necessarily mutually exclusive.[51,58] The reader is referred to these two excellent review articles for a more in-depth discussion of the pathogenesis of LQTS, which is beyond the scope of this chapter. In brief, one hypothesis suggests a sympathetic imbalance with a decrease in right cardiac sympathetic activity and higher-than-normal sympathetic activity on the left. The alternative hypothesis suggests an intracardiac abnormality—for example, dysfunction of potassium channel conductance. Obvious overlaps could occur with both hypotheses.

The mechanism of the torsade de pointes ventricular tachyarrhythmia is also controversial. Brachmann et al.[59] demonstrated in canine in vivo experiments that cesium chloride given intravenously could produce a polymorphic VT under certain experimental conditions. These authors also analyzed the effect of cesium chloride on canine ventricular myocardium using microelectrode techniques and showed the appearance of early afterdepolarizations (EAD). Cesium chloride blocks outward potassium currents, and the appearance of early afterdepolarizations was mechanistically linked to this observation. Tzivoni et al.[60] demonstrated that intravenous magnesium could suppress the acquired form of torsade de pointes VT, and Bailey et al.[61] subsequently confirmed this observation in the cesium dog model and demonstrated that magnesium suppressed early afterdepolarizations. Thus, a compelling argument could be made for early afterdepolarizations as the mechanism of torsade de pointes in either congenital or acquired LQTS, but many observations can still be explained by dispersion of repolarization with reentry as the mechanism.[62] It is interesting to note that early afterdepolarizations can be suppressed with overdrive pacing or faster heart rates, and one may wonder why all episodes of EAD-induced torsade de pointes should not be self-terminating if this were the only factor involved. It is possible that torsade de pointes is initiated by an EAD mechanism in many if not most patients with LQTS but that a sustained arrhythmia occurs via alternative mechanisms, possibly reentry. The only certain thing is that more data are needed to elucidate the mechanism of this arrhythmia in humans.

The idiopathic LQTS is characterized by a prolonged corrected QT interval on the ECG and the propensity to syncope or sudden death. Seizures of undefined etiology are a common presentation, often leading to a delay in the correct workup and therapy. As noted above, it is usually inherited as autosomal dominant without deafness but can be autosomal recessive and can also occur sporadically.[63]

As noted in Table 8-4, syncope or documented torsade de pointes ventricular arrhythmias are usually associated with intense emotions, vigorous physical activity, or awakening, especially with auditory stimuli.[63,64] Additional findings in some patients include ECG evidence of T-wave alternans, sinus bradycardia, and an abnormal ventricular contraction pattern by echocardiography.[58,65] The diagnosis of LQTS rests heavily on the definition of an abnormal QTc interval. In a report from the prospective study of LQTS by Moss and colleagues,[63] the patients were subdivided as "affected" if the QTc was greater than 440 ms and "unaffected" if the QTc was ≤440 ms. However, in a recent review of LQTS, Moss and Robinson[57] suggest that QTc is prolonged in adult men and women if it is greater than 450 ms and 470 ms, respectively, and borderline if it is 430 to 450 ms and 450 to 470 ms, respectively. It should also be remembered that the Bazett formula to correct for QT interval with rate changes has substantial problems in the presence of significant alterations of autonomic tone.[66]

### Therapy

Therapy for patients with idiopathic LQTS begins with beta-adrenergic blockers but can include implantation of a permanent pacemaker, left cervicothoracic sympathetic ganglionectomy, and—in very selected cases—implantation of a defibrillator (Table 8-4).[58,63] For beta blockers, we administer a large enough dose to demonstrate competitive blockade during exercise testing—for example, preventing exercise heart rates of greater than 120 to 130/min. Some patients may require pacemaker implantation if resting sinus bradycardia is marked. If symptoms continue, then alternative therapies will be necessary (Table 8-4). Recommendations for therapy of asymptomatic patients who have prolonged QTc are not as straightforward. Asymptomatic individuals who have long QTc apparently are at low risk for developing cardiac events and cardiac arrest is rare as an initial presentation.[57] Therapy may not be necessary, but it is recommended for the asymptomatic individual

with a strong family history of sudden death at a young age.[57]

### Acquired LQTS

The most common cause of acquired LQTS in our experience is associated with the use of antiarrhythmic agents such as quinidine, which can block outward potassium ions from cardiac cells and prolong the QT interval. These patients often undergo concomitant diuretic therapy and have hypokalemia. Other causes are noted in Table 8-4, which is not inclusive but lists many of the common etiologies. The mechanism of torsade de pointes in acquired LQTS is postulated to be triggered activity with EADs, but reentry is not discounted, as noted above under the discussion of congenital LQTS. The tachycardia commonly occurs with a short-long-short QRS complex sequence (Fig. 8-19). This ECG rhythm strip is taken from a patient receiving quinidine therapy. The patient has premature atrial complexes followed by pauses and a marked abnormality in repolarization, with a pronounced inverted T wave in the QRS complexes closing a pause. After the second premature atrial complex (fourth QRS complex), there is a relatively long pause, and the QRS complex ending the pause has a more marked inversion of the T wave and is followed by torsade de pointes. This short-long-short QRS complex sequence is very typical for the initiation of pause-dependent torsade de pointes in acquired LQTS.[51,67,68] The incidence of torsade de pointes secondary to antiarrhythmic drug therapy varies in the literature but accounted for 21 percent of iatrogenic causes of cardiac arrest.[69]

### Therapy

Probably the most important aspect of treatment for patients with acquired LQTS is a correct diagnosis. Not infrequently, patients with torsade de pointes due to hypokalemia or drugs will be given agents such as intravenous procainamide in an attempt to terminate the arrhythmia. This can obviously lead to a much worse situation. It is critically important

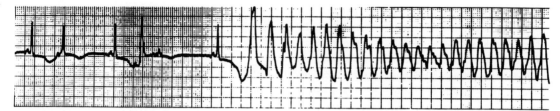

***Figure 8-19***   Typical initiation of torsade de pointes VT. The fourth QRS complex is premature and is followed by a relatively long pause. The QRS complex closing the pause is associated with a marked increase in the amplitude and duration of the inverted T and possibly U wave, and torsade de pointes tachycardia follows.

to obtain an ECG during baseline rhythm between episodes of torsade de pointes to evaluate the QTc interval. It is also necessary to review the electrolyte status and drugs the patient is receiving. As noted in Table 8-4, therapy consists of discontinuing the implicated drug and correcting any electrolyte abnormality. It is important to suppress subsequent episodes of torsade de pointes while the offending drug is being eliminated from the patient, and several methods are available to accomplish this. Temporary overdrive ventricular or atrial pacing is a proven, excellent method to prevent the recurrence of arrhythmia. It may not be possible to initiate pacing in a timely fashion, however, and other treatment options are available.

Tzivoni and colleagues[60] clearly demonstrated the success of intravenous magnesium sulfate to treat torsade de pointes. Using a 25% or 50% solution of magnesium sulfate, they suggested that a 2-g intravenous bolus be given over 1 to 2 min, which can be followed by a second 2-g bolus 5 to 15 min later if needed. A continuous infusion of 3 to 20 mg/min of magnesium sulfate can also be used. In 12 patients with acquired LQTS and torsade de pointes with a mean QTc of 0.64 s, they noted that 9 had no more torsade de pointes after the first dose of magnesium sulfate and the other 3 had a partial response.[60] Importantly, in 5 patients with coronary artery disease and polymorphic ventricular tachycardia with a normal QT interval, intravenous magnesium sulfate was ineffective and 3 patients responded to intravenous lidocaine and 2 to intravenous procainamide. This observation supports the concept that

torsade de pointes should be diagnosed only in the presence of a prolonged QTc interval, measured either immediately before the onset of ventricular tachycardia or at baseline, because therapy that can acutely exacerbate one type of arrhythmia—for example, procainamide in torsade de pointes—can be lifesaving in another patient. Temporary overdrive ventricular or atrial pacing or intravenous isoproterenol to increase the heart rate can effectively suppress torsade de pointes in acquired LQTS. Our bias is to avoid isoproterenol if possible.

The highest priority should be given to prevention of torsade de pointes. Drugs that are known to prolong the QT interval should be given cautiously to patients who have a propensity for conditions such as hypokalemia and avoided whenever possible in patients who have a baseline prolonged QTc interval. One should be careful when administering two or more agents that can prolong the QT interval in a given patient and preferably do this in-hospital during continuous ECG monitoring. Chapter 19 provides a more detailed discussion regarding when to hospitalize a patient to initiate antiarrhythmic drug therapy.

## Bidirectional Tachycardia

Bidirectional VT is usually a manifestation of digitalis toxicity. It is characterized by right bundle branch block morphology with alternating frontal-plane polarity.[70] It is important to recognize that this can be a digitalis toxic arrhythmia and to determine whether the patient is receiving digitalis. If digitalis toxicity is noted, methods to treat this—such as administration of potassium, lidocaine, or phenytoin—can be considered, but we recommend as initial therapy in this potentially life-threatening situation the administration of cardiac glycoside-specific Fab fragments.

# References

1.  Belhassen B et al: Idiopathic recurrent sustained ventricular tachycardia responsive to verapamil: An ECG-electrophysiologic entity. *Am Heart J* 108:1034, 1984.

2.  Ohe T et al: Idiopathic sustained left ventricular tachycardia: Clinical and electrophysiologic characteristics. *Circulation* 77:560, 1988.

3.  Page RL et al: Radiofrequency catheter ablation of idiopathic recurrent ventricular tachycardia with right bundle branch block, left axis morphology. PACE 16:327, 1993.

4.  Gallavardin L: Extrasystolie ventriculaire a paroxysmes tachycardiques prolonges. *Arch Mal Coeur* 15:298, 1922.

5.  Parkinson J, Papp C: Repetitive paroxysmal tachycardia. *Br Heart J* 9:241, 1947.

6.  Froment R et al: Paroxysmal ventricular tachycardia: A clinical classification. *Br Heart J* 15:172, 1953.

7.  Rahilly GT et al: Clinical and electrophysiologic findings in patients with repetitive monomorphic ventricular tachycardia and otherwise normal electrocardiogram. *Am J Cardiol* 50:459, 1982.

8.  Buxton AE et al: Repetitive, monomorphic ventricular tachycardia: Clinical and electrophysiologic characteristics in patients with and patients without organic heart disease. *Am J Cardiol* 54:997, 1984.

9.  Coumel P et al: Repetitive monomorphic idiopathic ventricular tachycardia, in Zipes DP, Jalife J (eds): *Cardiac Electrophysiology and Arrhythmias.* New York, Grune & Stratton, 1985, pp 457–468.

10. Morady F et al: Long-term results of catheter ablation of idiopathic right ventricular tachycardia. *Circulation* 82:2093, 1990.

11. Klein LW et al: Radiofrequency catheter ablation of ventricular tachycardia in patients without structural heart disease. *Circulation* 85:1666, 1992.

12. Follansbee WP et al: Nonsustained ventricular tachycardia in ambulatory patients: Characteristics and association with sudden cardiac death. *Ann Intern Med* 92:741, 1980.

13. Olshausen K et al: Ventricular arrhythmias in idiopathic dilated cardiomyopathy. *Br Heart J* 51:195, 1984.

14. Holmes J et al: Arrhythmias in ischemic and nonischemic dilated cardiomyopathy: Prediction of mortality by ambulatory electrocardiography. *Am J Cardiol* 55:146, 1985.

15. Meinertz T et al: Significance of ventricular arrhythmias in idiopathic dilated cardiomyopathy. *Am J Cardiol* 53:902, 1984.

16. Unverferth DV et al: Factors influencing the one-year mortality of dilated cardiomyopathy. *Am J Cardiol* 54:147, 1984.

17. DeMaria R et al: Ventricular arrhythmias in dilated cardiomyopathy as an independent prognostic hallmark. *Am J Cardiol* 69:1451, 1992.

18. Bigger JT Jr et al: Prevalence, characteristics and significance of ventricular tachycardia detected by 24-hour continuous electrocardiographic recordings in the late hospital phase of acute myocardial infarction. *Am J Cardiol* 58:1151, 1986.

19. Prystowsky EN: Antiarrhythmic therapy for asymptomatic ventricular arrhythmias. *Am J Cardiol* 61:102A, 1988.

20. Fananapazir L et al: Prognostic determinants in hypertrophic cardiomyopathy: Prospective evaluation of a therapeutic strategy based on clinical, Holter, hemodynamic, and electrophysiological findings. *Circulation* 86:730, 1992.

21. Kammerling JM et al: Characteristics of spontaneous nonsustained ventricular tachycardia poorly predict rate of sustained ventricular tachycardia. *Clin Res* 34:312A, 1986.

22.  Kennedy HL et al: Long-term follow-up of asymptomatic healthy subjects with frequent and complex ventricular ectopy. *N Engl J Med* 312:193, 1985.

23.  Wu D et al: Effects of atropine on induction and maintenance of atrioventricular nodal reentrant tachycardia. *Circulation* 59:779, 1979.

24.  Schwartz PJ et al: Autonomic mechanisms and sudden death: New insights from the analysis of baroreceptors reflexes in conscious dogs with and without a myocardial infarction. *Circulation* 78:969, 1988.

25.  LaRovere MT et al: Baroreflex sensitivity, clinical correlates and cardiovascular mortality among patients with a first myocardial infarction: A prospective study. *Circulation* 78:816, 1988.

26.  Sung RJ et al: Effects of β-adrenergic blockade on verapamil-responsive and verapamil-irresponsive sustained ventricular tachycardias. *J Clin Invest* 81:688, 1988.

27.  Sung RJ et al: Effects of verapamil on ventricular tachycardias possibly caused by reentry, automaticity, and triggered activity. *J Clin Invest* 72:350, 1983.

28.  Lerman BB et al: Adenosine-sensitive ventricular tachycardia: Evidence suggesting cyclic AMP-mediated triggered activity. *Circulation* 74:270, 1986.

29.  Woelfel A et al: Reproducibility and treatment of exercise-induced ventricular tachycardia. *Am J Cardiol* 53:751, 1984.

30.  Woelfel A et al: Efficacy of verapamil in exercise-induced ventricular tachycardia. *Am J Cardiol* 56:292, 1985.

31.  Sung RJ et al: Electrophysiologic mechanism of exercise-induced sustained ventricular tachycardia. *Am J Cardiol* 51:525, 1983.

32.  Wu D et al: Exercise-triggered paroxysmal ventricular tachycardia. *Ann Intern Med* 95:410, 1981.

33.  Palileo EV et al: Exercise provocable right ventricular outflow tract tachycardia. *Am Heart J* 104:185, 1982.

34.  O'Hara GE et al: Incidence, pathophysiology and prognosis of exercise-induced sustained ventricular tachycardia associated with healed myocardial infarction. *Am J Cardiol* 70:875, 1992.

35.  Mont L et al: Clinical and electrophysiologic characteristics of exercise-related idiopathic ventricular tachycardia. *Am J Cardiol* 68:897, 1991.

36.  Sokoloff NM et al: Plasma norepinephrine in exercise-induced ventricular tachycardia. *J Am Coll Cardiol* 8:11, 1986.

37.  Hong RA et al: Life-threatening ventricular tachycardia and fibrillation induced by painless myocardial ischemia during exercise testing. *JAMA* 257:1937, 1987.

38.  Amsterdam EA et al: Exercise and sudden death. *Cardiol Clin* 5:337, 1987.

39.  Wesley RC Jr et al: Catecholamine-sensitive right ventricular tachycardia in the absence of structural heart disease: A mechanism of exercise-induced cardiac arrest. *Cardiology* 79:237, 1991.

40.  McHenry PL et al: Comparative study of exercise-induced ventricular arrhythmias in normal subjects and patients with documented coronary artery disease. *Am J Cardiol* 37:609, 1976.

41.  Yang JC et al: Ventricular tachycardia during routine treadmill testing. *Arch Intern Med* 151:349, 1991.

42.  Milanes J et al: Exercise tests and ventricular tachycardia. *West J Med* 145:473, 1986.

43.  Codini MA et al: Clinical significance and characteristics of exercise-induced ventricular tachycardia. *Cathet Cardiovasc Diagn* 7:227, 1981.

44.  Fleg JL, Lakatta EG: Prevalence and prognosis of exercise-induced nonsustained ventricular tachycardia in apparently healthy volunteers. *Am J Cardiol* 54:762, 1984.

45.  Busby MJ et al: Prevalence and long-term significance of exercise-induced frequent or repetitive ventricular ectopic beats in apparently healthy volunteers. *J Am Coll Cardiol* 14:1659, 1989.

46.  Califf RM et al: Prognostic value of ventricular arrhythmias associated with treadmill exercise testing in patients studied with cardiac catheterization for suspected ischemic heart disease. *J Am Coll Cardiol* 2:1060, 1983.

47.  Sami M et al: Significance of exercise-induced ventricular arrhythmia in stable coronary artery disease: A coronary artery surgery study project. *Am J Cardiol* 54:1182, 1984.

48.  Mokotoff DM et al: Exercise-induced ventricular tachycardia: Clinical features, relation to chronic ventricular ectopy, and prognosis. *Chest* 1:10, 1980.

49.  Naccarelli GV et al: Role of electrophysiologic testing in managing patients who have ventricular tachycardia unrelated to coronary artery disease. *Am J Cardiol* 50:165, 1982.

50.  Dessertenne F: La tachycardie ventriculaire a deux foyers opposes variables. *Arch Mal Coeur* 59:263, 1966.

51. Jackman WM et al: The long QT syndromes: A critical review, new clinical observations and a unifying hypothesis. *Prog Cardiovasc Dis* 31:115, 1988.

52. Jervell A, Lange-Nielsen F: Congenital deaf mutism, functional heart disease with prolongation of the QT interval, and sudden death. *Am Heart J* 54:59, 1957.

53. Romano C et al: Aritmie cardiache rare dell'eta pediatrica. *Clin Pediatr (Phila)* 45:656, 1963.

54. Ward OC: A new familial cardiac syndrome in children. *J Irish Med Assoc* 54:103, 1964.

55. Keating M et al: Linkage of a cardiac arrhythmia, the long QT syndrome, and the Harvey *ras*-1 gene. *Science* 252:704, 1991.

56. Vincent GM et al: The spectrum of symptoms and QT intervals in carriers of the gene for the long-QT syndrome. *N Engl J Med* 327:846, 1992.

57. Moss AJ, Robinson JL: Long QT syndrome. *Heart Dis Stroke* 1:309, 1992.

58. Schwartz PJ et al: Pathogenesis and therapy of the idiopathic long QT syndrome, in Hashiba K, Moss AJ, Schwartz PJ (eds): *QT Prolongation and Ventricular Arrhythmias*. Ann NY Acad Sci 644:112, 1992.

59. Brachmann J et al: Bradycardia-dependent triggered activity: Relevance to the drug-induced multiform ventricular tachycardia. *Circulation* 68:846, 1983.

60. Tzivoni D et al: Treatment of torsade de pointes with magnesium sulfate. *Circulation* 77:392, 1988.

61. Bailey BS et al: Magnesium suppresses early afterdepolarizations and ventricular tachyarrhythmias induced in dogs by cesium. *Circulation* 77:1395, 1988.

62. Surawicz B: Electrophysiologic substrate of torsade de pointes: Dispersion of repolarization or early afterdepolarizations? *J Am Coll Cardiol* 14:172, 1989.

63. Moss AJ et al: The long QT syndrome: Prospective longitudinal study of 328 families. *Circulation* 84:1136, 1991.

64. Wellens HJJ et al: Ventricular fibrillation occurring on arousal from sleep by auditory stimuli. *Circulation* 46:661, 1972.

65. Nador F et al: Unsuspected echocardiographic abnormality in the long QT syndrome. *Circulation* 84:1530, 1991.

66. Browne KF et al: The influence of the autonomic nervous system on the Q-T interval in man. *Am J Cardiol* 50:1099, 1982.

67. Ejvinsson G, Orinius E: Prodromal ventricular premature beats preceded by a diastolic wave. *Acta Med Scand* 208:445, 1980.

68. Kay GN et al: Torsade de pointes: The long-short initiating sequence and other clinical features: Observations in 32 patients. *J Am Coll Cardiol* 2:806, 1983.

69. Bedell SE et al: Incidence and characteristics of preventable iatrogenic cardiac arrests. *JAMA* 265:2815, 1991.

70. Morris SN, Zipes DP: His bundle electrocardiography during bidirectional tachycardia. *Circulation* 43:32, 1973.

# Chapter 9

# Sustained Monomorphic Ventricular Tachycardia

Sustained monomorphic ventricular tachycardia (VT) is an arrhythmia that originates in the ventricles, does not require any supraventricular tissue for maintenance of the arrhythmia, and is of a uniform QRS configuration throughout the duration of tachycardia, which is 30 s or more. As was discussed in detail in Chap. 8, categorizing VT by mechanism or other specific characteristics is often difficult. The overwhelming majority of patients who have sustained monomorphic VT have some form of heart disease, usually coronary artery disease[1,2] although two specific forms of VT typically occur in patients without structural heart disease, as discussed later. This chapter is divided into subsections on sustained monomorphic VT that occur in various groups of patients. A general approach to patients with sustained monomorphic VT is presented first.

## History and Physical Examination

Patients who have sustained monomorphic VT may have a variety of symptoms that depend primarily on the hemodynamic effect of VT in a particular patient. The major determinants of hemodynamic response to VT are the rate of tachycardia, degree of myocardial dysfunction, and peripheral vascular adaptation. Common presenting symptoms range from palpitations and presyncope to syncope and cardiac arrest. In some patients symptoms may reflect concomitant organ disease—for example, angina in a patient with significant coronary artery obstruction. The level of myocardial dysfunction is not merely based on the left ventricular ejection fraction. Figure 9-1 shows examples of sustained monomorphic VT in two patients with a history of heart disease. Although the rates of tachycardia are similar, one patient (panel A) presented with palpitations whereas the other (panel B) had syncope. Note that the left ventricular ejection fraction was only 10 percent in the patient presenting with palpitations, but there was no history of congestive heart failure. In contrast, the patient who had syncope had an ejection fraction of 19 percent but was also ranked in New York Heart Association (NYHA) class II-III for congestive heart failure. In our experience syncope is more likely to occur in patients with a history of heart failure during sinus rhythm, which signifies a heart that will have limited compensatory ability during VT.

The most important historical information is determination of the presence of heart disease. Akhtar and colleagues[2] noted that structural heart disease occurred in 112 of 122 (92 percent) patients with VT compared with only 6 of 28 (21 percent) patients with supraventricular tachycardia (SVT). These authors also noted that VT was frequently misdiagnosed as SVT.[2] In our experience, this usually occurs when a patient presents with a wide QRS complex tachycardia and a relatively stable blood pressure (Figure 9-1A). It is critical to remember that hemody-

**No History of CHF**
**LVEF 10%**
**BP with VT-S 112/89 mmHg**

**NYHA II–III CHF**
**LVEF 19%**
**BP with VT-S**
**40 mmHg Sys., Syncope**

**A**

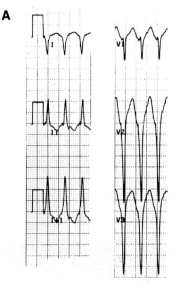

**B**

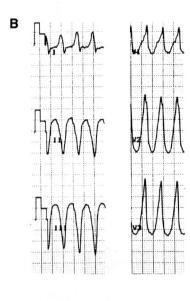

**VT$_{CL}$ 320 ms**

**VT$_{CL}$ 295 ms**

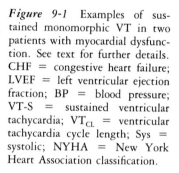

*Figure 9-1* Examples of sustained monomorphic VT in two patients with myocardial dysfunction. See text for further details. CHF = congestive heart failure; LVEF = left ventricular ejection fraction; BP = blood pressure; VT-S = sustained ventricular tachycardia; VT$_{CL}$ = ventricular tachycardia cycle length; Sys = systolic; NYHA = New York Heart Association classification.

namic stability during a wide QRS complex tachycardia does not exclude VT and hemodynamic instability during tachycardia does not exclude SVT.

Physical examination of the patient during tachycardia may disclose signs of ventriculoatrial dissociation, which rarely occur with SVT. During ventriculoatrial dissociation, the normal synchronized atrial to ventricular activation sequence is lost and the two chambers contract independently of each other. Thus, the relative position of the tricuspid and mitral valves in the ventricle at the time of ventricular contraction may vary from beat to beat and lead to cannon A waves in the neck veins, variable intensity of S$_1$, and variable systolic blood pressure. After restoration of sinus rhythm, the physical examination should be directed to uncovering signs of heart disease such as neck vein distension, pulmonary congestion, pathologic mur-

murs or gallops, and peripheral edema. The presence of decreased arterial pulsations or bruits over carotid or other arteries may suggest the presence of atherosclerotic disease.

## Electrocardiographic Evaluation

It is very important to obtain electrocardiographic (ECG) documentation of the wide complex QRS tachycardia, preferably a 12-lead ECG. An in-depth discussion of the differential diagnosis for wide complex QRS tachycardia is presented in Chap. 13, and only key points will be reviewed here. Electrocardiographic signs of ventriculoatrial dissociation are independent P waves and QRS complexes

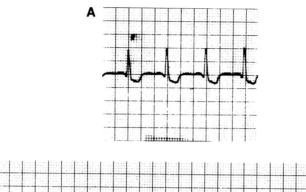

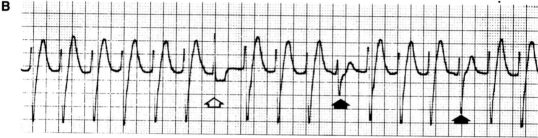

*Figure 9-2*  Fusion and capture QRS complexes during VT. (See text for details.)

and fusion and capture QRS complexes. Figure 9-2 demonstrates the normal QRS complex for this patient in panel A and the presence of capture (unfilled arrow) and fusion (filled arrow) QRS complexes in panel B. Note that the morphology of the fusion complexes is intermediate between the normal and VT QRS complexes. Fusion and capture QRS complexes occur when a supraventricular impulse activates all (capture) or part (fusion) of the ventricles during tachycardia. This may occur in patients who have slower VTs but, in our experience, are rarely seen in patients in whom the rate of tachycardia is 180 or greater. Figure 9-3 shows the electrophysiologic mechanism of fusion and capture QRS complexes. In Fig. 9-3A, the third QRS complex is narrow and generated from the sinus atrial impulse that captures the ventricles and yields a normal HV interval of 50 ms for this patient. In Fig. 9-3B, two fusion QRS complexes are noted with an HV interval of 40 ms, which is 10 ms shorter than that noted during sinus rhythm in this patient, and the QRS morphologies are intermediate between the sinus-generated complexes and those that occur during tachycardia. In some

patients, ventriculoatrial block but not total dissociation is present and may be identified on the ECG. In Fig. 9-4, 2:1 ventriculoatrial conduction is noted during VT. Note that a His bundle depolarization is present with each QRS complex regardless of the presence of an atrial depolarization. However, the His activation occurs within the QRS complex and represents retrograde activation of the His bundle during VT in this patient. The arrows in ECG lead III point to atrial activation on the ECG after every other QRS complex. Although the P waves are clearly seen in ECG lead III, they are not easily identified in several other leads, which reinforces the importance of obtaining a 12-lead ECG whenever possible during tachycardia.

Ventricular tachycardia can be left bundle branch block (Fig. 9-5) or right bundle branch block (Fig. 9-6) morphology, and the QRS duration is typically 120 ms or greater. Very uncommonly a relatively narrow QRS complex can occur during VT (Fig. 9-7). Hayes et al.[3] reviewed 12-lead ECGs of 106 patients with induced VT at electrophysiologic study. Of these patients, 5 (4.7 percent) had a QRS

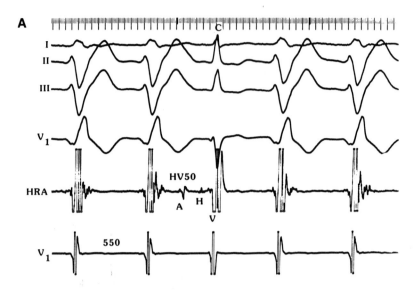

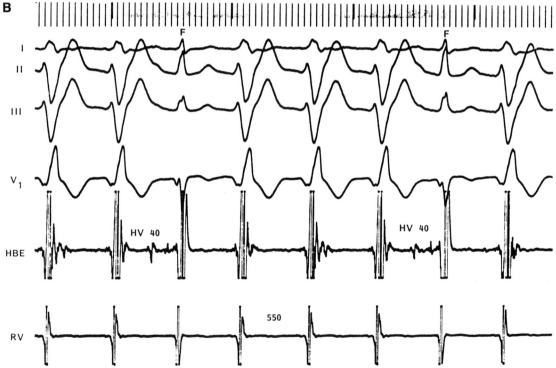

*Figure 9-3*   Electrophysiologic mechanism of fusion and capture QRS complexes during VT. *A*. The third QRS complex is narrow, with a HV interval of 50 ms, identical to that seen during sinus rhythm, and this represents a capture (C) QRS complex. *B*. the third and seventh QRS complexes are fusion (F) complexes with an intermediate QRS morphology between that of sinus rhythm and VT. The HV interval is 40 ms, less than that noted during sinus rhythm. For the time lines, each major division equals 50 ms.

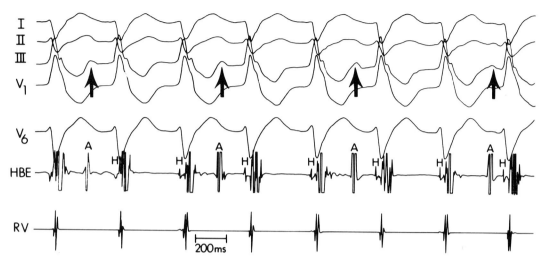

*Figure 9-4*   Ventricular tachycardia with 2:1 ventriculoatrial conduction. (See text for details.)

duration of 110 ms or less. Of the 5 patients, 4 had coronary artery disease and only one patient had no obvious structural heart disease. In patients with a relatively narrow QRS complex during VT it is possible that the origin of tachycardia is in the proximal His-Purkinje system, which would allow activation of most of the ventricles over the normal conduction system. Although this is theoretically possible, it is difficult to confirm even at electrophysiologic study. The fact that VT can occur with a QRS

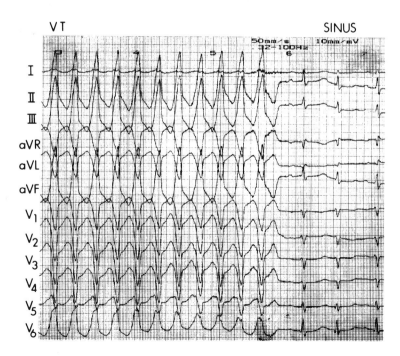

*Figure 9-5*   Left bundle branch block VT terminates spontaneously and sinus rhythm resumes for the last three QRS complexes in this tracing.

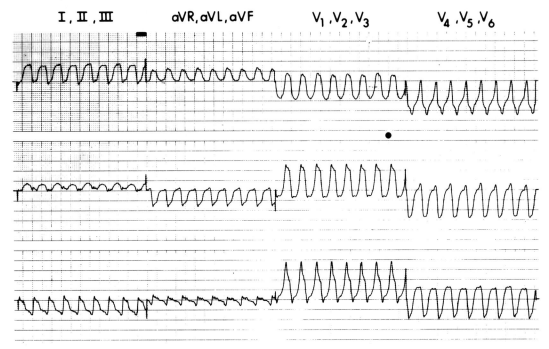

*Figure 9-6*    Right bundle branch block sustained monomorphic VT.

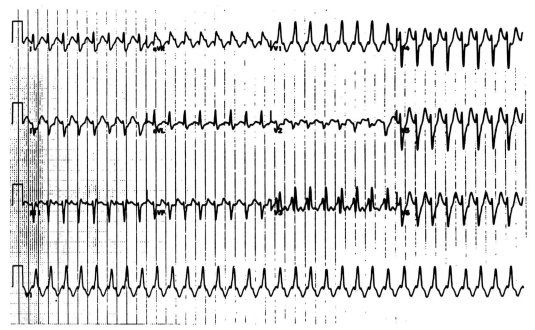

*Figure 9-7*    Relatively narrow QRS complex VT.

duration <120 ms emphasizes the importance of considering any relatively wide QRS complex tachycardia in a patient with structural heart disease as VT until proven otherwise. We recommend electrophysiologic testing in all such patients to confirm the diagnosis as well as to gauge the effects of therapy, as noted below.

## Electrophysiologic Testing

An in-depth review of methods of electrophysiologic testing is noted elsewhere.[1,4] Programmed electrical stimulation of the heart, in particular ventricular stimulation, is used to initiate sustained VT. Induction of VT using programmed stimulation techniques can occur in patients in whom the mechanism of tachycardia is due to reentry or triggered activity related to delayed afterdepolarizations but not when it is due to abnormal automaticity. Further, successful initiation of tachycardia at electrophysiologic testing depends on the type of arrhythmia and heart disease being studied as well as the stimulation techniques employed.[1,4] For example, in patients with a history

of sustained monomorphic VT, the frequency of initiation of sustained monomorphic VT is approximately 95 percent in patients who have coronary artery disease but only approximately 80 to 85 percent in patients with idiopathic dilated cardiomyopathy.[1,4]

Successful induction of sustained monomorphic VT depends on the pacing technique employed, with the use of three extrastimuli having a higher inducibility rate than that of one extrastimulus[5] (Fig. 9-8). However, as noted in Fig. 9-8, there is a tradeoff of specificity for sensitivity as more aggressive pacing techniques are employed. Thus, a very rapid—for example, with a cycle length <220 ms—monomorphic sustained VT initiated with triple extrastimuli may be a nonspecific arrhythmia in a patient who has documented hemodynamically stable slower VT. Unfortunately, some patients may have more than one clinical tachycardia, but only a slower VT has been documented. In these instances the more rapid VT initiated with triple extrastimuli might have important clinical consequences, and these decisions have to be made on an individual basis. We do consider sustained polymorphic VT or ventricular fibrillation initiated with triple extrastimuli in patients with a history of only sustained monomorphic

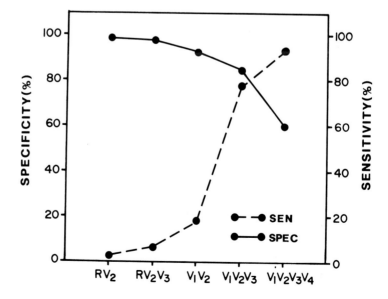

*Figure 9-8*  Schematic representation of the sensitivity and specificity of programmed ventricular stimulation techniques employed to induce VT. Specificity is noted on the left and sensitivity on the right. Techniques are as follows: $RV_2$ = one ventricular extrastimulus during sinus rhythm; $RV_2V_3$ = two ventricular extrastimuli in sinus rhythm; $V_1V_2$ = one ventricular extrastimulus during ventricular pacing; $V_1V_2V_3$ = two ventricular extrastimuli during ventricular pacing; $V_1V_2V_3V_4$ = three ventricular extrastimuli during ventricular pacing.

VT as nonclinical arrhythmias because of the lack of specificity of these tachycardias initiated with very aggressive pacing techniques.

Initiation of sustained monomorphic VT using various pacing techniques is demonstrated in Figs. 9-9 to 9-12. Multiple techniques should be attempted; we use an organized hierarchy of pacing techniques that proceeds from incremental atrial pacing to premature atrial stimulation; premature ventricular stimulation during sinus rhythm; premature ventricular stimulation using 1, 2, and then 3 ventricular extrastimuli during ventricular pacing; and burst ventricular pacing.

To increase yield of induction of VT, multiple pacing cycle lengths are employed as well as stimulation at two or more right ventricular sites.[1,4-6] In some individuals, infusion of isoproterenol is necessary as an adjunct for the induction of VT during programmed electrical stimulation.[7,8] In other patients, infusion of isoproterenol alone may initiate tachycardia.[9]

## Sustained Monomorphic Ventricular Tachycardia in Patients with Structural Heart Disease

### Coronary Artery Disease

The most common cause of sustained monomorphic VT is coronary artery disease.[1,2] When sustained VT occurs in a patient with chronic coronary artery disease, typically originating from an area of the ventricle associated with a healed myocardial infarction, the overwhelming evidence in experimental models as well as in humans suggests reentry as the mechanism for tachycardia.[10-14] The mechanisms of sustained monomorphic VT that occurs during the first 24 h of an acute myocardial infarction is not as clearly defined and may be due to several mechanisms, including reentry and forms of automaticity. Wellens et al.[10] failed to initiate sustained VT in 7 patients

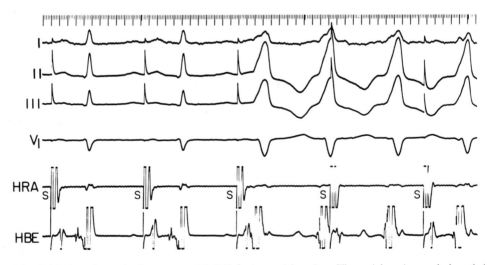

*Figure 9-9*   Initiation of sustained monomorphic VT during atrial pacing. The atrial pacing cycle length is fixed at 550 ms. Note that the first two QRS complexes are conducted from the high right atrial pacing site to the ventricle over the normal AV conduction system, with a His bundle electrogram preceding each QRS complex with the same HV interval identified during sinus rhythm. Ventricular tachycardia begins with the third QRS complex and was sustained in this individual. Ventricular tachycardia was initiated during incremental atrial pacing and only the last two normal QRS complexes are illustrated prior to the initiation of tachycardia. Note that the third atrial pacing stimulus to QRS interval is too short for this QRS complex to have been generated from the atrium.

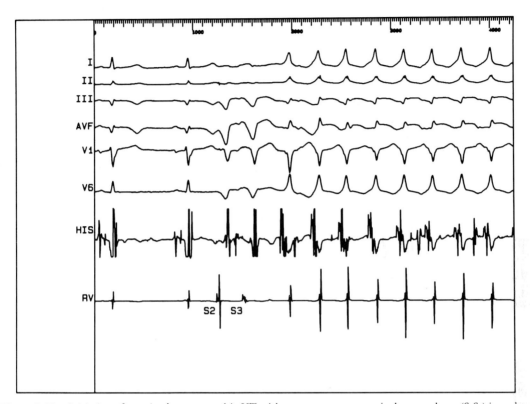

***Figure 9-10***   Initiation of sustained monomorphic VT with two premature ventricular complexes (S₂S₃) introduced during sinus rhythm. This is a left bundle branch block normal axis ventricular tachycardia. The first two sinus complexes demonstrate normal HV intervals as noted on the His bundle electrogram. Consistent His bundle depolarizations are not present before the wide QRS complexes during tachycardia confirming the ventricular origin of this arrhythmia.

in whom the arrhythmia presented in the first 24 h of acute myocardial infarction. In fact, all patients were in sustained VT when they entered the electrophysiology laboratory. In contrast, 18 of 21 patients in whom sustained VT occurred 5 weeks or later after acute myocardial infarction had their clinical arrhythmia initiated at electrophysiologic study.[10] Other investigators have shown that sustained monomorphic VT that occurs 3 to 14 days after myocardial infarction can be reproducibly initiated at electrophysiologic study. Marchlinski et al.[15] induced the clinical sustained VT in 15 of 20 (75 percent) of such patients and DiMarco and colleagues[16] initiated sustained VT in 16 of 20 (80 percent) patients. As stated earlier in this chapter, nearly 95 percent of

patients with sustained monomorphic VT that occurs months after myocardial infarction can have their arrhythmia reproducibly initiated at electrophysiologic study.[1] Although most electrophysiologists accept reentry as the cause of VT in the majority of patients in whom sustained VT can be initiated by programmed electrical stimulation, triggered activity often cannot be excluded.[17]

The QRS morphology during VT can either be right bundle branch block, left bundle branch block, or both in a patient in whom the interventricular septum is part of the tachycardia circuit. The morphology of VT will reflect the site of origin for the arrhythmia. For example, tachycardia originating in the posterior wall of the left ventricle near the

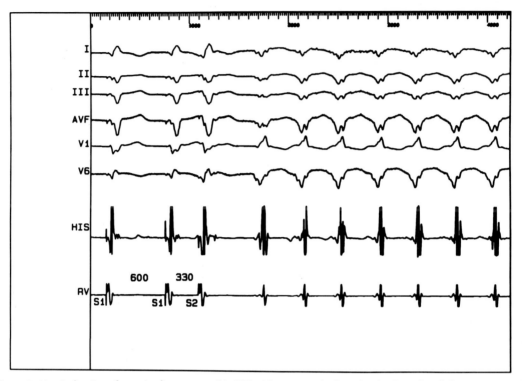

**Figure 9-11**    Induction of sustained monomorphic VT with one ventricular stimulus introduced during ventricular pacing. Pacing at the right ventricular apex at cycle length 600 ms and introduction of a premature ventricular complex with an $S_1S_2$ interval of 330 ms initiates sustained monomorphic VT of a right bundle branch block superior or northwest axis morphology.

interventricular septum that occurs after an inferior wall myocardial infarction commonly has a right bundle branch block, superior axis morphology. Often initiation of this arrhythmia is easier when pacing is performed from the right ventricular outflow tract compared with the right ventricular apex.[6] Initiation from the right ventricular outflow tract might be easier because the pacing catheter is presumably closer to the reentrant circuit in this situation.

### Therapy

#### Sustained Ventricular Tachycardia Occurring within 48 h of Acute Myocardial Infarction

Myocardial ischemia commonly initiates ventricular tachyarrhythmias, usually polymorphic VT or ventricular fibrillation (see Chap. 15). Few data are available concerning the appropriate therapy for patients who have their first episode of sustained monomorphic VT during the first 48 h of an acute myocardial infarction. In a study reported by Eldar et al.,[18] 28 of 4339 patients (0.6 percent) had sustained VT documented within the first 48 h of an acute myocardial infarction. However, one-half of these patients had polymorphic VT and therefore the actual incidence of sustained monomorphic VT was 0.3 percent in this series, illustrating the rarity of this event. There was no difference in 1-year mortality in patients discharged from the hospital who had sustained VT compared with those who did not.[18] However, a substantial number of patients were given antiarrhythmic drug therapy, and it is still unclear whether these patients require long-term treatment. Our current approach is to perform electro-

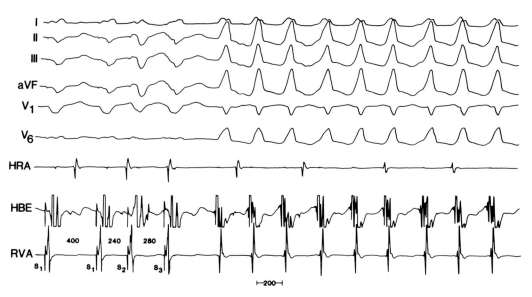

*Figure 9-12*   Initiation of sustained monomorphic VT with double extrastimuli during ventricular pacing. At a pacing cycle length of 400 ms, one ventricular extrastimulus did not induce tachycardia, but an $S_1S_2$ of 240 ms and $S_2S_3$ of 280 ms initiated sustained left bundle branch block normal axis VT. Note the lack of 1:1 ventriculoatrial conduction on the high atrial (HRA) electrogram during sustained wide QRS complex tachycardia.

physiologic studies in these individuals prior to hospital discharge. If sustained monomorphic VT is initiated using a standard pacing protocol without the addition of isoproterenol, these individuals are treated in a similar manner as patients who present with chronic coronary artery disease and sustained VT. Patients in whom tachycardia is not induced are not given any specific antiarrhythmic drug therapy but are treated as needed with anti-ischemic therapy and angiotensin converting enzyme inhibitors. We emphasize that insufficient data are available to identify which, if any, of these patients with sustained monomorphic VT occurring during the first 48 h of an acute myocardial infarction require specific antiarrhythmic treatment, and we present our method as merely one potential approach to these individuals.

*Sustained Monomorphic Ventricular Tachycardia Occurring 3 to 60 Days after Acute Myocardial Infarction*

Patients in whom sustained monomorphic VT occurs between 3 and 60 days after myocardial infarction typically have had a substantial myocardial infarction with a residual left ventricular ejection fraction of approximately 30 percent, and their original myocardial infarction was typically accompanied by complications.[15,16] Marchlinski et al.[15] retrospectively analyzed 40 patients who had sustained VT a mean of 20 days after myocardial infarction. One-, two-, and three-vessel coronary artery disease occurred in 26 percent, 44 percent, and 30 percent, respectively. The rate of VT was >220/min, 180 to 220/min, and <180/min in 33 percent, 38 percent, and 30 percent of patients, respectively. In 16 of 40 patients, sustained VT degenerated into ventricular fibrillation. Overall, 83 percent of patients had sustained VT initiated at electrophysiologic study and, like patients who have sustained monomorphic VT with chronic coronary artery disease[19] one or more sustained monomorphic VTs with a different QRS morphology than had been noted clinically were often induced. In this[15] series of patients, the outcome with serial drug testing as well as surgery was not very good, and several patients died suddenly during follow-up. In a more

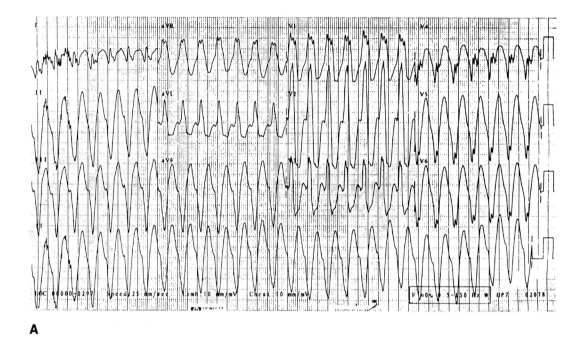

**A**

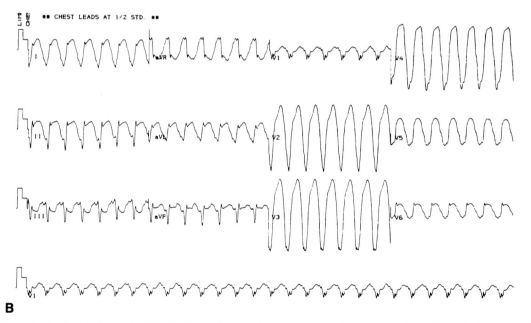

**B**

*Figure 9-13*  Serial electrophysiologic-electropharmacologic testing. *A.* Spontaneous hemodynamically stable VT with right bundle branch block morphology. *B.* At control electrophysiologic study sustained monomorphic left bundle branch block VT was initiated.

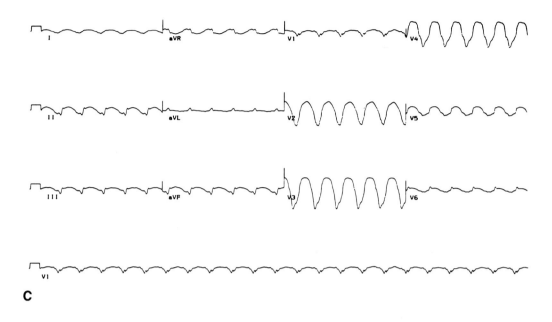

**C**

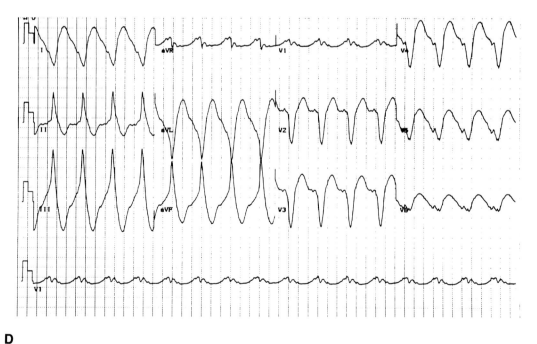

**D**

*Figure* 9-13 (*Continued*) *C.* Left bundle branch block sustained VT initiated during quinidine therapy with a morphology similar to but not the same as that noted at control electrophysiology study. *D.* Hemodynamically stable sustained right bundle branch block VT during amiodarone therapy.

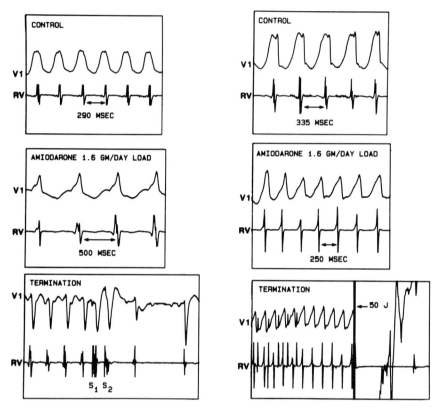

**Figure 9-14**   Effects of amiodarone treatment on two patients with inducible sustained VT at electrophysiologic study. (See text for details.)

but accelerates it to a cycle length of 270 ms, which is recognized by the device as an arrhythmia that will require more aggressive treatment and, as noted in the bottom panel, a 20-J shock is given that restores sinus rhythm. The use of these devices is covered in more detail in Chap. 21.

## Cardiomyopathy

Various forms of cardiomyopathy can be associated with sustained monomorphic VT. Bundle branch QRS morphology during tachycardia depends on the origin of the arrhythmia. A tachycardia focus in the free wall of the left and right ventricle will result in a right and left bundle branch block QRS morphology, respectively. When the origin is in the interventricu-

lar septum, QRS morphology can be either right or left bundle branch block. Many diseases may cause a cardiomyopathy, but in our experience idiopathic dilated cardiomyopathy is most frequently associated with sustained VT. Most patients with dilated cardiomyopathy can have their ventricular tachycardia initiated at electrophysiologic testing, although less frequently than with coronary artery disease.[4] Two specific entities that will be discussed separately are (1) arrhythmogenic right ventricular dysplasia with left bundle branch block sustained ventricular tachycardia and (2) bundle branch reentrant VT, which commonly but not exclusively occurs with markedly dilated cardiomyopathy.[38] Patients who have hypertrophic cardiomyopathy often have sustained polymorphic VT initiated at electrophysiologic testing

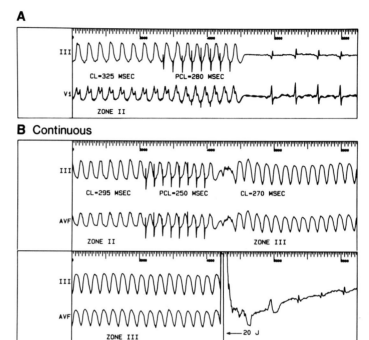

**A**

**B Continuous**

*Figure 9-15* Treatment of sustained VT by an implanted cardioverter defibrillator with antitachycardia pacing functions. (See text for details.) CL = cycle length of VT; PCL = pacing cycle length. Zone II and zone III are programmed rate zones, each of which has specific therapeutic modalities programmed to terminate the VT. In this device, zone III automatically requires high-energy defibrillation.

rather than sustained monomorphic ventricular tachycardia[39] (see Chap. 8).

### Therapy

Patients with sustained VT and dilated cardiomyopathy require therapy to prevent recurrences of the arrhythmia. If electrophysiologic testing initiates sustained VT, serial electrophysiologic-electropharmacologic testing can be performed. However, there is growing concern about the uncertainty of progression of this disease process, and we currently consider an implantable cardioverter defibrillator as early therapy in these patients. Pharmacologic treatment may be an important adjunct to decrease the frequency of tachycardia episodes and to slow the rate of tachycardia if it occurs. In the latter situation, better hemodynamic stability will be achieved during tachy-

cardia, and if an implantable device is chosen that is capable of antitachycardia pacing, the slower tachycardia rate will often increase the chance for successful pacing conversion to sinus rhythm.[40] Surgery is less likely to be successful because of the diffuse nature of this process, and it is usually not considered as prime therapy for these individuals.

### Bundle Branch Reentrant Ventricular Tachycardia

In most patients with VT, the presumed reentrant circuit is difficult to identify and most likely represents intramyocardial reentry. A specific type of VT exists that incorporates the right and left bundle branches in the tachycardia circuit and is termed bundle branch reentry.[38,41] Patients with bundle branch reentrant VT typically have substantial cardiac enlargement, a history of congestive heart failure, and either idiopathic dilated cardiomyopathy or coronary artery disease.[38] His-Purkinje dysfunction is usually present and manifested by a prolonged HV interval during supraventricular rhythm and nonspecific interventricular conduction delay, often with a pattern of the left bundle branch block type. Left bundle branch block morphology during tachycardia is most commonly observed, although macroreentrant VT can also have right bundle branch block morphology.[38]

Initiation of bundle branch reentrant VT in the clinical electrophysiology laboratory is demonstrated in Fig. 9-16 with a schematic representation in Fig. 9-17. In this patient two ventricular extrastimuli were necessary to initiate tachycardia. In Fig. 9-16, panel A, note that the $S_1S_2$ interval is 250 ms, which is kept constant in panels B and C. After the first premature complex $(S_2)$, a retrograde $H_2$ is present

with an $S_2H_2$ interval of 230 ms. Retrograde activation of the His bundle is presumably due to retrograde block in the right bundle branch with transseptal conduction and activation of the His bundle over the left bundle branch (Fig. 9-17, panel A). The $S_2S_3$ interval is 340 ms and yields an $S_3H_3$ interval of 180 ms without initiation of tachycardia. In Fig. 9-16, panel B, the $S_2S_3$ interval is shortened to 320 ms, and this results in an increased conduction delay from $S_3$ to $H_3$, which is now 200 ms. This is most likely due to slowing of conduction in the left bundle branch, ventricular myocardium, or both (Fig. 9-17, panel B). Bundle branch reentrant VT is finally initiated in Fig. 9-16, panel C when the $S_2S_3$ interval is shortened to 300 ms with a corresponding increase in $S_3H_3$ interval to 220 ms and completion of the reentrant circuit. Figure 9-17, panel C, depicts even more conduction delay than is noted in panel B, which allows enough time for the distal right bundle

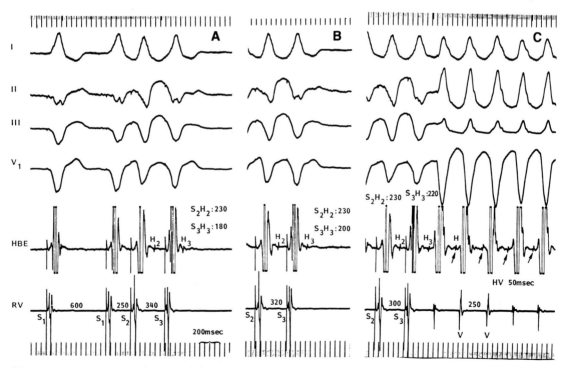

*Figure 9-16*    Initiation of sustained bundle branch reentrant VT. Arrows in panel C point to His bundle depolarizations. (See text for details.) *(From Lloyd et al.[41] Reproduced by permission from the American Heart Journal.)*

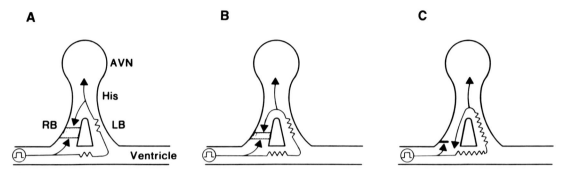

***Figure* 9-17**   Schematic representation of initiation of bundle branch reentrant VT. (See text for details.) The zigzag portion of the conduction line represents slowed conduction.

branch to recover from refractoriness and allow reexcitation of this area with completion of the reentrant circuit. The bundle branch macroreentrant circuit in this patient includes anterograde conduction over the right bundle branch, transseptal conduction, and retrograde conduction over the left bundle branch. Thus, the QRS morphology is left bundle branch block and will resemble a typical left bundle branch block morphology (Chap. 13). In this type of tachycardia the His bundle actively participates in the reentrant circuit. In contrast, other forms of VT may demonstrate retrograde His bundle depolarization, but His bundle conduction is not needed for maintenance of tachycardia (Fig. 9-4).

One should remember that there are many types of tachycardia other than bundle branch reentry that can have a left bundle branch block morphology (Table 9-1). Etiologies can include various forms of VT, SVT with bundle branch block or aberrancy, or preexcited tachycardia with anterograde conduction over an accessory pathway. Differentiation of these forms of tachycardia is critically important to the appropriate management of the patient, and in many if not most instances will require electrophysiologic study. In general, if the 12-lead ECG is identical during tachycardia and sinus rhythm, the mechanism is usually supraventricular. When the QRS complex resembles "typical" left bundle branch block morphology (Chap. 13), conduction usually proceeds over the right bundle branch to activate the ventricles; differential diagnosis includes bundle branch reen-

trant VT, SVT with left bundle branch block or aberrancy, and atriofascicular and nodofascicular reentry utilizing accessory pathways (see Chap. 7) (Fig. 9-18). The more "atypical" the left bundle branch block morphology, the more likely it is that VT is the mechanism, excluding various forms of preexcited tachycardias (Fig. 9-19). The electrophysiologic differentiation of the various forms of tachycardia noted in Table 9-1 is complex and beyond the scope of this discussion. However, several examples of left bundle branch block morphology tachycardia are illustrated in Figs. 9-20 to 9-23. Right ventricular outflow tract left bundle branch block VT is shown in Fig. 9-23 and endocardial catheter ablation of this

**Table 9-1   *Left Bundle Branch Block Tachycardia: Differential Diagnosis***

| Ventricular Tachycardia | Supraventricular Tachycardia |
| --- | --- |
| Coronary artery disease | SVT with aberrancy |
| | SVT with BBB |
| Arrhythmogenic RV dysplasia | Preexcited tachycardia |
| | Antidromic RT |
| RV cardiomyopathy | Atriofascicular RT |
| Bundle branch reentry | Nodoventricular RT |
| RV outflow tract | Nodofascicular RT |
| After TOF repair | Bystander participation |

*Abbreviations:* TOF = tetralogy of Fallot; SVT = supraventricular tachycardia; RV = right ventricle; RT = reentrant tachycardia; BBB = bundle branch block.

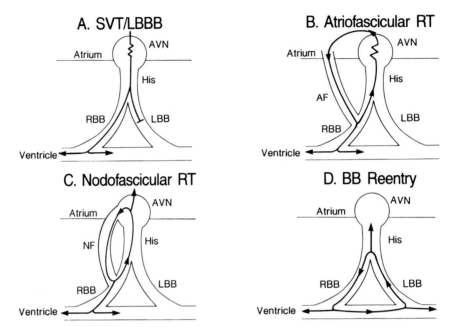

*Figure 9-18*   "Typical" left bundle branch block tachycardia mechanisms. As noted in the text, activation of the ventricles over the right bundle branch tends to give an ECG pattern of a typical left bundle branch block morphology. *A.* Any supraventricular tachycardia (SVT) with left bundle branch block aberrancy is one mechanism. *B.* Atriofascicular reciprocating tachycardia utilizes an accessory atrioventricular tract that connects the right atrium with the right bundle and subsequent conduction to the ventricle over the right bundle with retrograde conduction to the His bundle and AV node and then back to the right atrium. *C.* Nodofascicular reciprocating tachycardia in which the reentrant circuit utilizes a nodofascicular tract originating from the AV node and entering into the right bundle for anterograde conduction and retrograde conduction over the His bundle and through the AV node. This is clinically rare compared with atriofascicular reciprocating tachycardia. *D.* Bundle branch reentry with anterograde conduction over the right bundle branch and retrograde conduction over the left bundle branch can give a typical left bundle branch block morphology even though this is a form of VT. Abbreviations: AVN = atrioventricular node; AF = atriofascicular; NF = nodofascicular; LBB = left bundle branch; RBB = right bundle branch; RT = reentrant tachycardia.

tachycardia in Fig. 9-24; this will be discussed later in this chapter.

### Therapy

Antiarrhythmic drugs can be used to treat patients who have bundle branch reentrant VT, and serial electrophysiologic-electropharmacologic testing can be employed to test efficacy of therapy in these patients. More recently, endocardial catheter ablation techniques have been used to cure bundle branch reentrant VT. Several authors have demonstrated that ablation of the right bundle branch will

prevent both initiation of VT at electrophysiologic study and clinical recurrences of this arrhythmia.[42,43]

### *Arrhythmogenic Right Ventricular Dysplasia*

Arrhythmogenic right ventricular dysplasia (ARVD) is a myocardial disorder associated with left bundle branch block sustained monomorphic VT in association with a diffusely diseased right ventricle.[44] The musculature of the right ventricle is sparse and replaced by fibrous tissue and fatty infiltration. Uhl's anomaly differs from ARVD in that the former is often associated with congestive heart failure, whereas

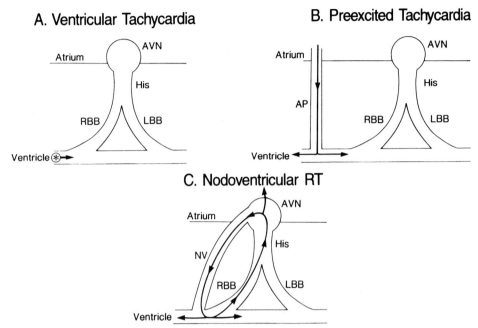

*Figure 9-19*   "Atypical" left bundle branch block mechanisms. *A*. Any VT originating in the right ventricular free wall or in some cases from the right ventricular septum can give a left bundle branch block morphology pattern, but it is usually atypical in form. *B*. Many forms of preexcited tachycardia that utilize a right free wall accessory pathway connecting to the right ventricle can yield an atypical left bundle branch block morphology. These include any atrial tachycardia with conduction over the accessory pathway as well as antidromic reciprocating tachycardia in which the accessory pathway is used for anterograde conduction and the normal ventriculoatrial conduction system for retrograde conduction, AV nodal reentry with anterograde conduction as a bystander over a right free wall pathway, and nodoventricular reciprocating tachycardia with an accessory pathway originating in the AV node and entering into the right ventricle *(C)*.

patients with ARVD usually present with symptoms of VT.[44] Nava et al.[45] reviewed information from family members of cases of juvenile death with demonstrated right ventricular dysplasia. These authors noted a familial occurrence of right ventricular dysplasia and suggested the possibility of a genetic origin for this disease in at least some patients.

Of particular importance is a history of exercise-related VT. In one study, 10 of 11 patients who died suddenly did so during exertion.[45] Further, Lascault et al.[46] noted a 36 percent occurrence of exercise triggering of VT, and Lemery et al.[47] reported that 8 of 11 (73 percent) patients had exercise-related VT. Most patients with ARVD have their arrhythmias prior to the fourth decade of life. Diagnosis should be suspected in any patient who

has no symptoms of cardiac dysfunction but presents with left bundle branch block tachycardia or with symptoms suggestive of tachycardia. Importantly, ARVD should be suspected in patients with multiple left bundle branch block tachycardia morphologies. During the workup of these individuals, signs of right ventricular disease will become apparent with noninvasive testing using techniques such as two-dimensional echocardiography, magnetic resonance imaging or nuclear imaging, or right ventricular angiography.[44,47,48] An important observation is T-wave inversion, often in ECG leads $V_1$ to $V_4$, or at least in several of these leads during sinus rhythm. In fact, repolarization abnormalities occurred in 19 of 22 patients with ARVD in the series published by Marcus et al.[44] At electrophysiologic testing, left

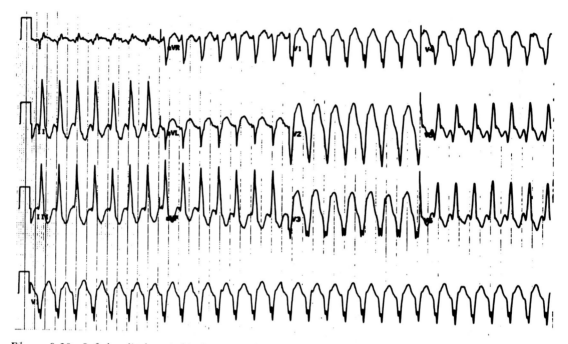

**Figure 9-20** Left bundle branch block sustained VT in a patient with coronary artery disease and previous myocardial infarction. Note the prolonged time from onset of the QRS complex to its nadir in ECG leads $V_1$ and $V_2$. This is consistent with VT.

bundle branch block tachycardia is initiated in the majority of patients.[44,47–49]

### Therapy

Therapy for patients with ARVD has included antiarrhythmic drugs, surgery, and endocardial catheter ablation,[44,46–51] and some patients may receive an implantable cardioverter defibrillator. Antiarrhythmic drugs appear to be effective in controlling VT in these patients.[46–48] Success has been achieved with several types of antiarrhythmic drugs, but Wichter et al.[48] demonstrated particular effectiveness with sotalol therapy. Surgery is reserved for patients who do not respond to antiarrhythmic drug therapy. Although ventriculotomy was initially proposed as a surgical method for patients with ARVD, more recently excellent results have been reported using disarticulation of the right ventricle.[49,50] Very preliminary results suggest the possibility of success with

endocardial catheter ablation, but too few data have been reported to judge the success of this modality.[51]

## Sustained Monomorphic Ventricular Tachycardia in Patients without Structural Heart Disease

### Right Bundle Branch Block/Left Axis Morphology

Many authors have presented data on patients with no demonstrable heart disease who have sustained monomorphic VT with right bundle branch block, left axis deviation morphology (Fig. 9-25; Table 9-2)[9,52–60] Very infrequently patients can have right bundle branch block, right axis deviation morphology during VT,[54,55,57] with electrophysiologic characteristics and responsiveness to verapamil therapy indistin-

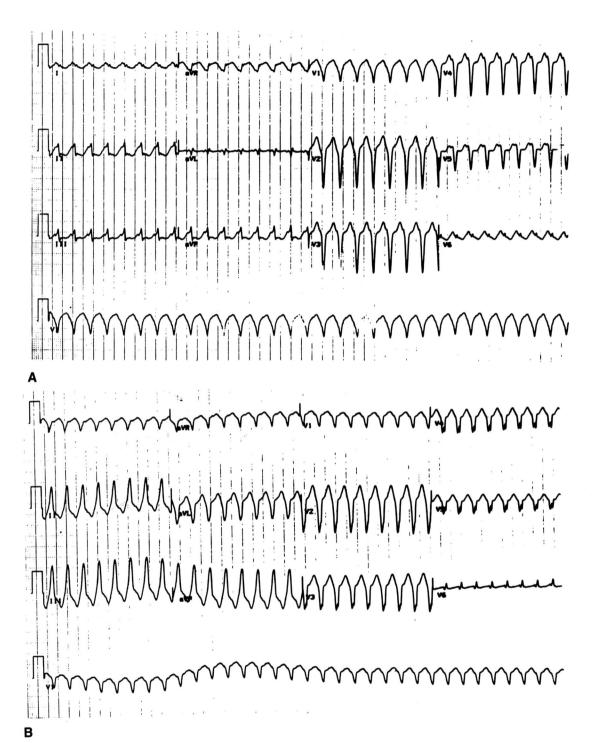

**A**

**B**

*Figure 9-21* Sustained left bundle branch block VT with two distinct morphologies (*A* and *B*). These tachycardias were initiated at electrophysiologic study in a young woman with a normal echocardiogram but in whom myocardial biopsy demonstrated thick endocardial fibrosis. Thus, this patient had some form of idiopathic cardiomyopathy. Note that the QRS duration is not very pronounced in either tachycardia.

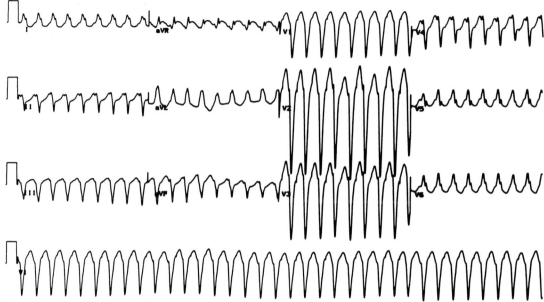

***Figure* 9-22**  AV nodal (AVN) reentrant tachycardia with left bundle branch block aberrancy initiated at electrophysiologic study. Note the rapid downstroke of the S wave in $V_1$ and $V_2$, with minimal duration of the r wave. This patient has "typical" left bundle branch block morphology during tachycardia, consistent with a supraventricular origin but not exclusive of some types of VT.

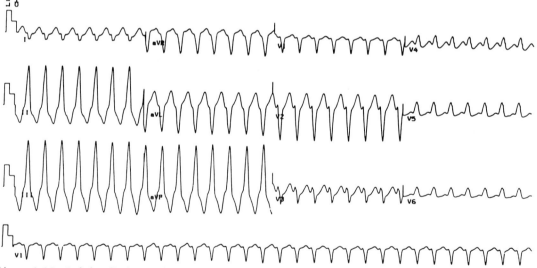

***Figure* 9-23**  Left bundle branch block morphology during VT that occurred in the right ventricular outflow tract in a patient with normal ventricular function. The QRS complexes are relatively narrow and not too dissimilar from "typical" left bundle branch block morphology. Patients with structurally normal ventricles who have right ventricular outflow tract tachycardia can have a left bundle branch block morphology that may mimic the typical form of left bundle branch block even though conduction to the ventricles does not proceed exclusively over the right bundle branch. *(From Prystowsky EN, Noble RJ: Electrophysiologic studies: Who to refer. Heart Dis Stroke 1:188, 1992. Reproduced by permission.)*

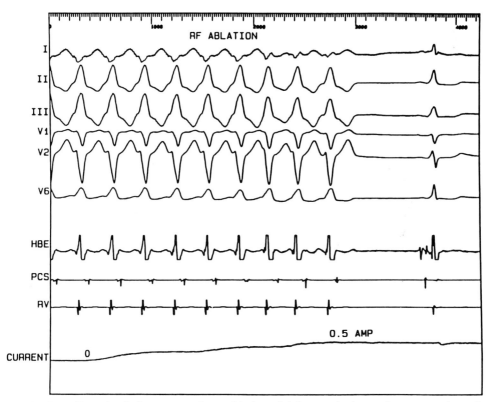

*Figure 9-24*   Recording of radiofrequency catheter ablation of right ventricular outflow tract tachycardia in the patient shown in Fig. 9-23. After less than 3 s of onset of radiofrequency energy, the tachycardia terminates and is no longer inducible. The last sinus QRS complex in this tracing shows minimal preexcitation. This patient had a very poorly functioning accessory pathway that could not be involved in any tachycardia; therefore ablation of the accessory pathway was not undertaken. *(From Prystowsky EN, Noble RJ: Electrophysiologic studies: Who to refer. Heart Dis Stroke 1:188, 1992. Reproduced by permission.)*

guishable from individuals with right bundle branch block, left axis deviation VT. Some investigators have observed inferior and/or inferolateral T-wave inversions after the termination of tachycardia[52,55] and others have reported T-wave inversions in ECG leads II, III, and aVF as well as in the lateral precordial leads during sinus rhythm.[56,60] However, these ECG findings in sinus rhythm have not been present in the majority of patients with this form of VT (Fig. 9-26). As noted in Table 9-2, patients are typically young and most are men, and symptoms during tachycardia are usually palpitations although occasionally syncope has been reported. Sudden death is rare in these patients.

The mechanism of tachycardia is unclear, but almost all patients can have their arrhythmia initiated at electrophysiologic study (Table 9-2), suggesting either a reentrant mechanism or possibly triggered activity. The method of tachycardia induction is variable and, although many patients have their arrhythmia initiated during rapid atrial or ventricular pacing, it is common for VT to be initiated with premature atrial or ventricular stimuli. It is difficult to define a mechanism of tachycardia based solely on its characteristics of induction at electrophysiologic study, yet, accepting these limitations, reentry appears to be present in most patients. Almost universal to this syndrome is the responsiveness of VT to

*Table 9-2   Right Bundle Branch Block/Left Axis Sustained VT in Patients without Overt Heart Disease*

| Author | Patients | Gender | Mean Age, years | Exercise-Provoked | PES Induction | Mean VTCL, ms | Therapy (IV) Effective Verapamil | Beta Blockers |
|---|---|---|---|---|---|---|---|---|
| Belhassen[52] | 3 | 2M; 1F | 20 | — | 2/3 | 392 | 3/3T | — |
| German[53] | 10 | 6M; 4F | 21[a] | — | 10 | — | 5/5T | — |
| Ohe[54] | 16 | 10M; 6F | 31 | — | 16 | 314 | 13/14T | — |
| Kasanuki[55] | 13 | 13M | 26 | — | 12/13 | 377 | 12T; 1SL | — |
| Lin[56] | 4 | 2M; 2F | 27 | 0/4 | 4 | 353 | 3T; 1SL | 0/4T; 1/4SL |
| Sung[9] | 6 | 3M; 3F | 30 | 4/6 | 6 | 423 | 6/6 SUPP | 6/6SL |
| Sethi[57] | 3 | 3M | 28 | 0/3 | 3 | 327 | 3/3T | — |
| Zipes[58] | 3 | 2M; 1F | 18 | 1/2 | 3 | 355 | — | — |
| Page[59] | 2 | 1M; 1F | 25 | 0/1 | 2 | 328 | — | — |
| Klein[60] | 4 | 3M; 1F | 27 | 1/4 | 1/2 | 353 | 3/3 | — |

[a]Age at onset of VT.

*Abbreviations:* M = male; F = female; PES = programmed electrical stimulation; VTCL = ventricular tachycardia cycle length; IV = intravenous; T = terminate; SL = slow rate; SUPP = suppress induction at PES.

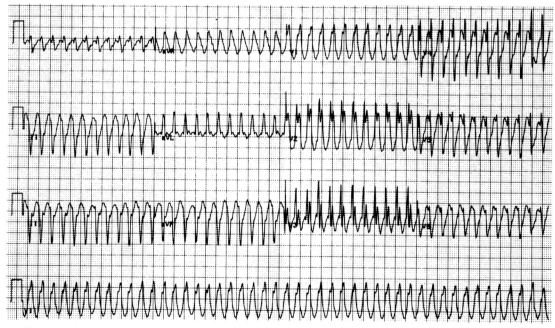

*Figure 9-25*  Sustained right bundle branch block, left axis deviation VT that occurred in a patient with no obvious structural heart disease. Isoproterenol infusion was necessary to help facilitate initiation of tachycardia with programmed ventricular stimulation at electrophysiologic study in this patient.

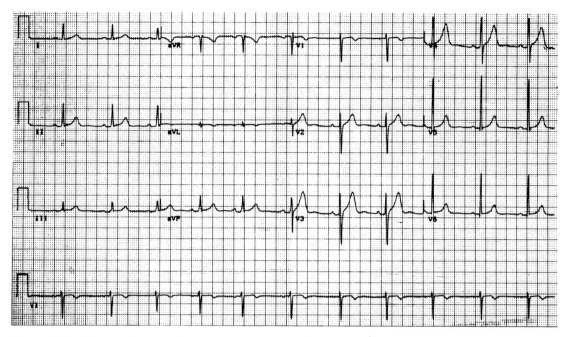

*Figure 9-26*   Electrocardiogram taken during sinus rhythm in the patient with ventricular tachycardia shown in Fig. 9-25. Note the lack of T-wave inversions in the inferior as well as anterior and anterolateral leads.

intravenous verapamil treatment (Table 9-2; Fig. 9-27). Almost all patients will have their tachycardia terminated when given 5 to 10 mg of intravenous verapamil, and slowing usually precedes termination. Beta-adrenergic blockers have been tested in only a few patients reported in the literature and appear to be relatively ineffective. Of note, VT is very uncommonly initiated during exercise testing, and most patients do not give a history of onset of tachycardia during exertion. Even so, in our experience some of these patients require intravenous isoproterenol in addition to programmed ventricular stimulation for induction of tachycardia at electrophysiologic testing.

### Therapy

We prefer oral verapamil therapy if drugs are needed to treat these patients. We usually begin with 240 to 360 mg/day, using sustained released

formulations. Nonpharmacologic treatment with endocardial radiofrequency catheter ablation should be considered for these patients. Page et al.[59] reported the successful elimination of this tachycardia in two patients using radiofrequency catheter ablation (Fig. 9-28). The site of origin of tachycardia was at the inferior septal region at the base of the posterior papillary muscle of the left ventricle. Introduction of radiofrequency energy terminated tachycardia and no recurrences have occurred in these two patients. Thus, we think that endocardial catheter ablation is an acceptable first-line treatment for these individuals.

### Left Bundle Branch Block/Right or Normal Axis

Unlike the syndrome of VT with right bundle branch block and left axis morphology that occurs in patients without structural heart disease, patients with normal ventricular function and left bundle branch block

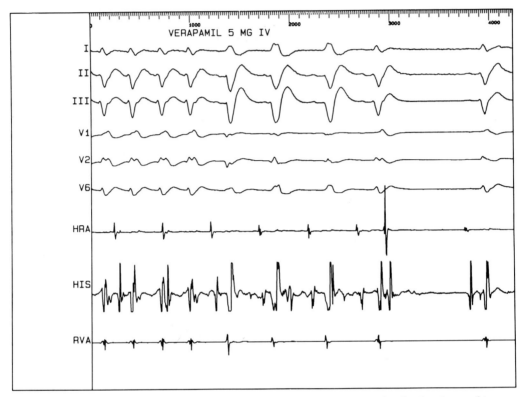

*Figure 9-27*   Termination of right bundle branch block, left axis deviation VT shortly after 5 mg of intravenous verapamil was given. (See text for details.)

VT form a more diverse group.[61-65] Most patients have an inferior or right axis during tachycardia, but a normal axis has also been described. The location of tachycardia is usually in the right ventricular outflow tract but, again, anatomic variations exist. The arrhythmia is usually inducible during programmed electrical stimulation at electrophysiologic study, but some patients require isoproterenol to initiate tachycardia with or without programmed electrical stimulation. In our experience and in most of the published patient series, sudden death rarely occurs in these patients.

Noninvasive evaluation and cardiac catheterization in these patients reveals no evidence of structural heart disease. The ECG during sinus rhythm is usually normal, which distinguishes these individuals from those with arrhythmogenic right ventricular dysplasia. During VT, the QRS duration is usually <140 ms and a more "typical" form of left bundle branch block pattern may occur in some patients (Fig. 9-23). When this happens, it is not surprising that the arrhythmia is often misdiagnosed as SVT with aberrancy. This underscores the importance of performing electrophysiologic studies in patients with wide complex QRS tachycardias.

*Therapy*

Several drugs have proved effective in the treatment of these patients. Success of certain agents may depend on the clinical presentation; for example, exercise-related arrhythmias more commonly will

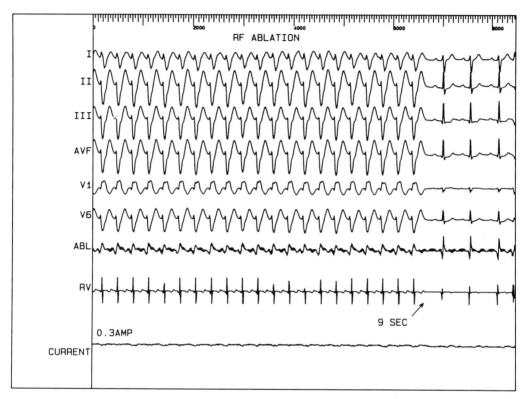

***Figure 9-28***   Endocardial radiofrequency (RF) catheter ablation of right bundle branch block, left axis deviation sustained VT. After 9 s of 0.3 A of energy delivered to the site of tachycardia in the left ventricle, the arrhythmia terminates and sinus rhythm is restored, as noted by the last three QRS complexes in this tracing. This patient has had no further episodes of tachycardia and tachycardia could no longer be initiated at electrophysiologic study. (*From Page et al.*[59] *Reproduced by permission from PACE.*)

respond to beta blockers or verapamil therapy. Endocardial catheter ablation frequently eliminates VT in these patients[66,67] (Fig. 9-24). Note that in Fig. 9-24 ventricular tachycardia terminates during upward titration of radiofrequency energy as 0.5 A is achieved. It is tempting to prescribe radiofrequency catheter ablation as first-line therapy in these relatively young individuals who otherwise will have to undergo years of antiarrhythmic drug therapy. Although we frequently utilize this technique to cure our patients with this form of VT, it must be remembered that few data are available regarding subsequent long-term complications of this technique in these patients.

## Commentary

It is clear that sustained monomorphic VT is not a monolithic diagnosis. The origin of tachycardia varies widely, depending in large measure on the underlying ventricular pathology. However, obvious structural heart disease is not present in all patients. The consequences of tachycardia depend on several factors, most importantly the degree of myocardial dysfunction, peripheral vascular adaptation, and tachycardia rate. Several types of therapy are available and need to be tailored for each patient.

# References

1. Prystowsky EN: Electrophysiologic-electropharma-cologic testing in patients with ventricular arrhythmias. *PACE* 11:225, 1988.
2. Akhtar M et al: Wide QRS complex tachycardia: Reappraisal of a common clinical problem. *Ann Intern Med* 109:905, 1988.
3. Hayes JJ et al: Narrow QRS ventricular tachycardia. *Ann Intern Med* 114:460, 1991.
4. Prystowsky EN et al: Induction of ventricular tachycardia during programmed electrical stimulation: Analysis of pacing methods. *Circulation* 73(II):32, 1986.
5. Buxton AE et al: Role of triple extrastimuli during electrophysiologic study in patients with documented sustained ventricular tachyarrhythmias. *Circulation* 69:532, 1984.
6. Klein LS et al: Electrophysiologic and anatomic characteristics of ventricular tachycardia induced at the right ventricular outflow tract but not at the apex. *Am Heart J* 122:464, 1991.
7. Reddy CP, Gettes LS: Use of isoproterenol as an aid to electric induction of chronic recurrent ventricular tachycardia. *Am J Cardiol* 44:705, 1979.
8. Freedman RA et al: Facilitation of ventricular tachyarrhythmia induction by isoproterenol. *Am J Cardiol* 54:765, 1984.
9. Sung RJ et al: Effects of β-adrenergic blockade on verapamil-responsive and verapamil-irresponsive sustained ventricular tachycardias. *J Clin Invest* 81:688, 1988.
10. Wellens HJJ et al: Observations on mechanisms of ventricular tachycardia in man. *Circulation* 54:237, 1976.
11. Josephson ME et al: Recurrent sustained ventricular tachycardia: 1. Mechanisms. *Circulation* 57:431, 1978.
12. El-Sherif N et al: Canine ventricular arrhythmias in the late myocardial infarction period: 8. Epicardial mapping of reentrant circuits. *Circ Res* 49:255, 1981.
13. Wit AL et al: Electrophysiologic mapping to determine the mechanism of experimental ventricular tachycardia initiated by premature impulses: Experimental approach and initial results demonstrating reentrant excitation. *Am J Cardiol* 49:166, 1982.
14. Dillon SM et al: Influence of anisotropic tissue structure on reentrant circuits in the epicardial border zone of subacute canine infarcts. *Circ Res* 63:182, 1988.
15. Marchlinski FE et al: Sustained ventricular tachyarrhythmias during the early post-infarction period: Electrophysiologic findings and prognosis for survival. *J Am Coll Cardiol* 2:240, 1983.
16. DiMarco JP et al: Sustained ventricular tachyarrhythmias within 2 months of acute myocardial infarction: Results of medical and surgical therapy in patients resuscitated from the initial episode. *J Am Coll Cardiol* 6:759, 1985.
17. Rosen MR, Reder RF: Does triggered activity have a role in the genesis of cardiac arrhythmias? *Ann Intern Med* 94:794, 1981.
18. Eldar M et al: Primary ventricular tachycardia in acute myocardial infarction: Clinical characteristics and mortality. *Ann Intern Med* 117:31, 1992.
19. Miller JM et al: Morphologically distinct sustained ventricular tachycardias in coronary artery disease: Significance and surgical results. *J Am Coll Cardiol* 4:1073, 1984.
20. Fisher JD et al: Cardiac pacing and pacemakers: II. Serial electrophysiologic-pharmacologic testing for control of recurrent tachyarrhythmias. *Am Heart J* 93:658, 1977.
21. Horowitz LH et al: Recurrent sustained ventricular tachycardia: 3. Role of the electrophysiologic study in selection of antiarrhythmic regimens. *Circulation* 58:986, 1978.
22. Mason JW, Winkle RA: Electrode-catheter arrhythmia induction in the selection and assessment of antiarrhythmic drug therapy for recurrent ventricular tachycardia. *Circulation* 58:971, 1978.
23. Waller TJ et al: Reduction in sudden death and total mortality by antiarrhythmic therapy evaluated by electrophysiologic drug testing: Criteria of efficacy in patients with sustained ventricular tachyarrhythmia. *J Am Coll Cardiol* 10:83, 1987.
24. Horowitz LN et al: Ventricular resection guided by epicardial and endocardial mapping for treatment of recurrent sustained ventricular tachycardia. *N Engl J Med* 302:589, 1980.
25. Frank R et al: Long-term experience of fulguration for the treatment of ventricular tachycardia (abstract). *PACE* 11:912, 1988.
26. Evans GT et al: The Percutaneous Cardiac Mapping

and Ablation Registry: Final summary of results. *PACE* 11:1621, 1988.

27. Borggrefe M et al: Catheter ablation of ventricular tachycardia using defibrillator pulses: Electrophysiological findings and long-term results. *Eur Heart J* 10:591, 1989.

28. Fitzgerald DM et al: Electrogram patterns predicting successful catheter ablation of ventricular tachycardia. *Circulation* 77:806, 1988.

29. Morady F et al: Concealed entrainment as a guide for catheter ablation of ventricular tachycardia in patients with prior myocardial infarction. *J Am Coll Cardiol* 17:678, 1991.

30. Mason JW et al: A comparison of electrophysiologic testing with Halter Monitoring to predict autiarrhythmic drug efficacy for ventricular tachyarrhythmias. *N Engl J Med* 392:445, 1993.

31. Prystowsky EN et al: Amiodarone: Interrelationship of dose and time of electrophysiologic and antiarrhythmic effects. *Circulation* 70(II):II-3, 1984.

32. Prystowsky EN et al: Factors associated with ventricular tachycardia suppression at electrophysiologic study during drug therapy. *Circulation* 70:II-56, 1984.

33. Spielman SR et al: Predictors of the success or failure of medical therapy in patients with chronic recurrent sustained ventricular tachycardia: A discriminant analysis. *J Am Coll Cardiol* 1:401, 1983.

34. Swerdlow CD et al: Clinical factors predicting successful electrophysiologic-pharmacologic study in patients with ventricular tachycardia. *J Am Coll Cardiol* 1:409, 1983.

35. Schoenfeld MH et al: Determinants of the outcome of electrophysiologic study in patients with ventricular tachyarrhythmias. *J Am Coll Cardiol* 6:298, 1985.

36. Naccarelli GV et al: Amiodarone: Risk factors for recurrence of symptomatic ventricular tachycardia identified at electrophysiologic study. *J Am Coll Cardiol.* 6:814, 1985.

37. Klein LS et al: Prospective evaluation of a discriminant function for prediction of recurrent symptomatic ventricular tachycardia or ventricular fibrillation in coronary artery disease patients receiving amiodarone and having inducible ventricular tachycardia at electrophysiologic study. *Am J Cardiol* 61:1024, 1988.

38. Caceres J et al: Sustained bundle branch reentry as a mechanism of clinical tachycardia. *Circulation* 79:256, 1989.

39. Fananapazir L et al: Prognostic determinants in hypertropic cardiomyopathy: Prospect evaluation of a therapeutic strategy based on clinical, Holter, hemodynamic, and electrophysiological findings. *Circulation* 86:730, 1992.

40. Naccarelli GV et al: Influence of tachycardia cycle length and antiarrhythmic drugs on pacing termination and acceleration of ventricular tachycardia. *Am Heart J* 105:1, 1983.

41. Lloyd EA et al: Sustained ventricular tachycardia due to bundle branch reentry. *Am Heart J* 104:1095, 1982.

42. Touboul P et al: Bundle branch reentrant tachycardia treated by electrical ablation of the right bundle branch. *J Am Coll Cardiol* 7:1404, 1986.

43. Tchou P et al: Transcatheter electrical ablation of right bundle branch: A method of treating macroreentrant ventricular tachycardia attributed to bundle branch reentry. *Circulation* 78:246, 1988.

44. Marcus F et al: Right ventricular dysplasia: A report of 24 adult cases. *Circulation* 65:384, 1982.

45. Nava A et al: Familial occurrence of right ventricular dysplasia: A study involving nine families. *J Am Coll Cardiol* 12:1222, 1988.

46. Lascault G et al: Ventricular tachycardia features in right ventricular dysplasia (RVD). *Circulation* 78:II-300, 1988.

47. Lemery R et al: Nonischemic sustained ventricular tachycardia: Clinical outcome in 12 patients with arrhythmogenic right ventricular dysplasia. *J Am Coll Cardiol* 14:96, 1989.

48. Wichter T et al: Efficacy of antiarrhythmic drugs in patients with arrhythmogenic right ventricular disease: Results in patients with inducible and noninducible ventricular tachycardia. *Circulation* 86:29, 1992.

49. Nimkhedkar K et al: Surgery for ventricular tachycardia associated with right ventricular dysplasia: Disarticulation of right ventricle in 9 of 10 cases. *J Am Coll Cardiol* 19:1079, 1992.

50. Guiraudon GM et al: Total disconnection of the right ventricular free wall: Surgical treatment of right ventricular tachycardia associated with right ventricular dysplasia. *Circulation* 67:463, 1983.

51. Leclercq JF et al: Results of electrical fulguration in arrhythmogenic right ventricular disease. *Am J Cardiol* 62:220, 1988.

52. Belhassen B et al: Idiopathic recurrent sustained

ventricular tachycardia responsive to verapamil: An ECG-electrophysiologic entity. *Am Heart J* 108:1034, 1984.

53. German LD et al: Ventricular tachycardia induced by atrial stimulation in patients without symptomatic cardiac disease. *Am J Cardiol* 52:1202, 1983.

54. Ohe T et al: Idiopathic sustained left ventricular tachycardia: Clinical and electrophysiologic characteristics. *Circulation* 77:560, 1988.

55. Kasanuki H et al: Idiopathic sustained ventricular tachycardia responsive to verapamil: Clinical electrocardiographic and electrophysiologic considerations. *Japan Circ J* 50:109, 1986.

56. Lin FC et al: Idiopathic paroxysmal ventricular tachycardia with a QRS pattern of right bundle branch block and left axis deviation: A unique clinical entity with specific properties. *Am J Cardiol* 52:95, 1983.

57. Sethi KK et al: Verapamil in idiopathic ventricular tachycardia of right bundle branch morphology: Observations during electrophysiologic and exercise testing. *PACE* 9:8, 1986.

58. Zipes DP et al: Atrial induction of ventricular tachycardia: Reentry versus triggered automaticity. *Am J Cardiol* 44:1, 1979.

59. Page RL et al: Radiofrequency catheter ablation of idiopathic recurrent ventricular tachycardia with right bundle branch block, left axis morphology. *PACE* 16:327, 1993.

60. Klein GJ et al: Recurrent ventricular tachycardia responsive to verapamil. *PACE* 7:938, 1984.

61. Buxton AE et al: Right ventricular tachycardia: Clinical and electrophysiologic characteristics. *Circulation* 68:917, 1983.

62. Pietras RJ et al: Chronic recurrent right ventricular tachycardia in patients without ischemic heart disease: Clinical, hemodynamic, and angiographic findings. *Am Heart J* 105:357, 1083.

63. Vetter VL et al: Idiopathic recurrent sustained ventricular tachycardia in children and adolescents. *Am J Cardiol* 47:315, 1981.

64. Wu D et al: Exercise-triggered paroxysmal ventricular tachycardia. *Ann Intern Med* 95:410, 1981.

65. Lerman BB et al: Adenosine-sensitive ventricular tachycardia: Evidence suggesting cyclic AMP-mediated triggered activity. *Circulation* 74:270, 1986.

66. Morady F et al: Long-term results of catheter ablation of idiopathic right ventricular tachycardia. *Circulation* 82:2093, 1990.

67. Klein LS et al: Radiofrequency catheter ablation of ventricular tachycardia in patients without structural heart disease. *Circulation* 85:1666, 1992.

# Chapter 10

# *Bradycardia: Causes of Pauses*

Bradycardia or transient asystole can result from a wide variety of disorders of the cardiac conduction system interacting with neural and humoral influences. Abnormalities may be discovered as incidental electrocardiographic (ECG) findings during screening or monitoring for other medical problems. Alternatively, they may be discovered after investigation for symptoms suggesting transient or persistent bradycardia. There is little difficulty when the abnormality is persistent and clearly related to presenting symptoms. Transient abnormalities, on the other hand, may be very difficult to demonstrate. A sudden and transient loss of consciousness or a feeling of impending unconsciousness (presyncope) are the major symptoms suggesting transient asystole. However, a wide variety of symptoms, possibly reflecting chronic or intermittent hypoperfusion of the central nervous system or other organ systems, may be caused by intermittent or chronic bradycardia, including dizzy or lightheaded spells, fatigue, cognitive disturbances, dyspnea, and so on. The diagnostic difficulties are compounded in the elderly, who frequently have mutliple chronic medical disorders and conduction system abnormalities that may be difficult to relate to symptoms.

## Diagnostic

The asymptomatic patient with unexpected ECG abnormalities is discussed in more detail in Chap. 11. In general, intervention is rarely indicated, although a reasonable search for silent cardiac disease and follow-up are usually warranted. The assessment of the patient presenting with symptoms suggesting bradycardia or conduction disorders can be guided by three general principles. First, a broad approach is necessary to understand the problem in its clinical context. Symptoms suggesting bradycardia are frequently nonspecific, with a wide variety of potential causes. A "reflex" focus on the cardiac conduction system without a thorough general assessment is inappropriate. Second, it must be appreciated that transient symptoms are an exercise in monitoring. The goal is to acquire ECG information, and direct correlation between these two variables—symptoms and data—is the desired end point. If a clear precipitating factor is described, it is important to try to reproduce the situation while the patient is monitored. Third, it may be impossible to obtain ECG data while the symptom is occurring. In such cases, inferences can be made using the presence of abnormalities detected even though they have not been associated with symptoms. For example, the detection of transient third-degree atrioventricular (AV) block strongly suggests that the patient's presenting light-headed spell was related to AV block, even though the episode recorded was not associated with symptoms. These inferences sometimes require considerable clinical judgment. For example, is the patient with a slightly prolonged sinus node recovery time blacking out from sinus arrest even though nothing has ever been documented? In general, the more striking the abnormality, the more confident the clinician is in making the inference that it is causing the symptoms.

### History and Physical Examination

A careful history taken from the patient or a good witness often provides a focus for subsequent investigations. The witness is especially important when the symptoms relate to presyncope or syncope, where the patient may be unable to provide important details. Transient bradycardia may cause a plethora of symptoms that are often nonspecific; therefore an open mind is required. The physical examination should be broad-based and should include attempts to reproduce symptoms if they are related to a specific physical activity. Careful carotid sinus massage during ECG monitoring may be part of the physical examination.

### Exercise Testing

Exercise testing is of value in assessing not only for coronary heart disease but also sinus node and AV node function. This may reveal chronotropic incompetence of the sinus node associated with sinus node dysfunction or it may reveal AV block or bundle branch block when the heart rate increases. It is particularly useful when the patient's symptoms are related to exercise.

### Ambulatory Monitoring

Ambulatory monitoring is the cornerstone for the investigation of suspected bradycardia as it provides the opportunity to monitor the patient during everyday activities and record the ECG during the occurrence of symptoms. The continuous 24-h Holter record is most frequently used and most useful when symptoms occur daily or almost daily. For patients with less frequent symptoms, event recorders are more useful. These can be applied by the patient and activated when symptoms appear, or they can record in a continuous-loop mode and provide ECG data around the time the device is activated by the patient. The latter devices require some competence and commitment from the patient, but they can be used by a close companion or relative if the patient is incapable of learning how to use them.

The ambulatory ECG may reveal abnormalities even if symptoms do not occur. Relating asymptomatic abnormalities to symptoms is not direct evidence but inference and must be done with caution. It must also be appreciated that healthy patients may have bradycardia of 40/min or less during sleep, Wenckebach AV block, sinus arrhythmia with 2-s pauses or greater, and sinus pacemaker shifts with slight changes in P-wave morphology and heart rate.

### Electrophysiologic Testing (See Chap. 17)

Electrophysiologic testing is considered when the patient's symptoms suggest a bradycardia (or other arrhythmia) but persistent attempts to obtain ECG documentation while symptoms occur have failed. The most optimistic expectation is to provoke a bradycardia that convincingly reproduces the patient's spontaneous symptoms. A more realistic aim is to uncover abnormalities of sinus node function or atrioventricular conduction that support bradycardia as an etiology but do not provide proof. This can provide a rationale for a therapeutic "trial" of permanent pacing if problematic symptoms persist without a firm diagnosis.[1] It must also be appreciated that a normal electrophysiology study does not rule out transient bradycardia.[2] Details of electrophysiologic testing are given in Chap. 17, with key points briefly reviewed below.

#### Conduction Intervals[3]

Intracardiac recordings can subdivide ECG intervals more specifically into intracardiac components. The PA interval is measured from the earliest onset of the P wave on the ECG to the first rapid deflection of the atrial electrogram at the His bundle recording. It reflects right intraatrial conduction (normal limits, 9 to $\leq$60 ms) and has minimal clinical use.

The atrio-His (AH) interval is measured from the rapid deflection on the atrial electrogram at the His bundle site to the onset of the His deflection. This approximates AV node conduction time (normal limits, 60 to 120 ms). The His–ventricle (HV) interval is measured from the onset of the His deflection to earliest recorded ventricular activation. This approximates His–Purkinje conduction time (normal limits, 35 to 55 ms). Incremental atrial pacing (pacing the atrium progressively faster) tests the conduction system in a dynamic way and assesses "margin of safety" for conduction. Incremental atrial pacing generally results in progressive prolongation of the AH interval followed by block proximal to the recorded His deflection (i.e., Wenckebach cycle length). The Wenckebach cycle length is usually between 350 and 500 ms and is very dependent on autonomic tone. The HV interval typically is constant, and block below the His at a cycle length > 350 ms is usually considered abnormal.

### Sinus Node Recovery Time

Spontaneous termination of a naturally occurring rapid heart rhythm results in a pause of variable duration due to overdrive suppression of the sinus node and subsidiary pacemakers. In the "tachycardia-bradycardia" syndrome, this pause is prolonged and results in symptoms. The sinus node recovery test is an attempt to measure this phenomenon in a systematic and reproducible way in the laboratory.[4-6]

Although intuitively the SNRT is a measure of overdrive suppression of automaticity, the test is also affected by conduction and refractoriness around the sinus node, autonomic tone, and the site of pacing. Overall, it can be said to reflect "sinus node function." The test is considered to be very specific for sinus node dysfunction (95 to 100 percent), although it can be normal in the presence of known sinus node dysfunction (sensitivity, 60 to 80 percent).[2]

### Sinoatrial Conduction Time (SACT)

Sinus node dysfunction may result from block of the sinus impulse to the atrium (sinus node exit block). This provided the rationale for measurement of the sinoatrial conduction by the indirect method.[7] Premature atrial stimuli are introduced throughout the sinus cycle and SACT is calculated from extrastimuli that result in reset of the sinus node. An alternative

method can also be used.[8] The validity of both methods depends on several assumptons that are debatable and subject to substantial error.[5] Direct methods to record SACT are also available.[9,10]

### Sinus Node Refractory Period

Introduction of premature atrial complexes during atrial pacing can result in interpolation. The sinus node effective refractory period (SNERP) is the longest $A_1A_2$ interval at which interpolation occurs[11] (Fig. 17-11). Abnormal SNERP values seem to correlate well with sinus node dysfunction.[11]

### Autonomic Testing

Sinus node dysfunction may be caused by intrinsic sinus node abnormality, abnormal autonomic innervation or reflex responsiveness, or combinations of the above. There have been two general approaches to assessing the contribution of autonomic abnormalities.

First, attempts have been made to assess responsiveness to standard agonists and antagonists.[4,5] Normalization of inappropriate bradycardia with atropine or an exaggerated response to atropine indicates that parasympathetic stimulation is contributing to sinus bradycardia, whereas a blunted response implicates intrinsic sinus node dysfunction. An exaggerated response to edrophonium suggests inappropriate responsiveness to normal parasympathetic stimulation. Similarly, a blunted response to isoproterenol suggests poor responsiveness to normal sympathetic stimulation. The intrinsic heart rate (IHR) is perhaps the most standardized test and is obtained by "total" autonomic blockade at rest with atropine (0.04 mg/kg) and propranolol (0.2 mg/kg).[12] The IHR adjusted for age has been determined as IHR = 118.1 − (0.57 × age) with 95 percent confidence limits of 14 percent for age 45 and under and 18 percent for age greater than 45. An abnormal IHR suggests intrinsic abnormality of the sinus node in the absence of autonomic influence. However, demonstration of intrinsic sinus node dysfunction does not equate with need for permanent pacemaker therapy, a clinical decision based on multiple factors.

The second approach is the use of physiologic or pharmacologic interventions aimed at assessing reflex responsiveness using a provocation known to initiate a series of changes. The response to standing involves decrease in vagal tone and increase in sympathetic tone. Carotid sinus massage (following precautions to evaluate carotid stenosis) assesses baroceptor response, with the end result being an increase in parasympathetic tone. A prolonged pause (greater than a 2.5 to 3.0-s) suggests an exaggerated response to normal parasympathetic drive or excessive parasympathetic drive.[13–15] The Valsalva maneuver assesses responsiveness to sympathetic stimulation (strain phase) and parasympathetic stimulation (poststrain phase). Passive tilt testing has become clinically useful, although the physiologic responses to this maneuver are incompletely understood.[16–19] Basically, passive tilt results in loss of parasympathetic tone and increase in sympathetic tone with pooling of blood volume in the lower torso. With continuation of tilt, normal subjects will maintain a relatively constant heart rate and blood pressure, while some will experience slowing of heart rate and loss of blood pressure (vasodepressor response). (See Chap. 18.)

# Classification of Causes of Bradycardia

Bradycardia may be classified broadly as spurious bradycardia, sinus node dysfunction, atrioventricular conduction disturbance, or neurally mediated ("reflex") bradycardia.

## Spurious Bradycardia

Spurious bradycardia refers to bradycardia or pauses mimicking sinus node or atrioventricular conduction disease clinically or electrocardiographically. A common example results from closely coupled ventricular ectopic activity not perceived as a pulse (pulse deficit). Closely coupled atrial premature depolarizations may not conduct to the ventricles (blocked atrial extrasys-

tole) and may mimic sinus arrest (Fig. 10-1). Technical difficulties with recording system or leads may result in brief "flat lines" which can mimic asystole or ventricular extrasystoles may have very low voltage in a monitored lead and simulate a pause. Rarely, His bundle extrasystoles may fail to conduct to either atria or ventricles but can still result in episodic AV block due to concealed conduction into the AV node.[20,21] (See Chap. 2.) This may be suspected clinically if manifest junctional extrasystoles are observed in conjunction with episodic AV block, but the diagnosis must be confirmed by His bundle recording.

## Sinus Node Dysfunction

The term *sick sinus syndrome*[4,5] refers to a constellation of ECG findings attributed to dysfunction of the sinus node and subsidiary pacemakers that results in symptomatic bradycardia or asystole. The term *sinus node dysfunction* refers to similar ECG abnormalities without symptoms. Several manifestations of sick sinus syndrome are recognized, although there may be considerable overlap in individuals.

### Sinus Bradycardia

By definition, a sinus rate less than 60/min is considered bradycardia. However, only "inappropriate" sinus bradycardia is considered to be sinus node dysfunction. A resting sinus rate of 40/min may be physiologic during sleep or in the well-conditioned athlete but is inappropriate in an individual during moderate activity. "Chronotropic incompetence" refers to a failure to increase sinus rate under appropriate physiologic circumstances as judged by comparison with normal age- and sex-matched individuals performing the same activity.

### Sinus Arrest

The term *sinus arrest* refers to an asystolic pause arbitrarily defined here as greater than 2s (Fig. 10-2). It may be terminated by a sinus cycle or a subsidiary pacemaker, frequently junctional. These pauses occur sporadically and the length of the pause is not an exact multiple of the P-P interval, suggesting that

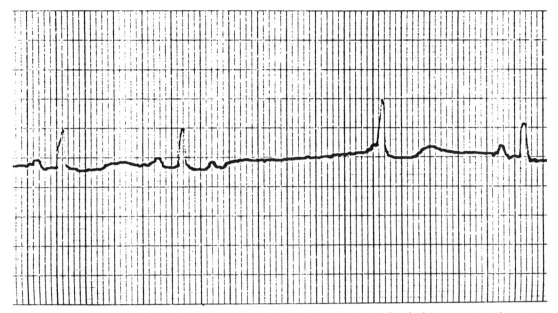

*Figure 10-1*   Pause due to blocked atrial extrasystole. In this example, the blocked P wave is evident in the deformed ST segment of the cycle prior to the pause.

the mechanism is a failure of automaticity of the sinus node. Since the actual mechanism (that is, failure of automaticity or conduction) usually cannot be determined from the ECG, some prefer the term sinus *pause* instead of *arrest*.

### Sinus Node Exit Block

Analysis of the sinus pause may suggest normal automaticity with intermittent exit block of the impulse from the sinus node to the surrounding atrium. A sudden pause where the length of the pause is an exact multiple of the P-P interval suggests

Mobitz type II sinus node exit block (Fig. 10-3). A progressive shortening of the P-P interval prior to the nonconducted P wave suggests Mobitz type I sinus node exit block. A definitive distinction between sinus arrest and exit block frequently cannot be made without recording the sinus node electrogram during the event. Practically, the distinction is not important.

### Bradycardia-Tachycardia Syndrome

As the name suggests, patients with this variant have episodes of both bradycardia and supraventricu-

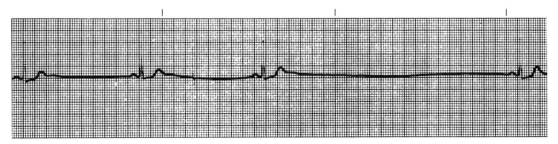

*Figure 10-2*   Pause due to sinus arrest.

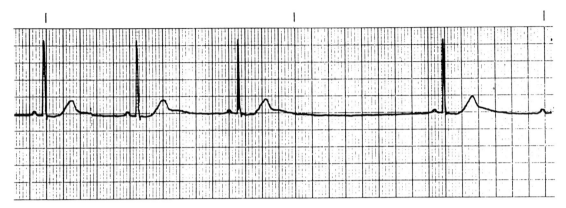

*Figure 10-3*   Pause compatible with sinus node exit block. The calculation is hampered by some sinus arrhythmia, but the asystolic pause closely approximates two sinus cycles, and other records in this patient showed this to be consistent.

lar tachycardia (Fig. 10-4). The most common tachycardia is atrial fibrillation. Pauses may be observed after abrupt cessation of tachycardia, presumably due to overdrive suppression of the sinus node and subsidiary pacemakers. Additionally, tachycardia may be initiated in the course of bradycardia or sinus arrest, possibly due to increased dispersion of refractoriness or early after depolarizations occurring with slower heart rates.

### Atrial Fibrillation

Lone atrial fibrillation, inability to cardiovert atrial fibrillation, and atrial fibrillation with a relatively slow ventricular response in the absence of drugs are frequently included in the spectrum of sick sinus syndrome in spite of the fact that the sinus node may not be the most prominent focus of abnormality with these arrhythmias.

### Pacemaker Shift

Slight changes in P-wave morphology with associated change in heart rate are frequently observed in asymptomatic individuals and reflect a shift in location of the dominant pacemaker in the sinus node region or possibly outside the sinus node (Fig. 10-5). This should be considered within the realm

of "normal" unless the alternate pacemaker site is associated with marked bradycardia.

### Symptoms

The cardinal symptoms of sick sinus syndrome are presyncope and syncope. However, cognitive dysfunction, fatigue, and other symptoms potentially related to hypoperfusion of organ systems can result. Finally, symptoms may be related to peripheral embolism associated with sick sinus syndrome.

### Incidence and Etiology [22]

Sick sinus syndrome is observed predominantly in the middle-aged and elderly. It accounts for 50 percent or more of pacemaker implants in North America. Sick sinus syndrome is associated with coronary heart disease, hypertension, and virtually any condition affecting the heart. It is frequently observed in the absence of any clinically identifiable heart disease. Acute myocardial infarction may be associated with sinus node dysfunction that may or may not resolve with time. Finally, it is important to remember that many drugs may cause sinus node dysfunction, usually aggravating preexisting sinus node dysfunction. These drugs include digitalis glycosides, beta blockers, calcium antagonists, anti-

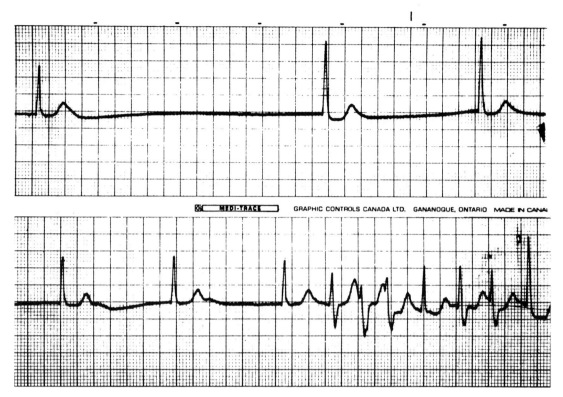

*Figure 10-4*   Tachycardia-bradycardia syndrome. This is a continuous record illustrating sinus arrest with a slow junctional escape rhythm followed by a paroxysm of atrial fibrillation. The reverse sequence was also seen in this patient, namely prolonged bradycardia after cessation of atrial fibrillation. Note the occurrence of bundle branch block during atrial fibrillation.

arrhythmics (especially amiodarone), sympatholytic antihypertensives such as alpha methyldopa and reserpine, and miscellaneous agents such as lithium carbonate and cimetidine.

### Therapy

Initial therapy is based on ECG abnormalities demonstrated or strongly suspected to be related to symptoms. Permanent pacing is the mainstay of therapy for sick sinus syndrome. Occasionally, supression of tachycardia with antiarrhythmic drugs in patients with tachycardia-bradycardia syndrome will also prevent bradycardia, although this strategy should be carried out with caution. Uncontrolled data support the use of atrial pacing to decrease the incidence of

atrial fibrillation and systemic embolization.[4] Atrial demand (AAI) pacing is adequate when there is no evidence of significant AV conduction disease (normal QRS, normal PR interval, atrial pacing with one-to-one conduction attainable at 120/min or greater). Although AV conduction disease often coexists with sinus node dysfunction, the rate of progression to complete AV block is low, 1 to 2 percent per year. Ventricular demand (VVI) pacing is indicated with chronic atrial fibrillation in patients with normal chronotropic response and infrequent bradycardia. Rate response should be considered as an additional feature in the presence of chronotropic incompetence. The high incidence of systemic embolization in sick sinus syndrome is probably related to atrial fibrillation. This provides a strong rationale for

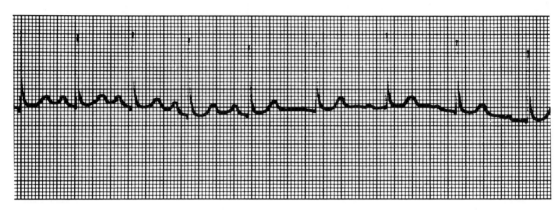

***Figure 10-5***   Sinus pacemaker shift. In this asymptomatic individual, there is a sudden slight prolongation of the cycle length accompanied by a change in the P-wave morphology, probably caused by a shift in the site of the primary pacemaker.

anticoagulation in addition to pacing in patients with demonstrated atrial fibrillation.

### Atrioventricular Block

Atrioventricular conduction disturbance can be associated with any process affecting the heart; consequently a detailed list of etiologies is not useful. Congenital AV block and AV block associated with surgery for congenital heart disease predominate in the young. Idiopathic fibrosis and calcification of the AV conduction system is predominantly a disease of the elderly. Ischemic and valvular heart diseases are also relatively common causes of conduction disease. Medications in therapeutic doses can result in clinical AV conduction disease, usually in patients with preexisting latent dysfunction. Digitalis glycosides, calcium channel blockers, and beta blockers affect the AV node, while the class 1 and 3 antiarrhythmic drugs can exacerbate block in the His-Purkinje system.

The ECG has traditionally provided the starting point for classifying patterns of AV block.[23,24] The ECG can usually provide accurate inferences on the site of AV block, namely the AV node, His bundle, or bundle branches. Recording of the intracardiac intervals during AV block is sometimes required to pinpoint the site of block in ambiguous cases (Fig.

10-6). Both the type of AV block and the site of block influence prognosis and the decision to pace. Block in the AV node is usually associated with a more stable junctional escape rate than block in the His bundle or bundle branches, which is associated with unstable escape pacemakers and unpredictable asystole.

### First-Degree AV Block

First-degree AV block, defined as PR interval greater than 0.2 s, can result from intraatrial delay, AV nodal delay, infranodal delay (His bundle or bundle branches), or combinations of the above. The AV node conduction time is the predominant influence on the PR interval and is almost invariably prolonged in first-degree AV block. Of node, no P waves are actually "blocked" and some prefer the term first-degree *conduction delay*.

### Second-Degree AV Block

Second-degree AV block is usually classified as Mobitz type I or II. The descriptor "high-grade" or "advanced" AV block is added with Mobitz type II block and a slow ventricular response (greater than 2 to 1 AV conduction ratio).

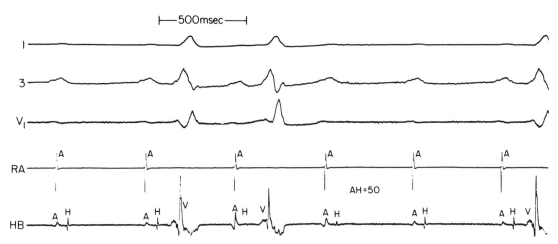

*Figure 10-6*   Atrioventricular block due to failure of conduction in the His-fascicular system. The surface ECG shows intraventricular conduction delay and a constant PR interval of conducted QRS complexes. The nonconducted P wave is associated with a normal A and H deflection without a subsequent QRS, denoting block below the level of the recorded His potential. 1, 3, V₁ = surface ECG leads, HB = His bundle electrogram, RA = high right atrial electrogram.

Mobitz type I AV block (Wenckebach block) requires prolongation of the PR interval prior to the blocked cycle and shortening of the PR interval in the first conducted cycle after block.[25] In "classic" Wenckebach periodicity, the R-R interval shortens prior to the blocked cycle, since maximum prolongation of the PR interval occurs between the first and second cycle of the sequence. The site of block in the majority of Mobitz type I sequences is the AV node (Fig. 10-7). Mobitz type I block is considered physiologic, with high vagal tone seen in athletes and during sleep.

Mobitz type II block requires a constant PR interval prior to and following the blocked cycle. The site of block is generally the His–Purkinje system. It is impossible to designate fixed 2 to 1 AV block as Mobitz type I or II since this requires seeing at least two conducted cycles prior to block. Maneuvers to alter sinus rate will usually clarify this. Atropine will increase sinus rate and improve AV nodal conduction but will worsen His-Purkinje block. Vagal maneuvers will decrease sinus rate and prolong AV nodal conduction and tend to improve block at or below the His. Appearance or worsening of block during exercise strongly suggests block below the

AV node. Enhanced sympathetic and decreased parasympathetic tone occur with exercise and facilitate AV node conduction.

Site of block in the AV node is favored by a Mobitz type I pattern, a narrow QRS, and a prolonged PR interval of conducted beats. Site of block in the His bundle or bundle branches is favored by a Mobitz type II pattern, bundle branch block or intraventricular conduction delay, and a relatively normal PR interval of conducted cycles.

### Third-Degree AV Block

Third-degree or complete AV block results in atrioventricular dissociation. The site of block can usually be inferred by the characteristics of the escape pacemaker emerging distal to the block site. Block in the AV node is characterized by the following:

- A narrow QRS escape pacemaker (i.e., supraventricular morphology)
- Escape rate of 40 or greater
- Acceleration of the escape rate after atropine and exercise.

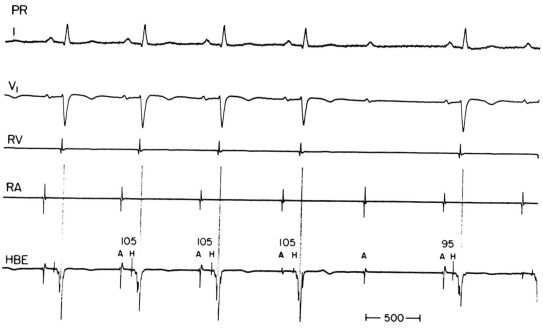

*Figure 10-7*   Apparent Mobitz 2 block due to failure of conduction over the AV node. The surface QRS complex and PR interval are normal and there is no prolongation of the PR interval prior to the nonconducted P wave. The nonconducted P wave is associated with an atrial deflection without a subsequent His deflection denoting block in the AV node. The PR and AH intervals following the block cycle are slightly shorter than the preceding conducted ones, providing a clue that the level of block is in the AV node. There is also an increase in the P-P interval prior to the blocked P wave, suggesting an increase in vagal tone as a possible mechanism for block.

Block in the His bundle or bilateral bundle branch block is characterized by the following:

- A wide QRS escape pacemaker
- Escape rate frequently of 40/min or less
- Failure to accelerate after atropine

In addition, junctional pacemakers are more stable and less prone to overdrive suppression and sudden asystole than are distal pacemakers.

### Congenital AV Block

Congenital AV block is observed in approximately 1 per 20,000 live births.[26–28] It occurs in association with overt congenital heart disease (endocardial cushion defect, corrected transposition) or without congenital heart disease. The latter has been associated with maternal lupus and other collagen disease.[29] Congenital AV block is usually at the level of the AV node and is felt to be related to a developmental failure of the atrium to contact the AV node or failure of the AV node to contact the His bundle. Pacing is usually indicated for symptoms (presyncope, syncope, poor exercise tolerance). The decision to pace asymptomatic individuals is considerably more controversial, but guidelines proposed have included resting heart rate less than 40/min with failure to increase rate substantially with exercise, occurrence of ventricular ectopy with exercise, demonstrated block below the His bundle, and prolonged junctional recovery time (corrected junctional recovery time greater than 200 ms).[25]

### Decision to Pace

The decision to pace is related to symptom status, the degree of block, and the site of block. Pacing is indicated in the symptomatic individual regardless of the site of block. In the asymptomatic individual, pacing is indicated in both second- and third-degree AV block at the level of the His bundle or bundle branches because of the potential for sudden asystole.[30] Pacing may be indicated in third-degree AV block at the AV node level for considerations discussed in congenital AV block. Electrophysiologic testing for bifascicular block with the intent of predicting symptoms is not helpful. The incidence of progression to complete heart block is low (1 to 3 percent per year) and not accurately predicted by test results.

### Role of Electrophysiologic Testing

Most decision making in patients with AV block is determined by clinical and ECG variables. Electrophysiologic testing is indicated to determine the site of block in second- or third-degree block if this is equivocal and if the information is necessary for clinical decision making. It may be useful in third-degree AV nodal block to determine the properties of the junctional escape pacemaker if the decision to pace is equivocal. Finally, it may be useful if symptoms of presyncope or syncope are suspected to be related to AV block, but clinical documentation is not available.

### Neurally Mediated Bradycardia

Both sinus arrest and AV block can occur in the absence of resting sinus or AV node dysfunction as a result of autonomic stimulation. Various syndromes have been described, including carotid sinus hypersensitivity, vasodepressor ("neurally mediated") syncope, cough syncope, swallow syncope, glossopharyngeal neuralgia syncope, micturition syncope, and defecation syncope. These entities have in common various recognized precipitating factors triggering a reflex that culminates in a vasodepressor response and/or bradycardia (cardioinhibitory) mediated at least in part by the parasympathetic nervous system. The cardioinhibitory but not the vasodepressor response is attenuated or inhibited by atropine. The most common and best-studied syndromes are the hypersensitive carotid sinus syndrome and vasodepressor (vasovagal, neurally mediated) syncope. In addition, an ill-defined syndrome of persistent, inappropriate hypervagotonia has been described, where resting abnormalities of sinus node and AV node conduction are reversed by atropine.

### Carotid Sinus Hypersensitivity[13–15]

Pressure on the right or left carotid sinus (after clinical or laboratory exclusion of carotid artery disease) produces a reflex slowing of the sinus rate and decrease in blood pressure mediated by activation of carotid baroreceptors. An "exaggerated" reflex is generally defined arbitrarily as cardiac asystole of 3 s or more or a drop in blood pressure of 30 to 50 mmHg.[31] An abnormal reflex is more frequently observed in the elderly and in association with hypertension, coronary artery disease, or in the presence of beta blockers. An abnormal response may be observed in asymptomatic individuals. The classic presentation in symptomatic patients is presyncope or syncope produced by maneuvers that stimulate the carotid baroreceptors, such as stretching the neck while shaving, reaching for a high object, or wearing a tight collar. Probably more frequently, there are no obvious precipitating factors prior to symptoms. The diagnosis of carotid sinus syndrome depends on the demonstration of the abnormal reflex with a convincing reproduction of symptoms or, more frequently, exclusion of other potential causes of the symptoms.

The carotid sinus response usually results in both a cardioinhibitory (bradycardia) component and a vasodepressor component, with the former being the most frequent and dominant. The cardioinhibitory component but not the vasodepressor component is blocked by atropine. Patients with recurrent symptoms may require permanent pacing, and atrioventricular pacing may be preferable to ventricular pacing.

Prior to institution of permanent pacing, it is useful to demonstrate that temporary pacing prevents syncope (cardioinhibitory component dominant) during carotid sinus stimulation.

*Vasodepressor (Vasovagal, Neurally Mediated) Syncope* [16–19]

The classic "faint" has long been recognized as a clinical entity. Typically, symptoms will begin in childhood or adolescence and may recur for many years. The precipitating event is often an emotional upset, physical pain, a hot, uncomfortable environment, or prolonged standing. There is frequently a prodrome of visceral symptoms such as nausea, cold sweat, or epigastric distress followed by presyncope or syncope. The episode may be attenuated or aborted by supine posture. The patient is observed to be pale, clammy, and pulseless with dilated pupils during syncope.

It is now appreciated that this classic presentation may be only the tip of the iceberg. Many patients with unexplained syncope in the absence of the typical prodrome are observed to have vasodepressor syncope when submitted to passive upright tilt and/or isoproterenol infusion (see Chap. 18). While "normals" maintain heart rate and blood pressure with this maneuver, abnormals will experience a slowing of the heart rate and hypotension accompanied by presyncope or syncope and reproduction of their unique prodrome. The cardioinhibitory but not the vasodepressor component is prevented by atropine or pacing. Initiation of the reflex is thought to occur via cardiac receptors activated by aggressive cardiac contraction in the presence of a decreased afterload. The response may be attenuated or eliminated by pretreatment with beta blockers or disopyramide, possibly related to the negative inotropic effect of both agents.

## Commentary

Clinical correlation of documented ECG abnormalities with symptoms is the crux of assessing bradycardia. Invasive electrophysiologic testing has contributed greatly to our understanding of bradycardia and remains helpful in selected individuals. Institution of therapy in asymptomatic individuals is infrequently considered. It is important to have a high index of suspicion for "neurally mediated" or "reflex" bradycardia, since pacing may not prevent associated symptoms related to vasodepression.

## References

1. Rattes MF et al: Efficacy of empirical cardiac pacing in syncope of unknown cause. *Can Med Assoc J* 140:381, 1989.
2. Fujimura O et al: The sensitivity of electrophysiological testing in patients with syncope caused by transient bradycardia. *N Engl J Med* 21:1703, 1989.
3. Josephson ME, Seides SF: Electrophysiologic investigation: General concepts, in Josephson ME, Seides SF (eds): *Clinical Cardiac Electrophysiology; Techniques and Interpretations*. Lea and Febiger, Philadelphia, 1979, pp 23–59.
4. Benditt DG et al: Sinus node dysfunction: Pathophysiology, clinical features, evaluation and treatment, in Zipes DP, Jalife J (eds): *Clinical Electrophysiology From Cell to Bedside*. Saunders, Philadelphia, 1990, pp 708–734.
5. Jordan AL, Mandel WJ: Disorders of sinus function, in Madel WJ (ed): *Cardiac Arrhythmias Their Mechanisms, Diagnosis, and Management*. Lippincott, Philadelphia, 1987, pp 321–342.
6. Benditt DG et al: Analysis of secondary pauses following termination of rapid atrial pacing in man. *Circulation* 54:436, 1976.
7. Strauss HC et al: Premature atrial stimulation as a key to the understanding of sinoatrial conduction in man. *Circulation* 47:86, 1973.
8. Narula OS et al: A new method for measurement of sinoatrial conduction time. *Circulation* 58:806, 1978.

9.  Gomes JAC et al: New application of direct sinus node recordings in man: Assessment of sinus node recovery time. *Circulation* 70:663, 1984.

10. Gomes JAC et al: The sinus node electrogram in patients with and without sick sinus syndrome: Techniques and correlation between directly measured and indirectly estimated sinoatrial conduction time. *Circulation* 66:864, 1982.

11. Kerr CR, Strauss HC: The measurement of sinus node refractoriness in man. *Circulation* 68:1231, 1983.

12. Jose AD, Gollison D: The normal range and the determinants of the intrinsic heart rate in man. *Cardiovasc Res* 4:160, 1970.

13. Sagie A et al: Carotid sinus hypersensitivity and the carotid sinus syndrome. *Prog Cardiovasc Dis* 31:379, 1989.

14. Wenger TL et al: Hypersensitive carotid sinus syndrome manifested as cough syncope. *PACE* 3:332, 1980.

15. Davies AB et al: Carotid sinus hypersensitivity in patients presenting with syncope. *Br Heart J* 42:583, 1979.

16. Waxman MB et al: Isoproterenol induction of vasodepressor-type reaction in vasodepressor-prone persons. *Am J Cardiol* 63:58, 1989.

17. Milstein S et al: Cardiac asystole: A manifestation of neurally mediated hypotension-bradycardia. *J Am Coll Cardiol* 49:1626, 1989.

18. Almquist A et al: Provocation of bradycardia and hypotension by isoproterenol and upright posture in patients with unexplained syncope. *N Engl J Med* 320:346, 1989.

19. Rea RF: Neurally mediated hypotension and bradycardia: Which nerves? How mediated? *J Am Coll Cardiol* 49:1633, 1989.

20. Langendorf R: Concealed AV conduction: the effect of blocked impulses on the formation and conduction of subsequent impulses. *Am Heart J* 35:542, 1948.

21. Anderson GJ et al: Concealed junctional bigeminy inducing pseudo 2:1 AV block. *J Electrocardiol* 14:91, 1981.

22. Kerr CR et al: Sinus node dysfunction. *Cardiol Clin* 1:187, 1983.

23. Kastor JA: Atrioventricular block (part 1). *N Engl J Med* 292:462, 1975.

24. Kastor JA: Atrioventricular block (part 2). *N Engl J Med* 292:572, 1975.

25. Narula OS: Clinical concepts of spontaneous and induced atrioventricular block, in Mandel WJ (ed): *Cardiac Arrhythmias Their Mechanisms, Diagnosis and Management.* Lippincott, Philadelphia, 1987, pp 321–342.

26. Patton JN et al: Conduction system of the heart, in Brandenburg RO, Fuster V, Giuliani ER (eds): *Cardiology: Fundamentals and Practice.* Year Book, Chicago, 1987, pp 828–850.

27. Dewey RC et al: Use of ambulatory electrocardiographic monitoring to identify high-risk patients with congenital complete heart block. *N Engl J Med* 316:835, 1987.

28. Waxman MB et al: Familial atrioventricular heart block: An autosomal dominant trait. *Circulation* 51:226, 1975.

29. Chameides L et al: Association of maternal lupus erythematosus with congenital complete heart block. *N Engl J Med* 297:1204, 1977.

30. Strasberg B et al: Natural history of chronic second-degree atrioventricular nodal block. *Circulation* 63:1043, 1981.

31. Thomas JE, Hammill SC: Syncopal disorders, in Brandenburg RO, Fuster V, Giuliani ER (eds): *Cardiology: Fundamentals and Practice.* Year Book, Chicago, 1987, pp 689–700.

# Part III
## Clinical Presentations

# Chapter 11

# Electrocardiographic Abnormalities in Asymptomatic Individuals

Physicians are frequently confronted by electrocardiographic (ECG) abnormalities that are discovered incidentally during screening or during the course of investigating an unrelated problem. These are more frequent in the elderly,[1] reflecting to some degree an increasing prevalence of subclinical heart disease. Appropriate advice to the patient requires a knowledge of the natural history of the abnormality and potential favorable effects of a contemplated intervention. An intervention in an asymptomatic individual should be undertaken only with clear information supporting a decrease in morbidity and mortality.

## Bradyarrhythmias

### Sinus Node Dysfunction

Sinus node "dysfunction" is said to be present when the electrocardiographic criteria of sick sinus syndrome (severe inappropriate bradycardia, sinus pause, chronic atrial fibrillation with a slow ventricular response, alternating tachycardia and bradycardia) are present in the absence of symptoms.[2] The diagnosis must be made with caution, since sinus bradycardia to 40/min or less and sinus pauses to 1.5 s or greater can be observed in normal individuals during sleep and at rest.[3] There are no data to support the efficacy of permanent pacing in patients with asymptomatic sinus node dysfunction.[2,4–6] Patients followed for asymptomatic sinus node dysfunction may ultimately develop symptoms requiring pacing, but mortality is dependent on the presence and severity of coexistent disease.

The decision to pace becomes more complex in the patient with sinus node dysfunction who has vague or nonspecific symptoms (fatigue, personality change, memory impairment, dizzy spells) which could potentially be due to bradycardia. The relationship of these symptoms to bradycardia may be established by ambulatory monitoring or treadmill testing, but frequently the link is difficult to clarify and the decision to pace must be guided by clinical judgment.

### Atrioventricular Block

The risk of syncope or death in patients with atrioventricular (AV) block depends both on the presence of concomitant heart disease and the site of block. In asymptomatic individuals, first-degree AV block and Mobitz type I second-degree AV block are relatively common,[7] the latter usually reflecting vagal tone. Pacing is not indicated. The situation is more complex with Mobitz type II second-degree AV block. Knowledge of the site of the block is helpful, as AV nodal block is generally benign, while block at the His–Purkinje level is more likely to progress and become symptomatic.[8] The level of block can frequently be approximated by ECG criteria, with intracardiac electrophysiologic assessment useful for equivocal cases (Chap. 10). Pacing is arguably justified in patients with proven infranodal block, but the decision in an individual is open to clinical judgment.

Complete AV block is uncommon in asymptomatic individuals,[7] and acquired AV block is almost invariably associated with symptoms. More difficult therapeutic decisions arise in the pediatric or younger patient with complete congenital AV block.[9] The level of block in these individuals in usually at the AV node, and the escape pacemaker may be stable and responsive to autonomic influences. Although many of these patients may remain asymptomatic throughout their lives, some will develop syncope and sudden death. Efforts to predict this outcome have not led to unequivocal guidelines, but several risk factors have been identified which generally indicate a more sluggish and unpredictable escape pacemaker. These include the following:

1. Mean heart rate <50/min while awake with little variability on ambulatory monitoring
2. Absence of heart rate increase during exercise
3. Associated ventricular arrhythmias
4. Exit block of the junctional escape rhythm
5. Wide QRS
6. Prolonged QT interval
7. Associated heart disease
8. Prolonged junctional recovery time at electrophysiologic testing

These observations have not been rigorously evaluated in large numbers of individuals but are supported by smaller studies and are intuitively reasonable. They may assist in the clinical decision to institute pacing until more clear-cut guidelines are available.

### Bundle Branch Block

The prevalence of bundle branch block (see Chap. 3) in asymptomatic individuals depends on the popula-

tion tested, but it is generally in the range of 0.1 to 2 percent.[7] Bundle branch block may be an isolated abnormality or may be a marker of coexistent heart disease. Mortality is related to the accompanying heart disease and is not increased in the otherwise healthy individual. A key issue is potential progression to complete heart block, and this is too infrequent and unpredictable to justify prophylactic pacing.[10,11]

Bifascicular block with or without prolongation of the PR interval would intuitively suggest more severe conduction system abnormalities than simple bundle branch block. Nonetheless, the risk of progression to complete heart block is in the range of 1 percent per year,[12] which is too low to justify pacing in the asymptomatic individual. Bifascicular block may indicate coexistent heart disease, but the increased mortality in this group is generally not related to bradycardia and there is no firm evidence that prophylactic pacing prolongs survival.[8,13,14] Electrophysiologic testing is generally not helpful in this context. A prolonged HV interval is frequently a marker of more extensive disease but does not reliably predict progression to complete heart block.[8] In summary, the finding of bundle branch block in an asymptomatic individual merits clinical assessment to uncover potential associated heart disease but not prophylactic pacing.

## Tachyarrhythmias

### Atrial Ectopy and Supraventricular Tachycardia

The prevalence of atrial extrasystoles in normal populations may be as high as 3 percent by 12-lead electrocardiography[7] and 50 percent by 24-h ambulatory monitoring.[3] Atrial ectopy may be a manifestation of occult heart disease, pulmonary embolism, or thyrotoxicosis, but the ubiquity of the finding in normals makes it very nonspecific. Treatment is not indicated. Nonsustained supraventricular tachycardia (SVT) is also relatively common in normal populations[15] and similarly has poor specificity as a marker for occult disease.

Sustained SVT other than atrial fibrillation is rarely seen in the absence of symptoms. Interestingly, some patients may have incessant SVT (Chap. 6) and be totally unaware of their rapid heartbeat. This may lead to cardiomyopathy and congestive heart failure in some individuals. The general strategy is to assess exercise tolerance and ventricular size and function. Patients with impaired ventricular function should be treated, while those with normal ventricular function may be followed carefully with serial assessment of ventricular performance.[16]

### Atrial Fibrillation

The prevalence of atrial fibrillation in asymptomatic individuals varies with the age group under study, with estimates of 0.01 to 4 percent in patients over age 60.[7,17–19] It generally occurs in the context of cardiac abnormality or other medical disease and less frequently in the absence of cardiac disease ("lone" atrial fibrillation). Two percent of a study cohort in the Framingham experience[20] developed atrial fibrillation over a follow-up of two decades, with approximately two-thirds of these occurring in the context of overt heart disease. While coexistent heart disease is the most powerful prognostic indicator, the appearance of atrial fibrillation was associated with a mortality double that of controls. An important cause of morbidity and mortality in both chronic and paroxysmal atrial fibrillation is systemic embolism and stroke,[17,20] with an incidence in the order of 5.46 per 100 patient-years of follow-up.[21] This incidence can be reduced with prophylactic anticoagulation with warfarin and possibly aspirin (see Chap. 6).

The asymptomatic patient found to have atrial fibrillation merits assessment to determine the presence and extent of coexistent cardiac and medical disease. Further management is less clear with regard to options of chronic anticoagulation or attempts to restore and maintain sinus rhythm with antiarrhythmic drugs. The inconvenience, expense, and morbidity of the latter must be weighed against the potential for systemic embolism in an individual, even though anticoagulation appears to be beneficial for groups as a whole.[18,22] There are few data supporting

maintenance of sinus rhythm with antiarrhythmic drugs to reduce the risk of systemic emboli. In general, we recommend an attempt to reduce the incidence of systemic embolism with anticoagulation. In selected individuals, antiarrhythmic drugs are given to restore sinus rhythm.

### Ventricular Ectopy and Tachycardia

Ventricular ectopy (see Chap. 8) is very common and may be found in 40 to 75 percent of normal individuals, with complex ectopy in 5 to 10 percent.[7] The only justification to treat an asymptomatic individual is to improve survival. Consequently, treatment with antiarrhythmic drugs should be preceded by a demonstration of increased mortality in the population in question and proof that treating this group reduces mortality.

In the asymptomatic individual with minimal or no cardiac abnormality, the finding of ventricular ectopy or even ventricular tachycardia (VT) carries no demonstrable increased risk of sudden death.[22,23] On the other hand, there is little doubt that frequent (>5 to 10/h) ectopy and nonsustained VT correlates with an increased risk of sudden death in patients after acute myocardial infarction,[24–28] and those with dilated cardiomyopathy,[29] and probably any cardiac abnormality associated with severe left ventricular dysfunction.[22,30] This increased risk appears to be additive to the contribution of left ventricular dysfunction.[27] This information has provided an intuitive rationale for the suppression of ectopic activity with antiarrhythmic drugs in these individuals. The difficulties with this strategy are as follows:

1. Ventricular ectopic activity lacks specificity for identifying the potential victim of sudden death. This subjects many individuals to the unnecessary cost, inconvenience, and potential hazards of antiarrhythmic therapy.[31]
2. Is is not clear whether ventricular ectopy causes sudden death or is merely a marker for the individual prone to have this complication by other mechanisms. Even if ventricular ectopy is causative, it is not certain that elimination of ectopy is an adequate end point of therapy.

3. Finally, reduction of mortality with antiarrhythmic drugs in the individual with ectopy has not been demonstrated. Indeed, therapy with mexiletine in one trial was associated with a trend toward increased mortality in the treated group.[32] Therapy with encainide and flecainide in the Cardiac Arrhythmia Suppression Trial (CAST)[33] and moricizine in CAST II[34] was associated with increased mortality compared to controls. This raises the possibility that proarrhythmia may be a dominant factor limiting the usefulness of the drugs tested to this date in this context.

There are inadequate data to make definitive recommendations regarding antiarrhythmic therapy in so called high-risk patients with ventricular ectopy. Nonetheless, it would seem that prophylactic antiarrhythmic therapy of these patients requires more specific identification of the patient at risk for sudden death, perhaps using multiple clinical and laboratory variables in addition to promising indicators provided by signal averaging techniques or programmed electrical stimulation. Finally, it must be demonstrated that antiarrhythmic therapy directed at the suppression of ectopy improves survival. If so, specific drugs and specific end points remain to be identified.

## Arrhythmias during Sleep

Sleep is associated with vagal predominance. Sinus arrhythmia is frequent; sinus bradycardia to <40/min and sinus pauses >1.75 s are not unusual in normal individuals during sleep[3] (Fig. 11-1). Similarly, atrioventricular Wenckebach is relatively common and may be considered physiologic. Ventricular arrhythmias are not a predominant feature during sleep in either normal individuals or patients with ischemic heart disease.[35]

The sleep apnea syndrome[36,37] is characterized by hypoventilation, somnolence, and cor pulmonale, with occurrence of obstructive apnea during sleep. One study showed a higher prevalence of extreme bradycardia and ventricular ectopic activity[37] during sleep, whereas another[36] found nothing to distinguish these patients from normal individuals. Nonetheless, the findings in sleep apnea syndrome have not been related to mortality and the clinical significance of observed arrhythmias has not been established.

## Ventricular Preexcitation

A short PR interval in the absence of ventricular preexcitation is of no significance in the asymptomatic individual and probably reflects part of the spectrum of normal atrioventricular nodal physiology (Chap. 7). On the other hand, the Wolff-Parkinson-White pattern may be associated with sudden death, and this is usually related to the occurrence of atrial fibrillation with a rapid ventricular response over an accessory atrioventricular pathway (the so-called Kent bundle). Patients resuscitated from ventricular fibrillation are invariably found to have inducible atrial fibrillation with a rapid ventricular response and a shortest R-R interval (SRR) between preexcited beats <250 ms.[38]

The latter finding raises the possibility of screening asymptomatic subjects by elective induction of atrial fibrillation and targeting the group at risk (SRR < 250 ms) for prophylactic therapy. There are two serious logistic difficulties to this strategy. First, the prevalence of the Wolff-Parkinson-White pattern is on the order of 0.1 to 0.3 percent of the general population, while the incidence of sudden death in asymptomatic individuals is exceedingly low, on the order of 1 per 1000 years of patient follow-up at the most pessimistic estimate.[39]

Second, the prevalence of a rapid ventricular response (SRR < 250) when atrial fibrillation is induced in the asymptomatic individual is far too high (approximately 17 percent!) to make this a specific marker for targeting interventions.[40] In other words, a high percentage of asymptomatic individuals are at theoretical risk, but the occurrence of ventricular fibrillation as the first symptom in the asymptom-

## A. 2:16 am

## B. 2:19 am

## C. 4:33 am

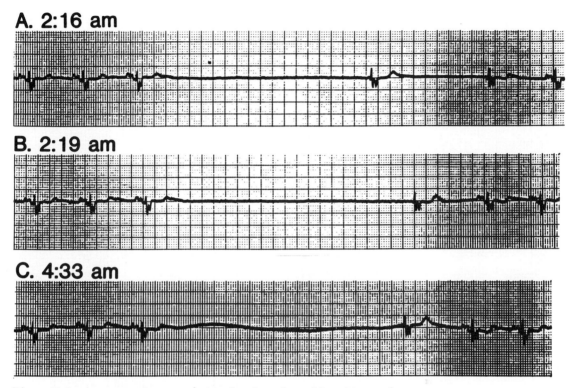

*Figure 11-1* Asymptomatic pauses during sleep in patient with no history of syncope or presyncope.

atic individual is rare and sporadic. These facts make it difficult to recommend mass screening and aggressive management of the asymptomatic individual with the Wolff-Parkinson-White pattern. Nonetheless, some individuals may wish to pursue investigation even though the risk of ventricular fibrillation is very low. An example might be the airline pilot, in whom even a remote risk of ventricular fibrillation may be unacceptable. These difficult decisions must be made on an individual basis.

Noninvasive testing may be helpful in approximating the ventricular response in the event of atrial fibrillation. The patient found to have sudden or intermittent normalization of a prominent delta wave will invariably *not* have a rapid preexcited ventricular response during atrial fibrillation. This observation may be made with multiple 12-lead ECGs, ambulatory electrocardiography, or exercise testing. It is

important not to consider apparent loss of preexcitation in patients with subtle preexcitation, since the latter may only represent a slight shift in ventricular fusion and not true block in the accessory pathway. Only loss of a prominent delta wave with concomitant prolongation of the PR interval should be considered as accessory pathway block (Fig. 11-2).[39] Noninvasive pharmacologic tests have also been proposed to approximate accessory pathway refractoriness. For example, loss of preexcitation after intravenous procainamide[41] has been correlated with a long refractory period of the accessory pathway and a slow ventricular response during atrial fibrillation. The accuracy of such tests has been seriously questioned.[42,43] Even if they prove to be reasonably predictive of SRR during atrial fibrillation, the clinician will be left with the same therapeutic dilemmas as if atrial fibrillation had actually been induced.

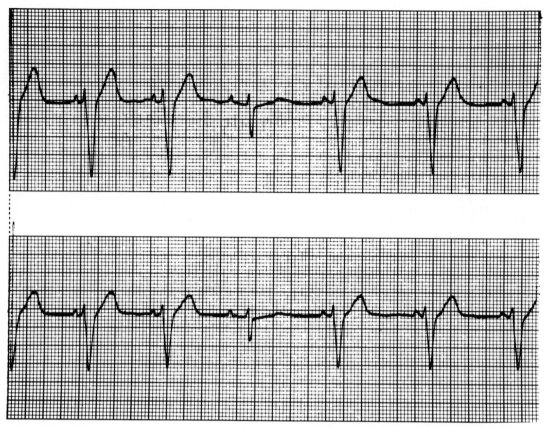

*Figure 11-2*    Sudden loss of preexcitation in a patient with Wolff-Parkinson-White pattern. Two leads of an ambulatory record are shown. The first three complexes have a typical preexcitation pattern. Preexcitation is abruptly lost in the fourth complex, with normalization of the QRS complex and prolongation of the PR interval. This represents a precarious margin of safety for conduction over the accessory pathway and predicts a slow preexcited ventricular response during atrial fibrillation.

## Commentary

A few generalizations may be made about ECG abnormalities in asymptomatic individuals. Electrocardiographic abnormalities may be markers for associated cardiac or medical disease. The ultimate prognosis is usually that of the associated disease. It is always appropriate to conduct a thorough clinical evaluation with reasonable investigations to clarify the problem. It is always appropriate to follow up any abnormality that may ultimately be progressive. It is impossible to improve the symptomatic status of an asymptomatic individual, and any intervention must be made with the intent of preventing impending morbidity or mortality. There should be reasonable evidence in the literature to support both this impending mortality as well as a reasonable expectation that therapy will improve this. Since both these criteria are rarely met, a conservative noninterventional approach is usually appropriate.

# References

1. Fisch C: Electrocardiogram in the aged: An independent marker of heart disease? *Am J Med* 70:4, 1981.

2. Kerr CR et al: Sinus node dysfunction. *Cardiol Clin* 1:187, 1983.

3. Brodsky M et al: Arrhythmias documented by 24 hour continuous electrocardiographic monitoring in 50 male medical students without apparent heart disease. *Am J Cardiol* 39:390, 1977.

4. Mazuz M, Friedman HS: Significance of prolonged electrocardiographic pauses in sinoatrial disease: Sick sinus syndrome. *Am J Cardiol* 52:485, 1983.

5. Hilgard J et al: Significance of ventricular pauses of 3 seconds or more detected on 24 hour Holter recordings. *Am J Cardiol* 55:1005, 1985.

6. Gann D et al: Electrophysiologic evaluation of elderly patients within sinus bradycardia: A long term follow-up study. *Ann Intern Med* 90:24, 1979.

7. Barrett PA et al: Frequency and prognostic significance of electrocardiographic abnormality in clinically normal individuals. *Progr Cardiovasc Dis* 23:299, 1981.

8. Surawicz B: Prognosis of patients with chronic bifascicular block. *Circulation* 60:40, 1979.

9. Dewey RC et al: Use of ambulatory electrocardiographic monitoring to identify high risk patients with congenital complete heart block. *N Engl J Med* 316:835, 1987.

10. Rotman M, Triebivasser JH: A clinical and follow-up study of right and left bundle branch block. *Circulation* 51:477, 1975.

11. Fisch GR et al: Bundle branch block and sudden death. *Progr Cardiovasc Dis* 23:187, 1980.

12. Dhingra RC et al: Significance of chronic bifascicular block without apparent organic heart disease. *Circulation* 60:33, 1979.

13. McAnulty JH et al: A prospective study of sudden death in "high risk" bundle branch block. *N Engl J Med* 299:209, 1978.

14. Peters RW et al: Prophylactic permanent pacemakers for patients with chronic bundle branch block. *Am J Med* 66:978, 1979.

15. Clarke JM et al: The rhythm of the normal human heart. *Lancet* 2:508, 1976.

16. O'Neill BJ et al: Results of operative therapy in the permanent form of junctional reciprocating tachycardia. *Am J Cardiol* 63:1074, 1989.

17. Petersen P et al: Placebo-controlled, randomized trial of warfarin and aspirin for prevention of thromboembolic complications in chronic atrial fibrillation. *Lancet* 8631:175, 1989.

18. Shimomura K et al: Significance of atrial fibrillation as a precursor of embolism. *Am J Cardiol* 63:1405, 1989.

19. Kerr CR et al: Atrial fibrillation: Fact, controversy and future. *Clin Progr Electrophysiol Pacing* 3:319, 1985.

20. Kannel WB et al: Epidemiologic features of chronic atrial fibrillation: The Framingham study. *N Engl J Med* 306:1018, 1982.

21. Roy D et al: Usefulness of anticoagulant therapy in the prevention of embolic complications of atrial fibrillation. *Am Heart J* 112:1039, 1986.

22. Morganroth J, Horowitz LN: Antiarrhythmic drug therapy 1988: For whom, how and where? *Am J Cardiol* 62:461, 1988.

23. Kennedy HL, Underhill SJ: Frequent or complex ventricular ectopy in apparently healthy subjects. *Am J Cardiol* 38:141, 1976.

24. Buxton AE et al: Prognostic factors in nonsustained ventricular tachycardia. *Am J Cardiol* 53:1275, 1984.

25. Ruberman W et al: Repeated 1 hour electrocardiographic monitoring of survivors of myocardial infarction at 6 month intervals: Arrhythmia detection and relation to prognosis. *Am J Cardiol* 47:1197, 1981.

26. Bigger JT Jr: Relation between left ventricular dysfunction and ventricular arrhythmias after myocardial infarction. *Am J Cardiol* 57:8B, 1986.

27. Bigger JT Jr et al: Prevalence, characteristics and significance of ventricular tachycardia detected by 24-hour continuous electrocardiographic recordings in the late hospital phase of acute myocardial infarction. *Am J Cardiol* 58:1151, 1986.

28. Kostis JB et al: Prognostic significance of ventricular ectopic activity in survivors of acute myocardial infarction. *J Am Coll Cardiol* 10:231, 1987.

29. Meinertz T et al: Significance of ventricular arrhythmias in idiopathic dilated cardiomyopathy. *Am J Cardiol* 53:902, 1984.

30. Maron BJ et al: Prognostic significance of 24 hour ambulatory electrocardiographic monitoring in pa-

tients with hypertrophic cardiomyopathy: A prospective study. *Am J Cardiol* 48:252, 1981.

31. Brugada P, Wellens HJJ: Arrhythmogenesis of antiarrhythmic drugs. *Am J Cardiol* 61:1108, 1988.

32. IMPACT Research Group: International mexiletine and placebo antiarrhythmic coronary trial: 1. Report on arrhythmia and other findings. *J Am Coll Cardiol* 4:1148, 1984.

33. Echt DS et al: Mortality and morbidity in patients receiving encainide, flecainide or placebo: The Cardiac Arrhythmia Suppression trial. *N Engl J Med* 324:781, 1991.

34. Effect of the antiarrhythmic agent moricizine on survival after myocardial infarction: The Cardiac Arrhythmia Suppression Trial II Investigators. *N Engl J Med* 327:227, 1992.

35. Lown B et al: Sleep and ventricular premature beats. *Circulation* 48:691, 1973.

36. Miller WP: Cardiac arrhythmias and conduction disturbances in the sleep apnea syndrome: Prevalence and significance. *Am J Med* 73:317, 1982.

37. Guilleminault C: Cardiac arrhythmia and conduction disturbances during sleep in 400 patients with sleep apnea syndrome. *Am J Cardiol* 52:490, 1983.

38. Klein GJ et al: Ventricular fibrillation in the Wolff-Parkinson-White syndrome. *N Engl J Med* 301:1080, 1979.

39. Klein GJ et al: Asymptomatic Wolff-Parkinson-White: Should we intervene? *Circulation* 80:1902, 1989.

40. Leitch JW et al: Prognostic value of electrophysiology testing in asymptomatic patients with Wolff-Parkinson-White pattern. *Circulation* 82:1718, 1990.

41. Wellens HJJ et al: Use of procainamide in patients with the Wolff-Parkinson-White syndrome to disclose a short refractory period of the accessory pathway. *Am J Cardiol* 50:1087, 1982.

42. Fananapazir L et al: Procainamide infusion test: Inability to identify patients with Wolff-Parkinson-White syndrome who are potentially at risk of sudden death. *Circulation* 77:1291, 1988.

43. Boahene KA et al: Value of a revised procainamide test in the Wolff-Parkinson-White syndrome. *Am J Cardiol* 65:195, 1990.

# Chapter 12

# *Narrow QRS Tachycardia*

The supraventricular tachycardias are classified by mechanism in Chaps. 6 and 7, where the specific entities are discussed in more detail. This chapter is intended to provide a practical diagnostic and therapeutic approach to the patient presenting with supraventricular tachycardia of unknown mechanism. It will become evident that simple guidelines can narrow the diagnostic possibilities and suggest appropriate therapy in most patients.

## *Definition and Classification*

Supraventricular tachycardia may be defined as tachycardia in which the "atrium or atrioventricular junction above the bifurcation of the His bundle is the origin or a critical link in the perpetuation of tachycardia."[1] The QRS morphology is normal or aberrant, the latter generally being functional right or left bundle branch block. A classification based on mechanism as presented in Fig. 12-1 is useful for cataloging and discussing tachycardia, but it is less helpful when a supraventricular tachycardia of unknown mechanism presents itself.

A more useful working classification should be simple and helpful for guiding therapy. In one such classification, all the supraventricular tachycardias can be placed into one of two categories based on the requirement of the atrioventricular (AV) node for the perpetuation of tachycardia (Fig. 12-2). The tachycardia is "independent" of the AV node when the arrhythmia "generator" is above the level of the AV node. The AV node–independent tachycardias

are not influenced by AV block and comprise all forms of atrial tachycardia, including atrial reentrant tachycardia, atrial flutter, and atrial fibrillation. With rare exceptions,[2] continuation of supraventricular tachycardia in the presence of AV block classifies the tachycardia as AV node–independent (Fig. 12-3). On the other hand, the tachycardia is "dependent" on the AV node when the node is a critical component

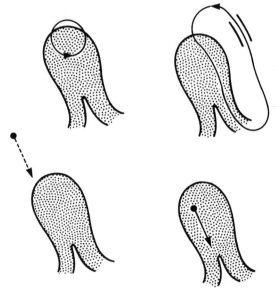

*Figure 12-1* Classification of supraventricular tachycardia by mechanism. Mechanisms include AV node reentry (top left), AV reentry utilizing an accessory pathway (top right), nonparoxysmal junctional tachycardia (lower right), and atrial tachycardia due to atrial reentry or abnormal automaticity (lower left). Atrial tachycardia also includes rhythms such as atrial flutter and atrial fibrillation.

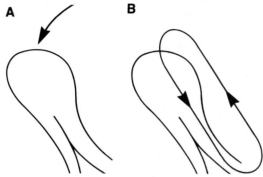

*Figure 12-2* Classification based on the requirement or lack of requirement of the AV node in the tachycardia mechanism. Panel *A* represents AV node–independent tachycardia such as atrial flutter, atrial fibrillation, or ectopic atrial tachycardia. Panel *B* represents AV node–dependent tachycardia such as AV reentry using the AV node for anterograde conduction and an accessory pathway for retrograde conduction (as illustrated) or AV node reentry.

of the tachycardia mechanism. AV node–dependent tachycardias include those due to AV node reentry or AV reentry utilizing an accessory pathway. With rare exceptions in some patients with AV node reentry,[2] AV node–dependent tachycardias cannot continue in the presence of AV block. Most supraventricular tachycardias can be readily classified into AV node–"dependent" or "independent," and this can direct appropriate pharmacologic strategy.

## History and Physical Examination

As with all tachycardias, the clinical assessment can provide important clues to the tachycardia mecha-

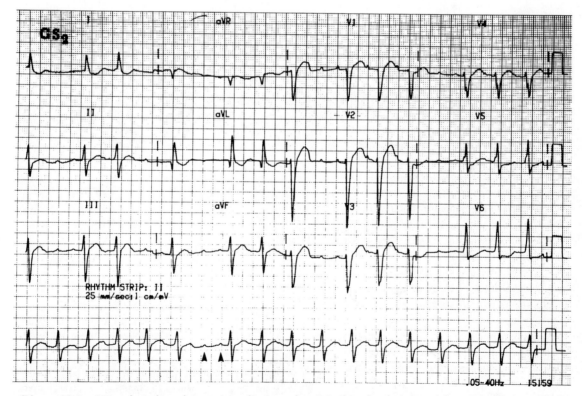

*Figure 12-3* AV node–independent tachycardia later determined to be due to atrial reentry. Tachycardia is unaffected by transient AV block clearly evident in the rhythm strip (arrowheads).

# The Color Plates

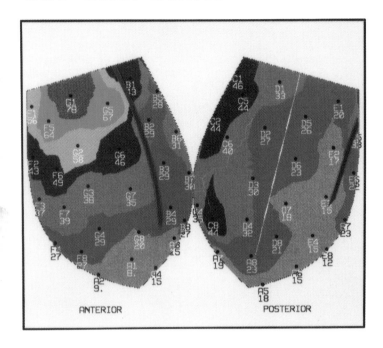

ANTERIOR     POSTERIOR

Plate 1. Normal epicardial ventricular activation. The format for Figs. 1-3, 1-4, and 1-5 is the same. At the time of surgery, a 56-electrode array sock was positioned on the epicardial surface of the heart; during one QRS complex, ventricular activation was obtained at all sites. Each site is noted by a letter and number that designate the electrode position and, underneath, by the local activation time, using the initiation of the surface QRS complex as time 0. The left anterior descending (LAD) coronary artery is schematically represented in the anterior view and the posterior descending (PDA) coronary artery is represented similarly in the posterior view. These are approximate positions as noted during surgery. In this figured, note the rapid activation of the entire right and left ventricles. The last area activated is the base of the right ventricle, and activation time is complete within 78 ms. The right ventricle in the anterior view is to the left of the LAD and in the posterior view to the right of the PDA. This method of displaying the heart assumes that the posterior crux of the heart is divided and the ventricles are then laid out flat. The base of the heart with the atria removed is at the top of the figure and the apex (electrodes A1 through A8) is at the bottom. It is not that critical to analyze each point but rather to realize that the entire epicardial surface of the ventricle is activated relatively quickly.

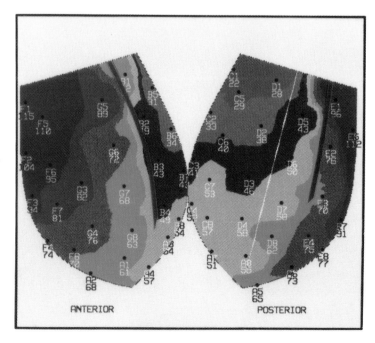

ANTERIOR     POSTERIOR

Plate 2. Epicardial ventricular activation during right bundle branch block. (See Fig. 1-3 for details of mapping methods.) Note that the left ventricle, represented by electrodes B through D, is activated in a normal fashion and relatively quickly. However, the right ventricle, represented by electrodes E through G, is activated late, as would be expected in right bundle branch block. Point $F_1$ is activated 115 ms after the initiation of the surface QRS complex. Compare this activation with that noted in Fig. 1-3.

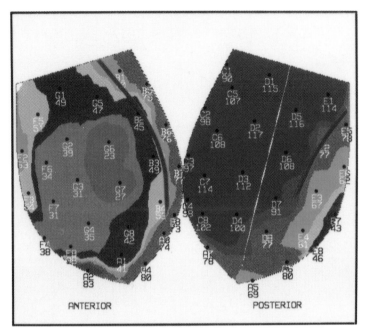

Plate 3. Epicardial ventricular activation in left bundle branch block. (See Fig. 1-3 for details of mapping.) In contrast to Fig. 1-4, the earliest activated sites in this patient are on the right ventricle and the latter activated points on the left ventricle, as expected with left bundle branch block. Right ventricular points are primarily noted by G and E, which are left of the LAD in the anterior view and right of the PDA in the posterior view. Note that the last area to be activated is on the left ventricle at D2 (117 ms), in contrast to the last area activated during right bundle branch block, which is on the right ventricular epicardial surface (see Fig. 1-4).

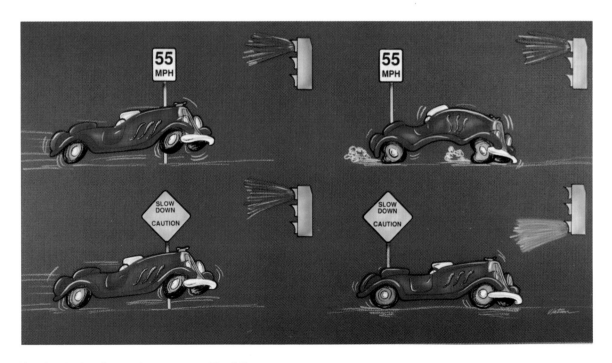

Plate 4.  Analogy for gap phenomenon (see Fig. 4-2).

nism. The AV node–dependent tachycardias, such as AV node or AV reentry, involve a tachycardia substrate present from birth and are, in essence, congenital abnormalities. Accordingly, a long history of paroxysmal (sudden in onset) tachycardia since childhood or early adulthood would suggest these latter mechanisms. On the other hand, AV node–independent tachycardias—such as atrial flutter, atrial fibrillation, or atrial tachycardia—are probably "acquired" in the majority of patients and frequently associated with organic heart disease.[3,4] For example, the occurrence of supraventricular tachycardia in a 60-year-old man with chronic obstructive lung disease should suggest AV node–independent tachycardia, such as atrial flutter, rather than AV (accessory pathway) reentry. The AV node–independent tachycardias, such as those due to intraatrial reentrance, are also more likely with congenital heart disease such as atrial septal defect or after operative repair of such lesions. An exception may be Ebstein's anomaly, which is associated with a higher than expected frequency of the Wolff-Parkinson-White syndrome.

Other clues can be obtained from the history, although it must be appreciated that they are fallible. Perception of irregularity suggests atrial fibrillation. The converse is not helpful, since even atrial fibrillation can be perceived as regular if sufficiently rapid. Regular constant neck pulsations, presumably due to simultaneous atrial and ventricular contraction, suggest AV node reentry. Sudden termination with maneuvers such as Valsalva, quiet breathing, squatting, or lying down suggests AV node dependence. Finally, consistent onset with exertion suggests AV node dependence.

The physical examination during tachycardia or otherwise is usually not helpful. Findings of cardiac dysfunction or pulmonary disease are more common with AV node–independent tachycardia. The hemodynamic status of the patient depends on such factors as ventricular function, tachycardia rate, and peripheral vascular resistance and gives no clue to the tachycardia mechanism. Of course, the physical findings of AV dissociation (cannon A waves, variable $S_1$, variable pulse pressure) overwhelmingly point to a diagnosis of ventricular tachycardia.

## Electrocardiographic Diagnosis

A good quality 12 lead electrocardiogram (ECG) with rhythm strip using the lead best showing P waves is essential. Identification of P waves may be facilitated in several ways:

1. A careful comparison with a previous 12-lead ECG may help identify P waves "buried" in the QRS complex or ST segment.
2. Nonstandard ECG leads such as the "Lewis" lead may identify P waves. For example, positioning the right-arm lead in the upper sternum and the left-arm lead in the lower sternum may provide a larger-amplitude P wave.
3. Positioning an esophageal lead[5–7] will usually provide a good atrial electrogram. This lead may also be used for programmed atrial stimulation (see Chap. 18).
4. Atrial activity may also be recorded using signal-averaged electrocardiography,[8] and atrial mechanical activity may sometimes be identified using echocardiography.[9]

There are several points of focus to aid diagnosis using the 12-lead ECG:

1. The P wave morphology may provide an approximation to the atrial activation sequence and suggest a site of origin of atrial activation.[10,11] For example, a negatively oriented P wave in lead 1 suggests activation from left atrium to right atrium (AV reentry utilizing a left lateral accessory pathway or left atrial tachycardia), while negative P waves in the inferior leads 2, 3, and AVF suggest activation beginning in the posterior right or left atrium at or near the coronary sinus orifice. Unfortunately, the P wave is frequently obscured by ventricular depolarization and repolarization, making this a technically difficult exercise.
2. By definition, an atrial rate of 250 cycles per minute or faster is atrial flutter. A ventricular rate of 150 to 160/min should suggest the possibility of atrial flutter with 2-to-1 AV

block. Otherwise, there is too much overlap in ventricular rates observed with different mechanisms for rate to be useful.

3.  A change in rate with transition from normal QRS to a bundle branch block pattern points to a mechanism of AV reentry utilizing an accessory pathway (Chap. 7). The latter observation obviously suggests that one of the bundle branches is part of the reentrant circuit, with block in that bundle branch prolonging circuit size. Atrioventricular reentry is the only supraventricular tachycardia that incorporates ventricular and His-Purkinje tissue in the circuit.

4.  A phasic alternation in QRS amplitude ("QRS alternans") during stabilized tachycardia has been suggested by some[12] but not others[13] to support the diagnosis of AV reentry using an accessory pathway. Our experience and that of others[14] suggests that QRS alternans is probably a function of a faster tachycardia rate and not of a specific mechanism. However, QRS cycle alternans, a regular alternating long-short R-R interval during tachycardia, strongly suggests AV node dependence.

5.  Observations during spontaneous tachycardia termination may be helpful (Figs. 12-4 and 12-5). In Fig. 12-5, tachycardia terminates, with the last event being a P wave. This strongly suggests that the AV node is part of the reentrant circuit (AV node dependent), as in atrioventricular reentry. AV node–independent tachycardia, such as atrial tachycardia, will not terminate in this way, since AV block would have to occur fortuitously on the very last atrial cycle of the tachycardia.

6.  The AV relationship is very helpful if P waves can be identified. If atrial tachycardia persists in the presence of AV block, the tachycardia can be classified as AV node-independent. With AV node-dependent tachycardia, the position of the P wave relative to the QRS can be helpful (Fig. 12-6).[3,10,11,14] The presence of a P wave simultaneous or nearly simultaneous with the QRS favors the diagnosis of AV node reentry. If the P wave is clearly past the QRS complex, with the RP interval less than the PR interval, a diagnosis of atrioventricular reentry utilizing an accessory pathway is probable (Fig. 12-7). In an uncommon type of tachycardia, with the RP greater than the PR interval, the mechanism is generally AV reentry utilizing an atypical accessory pathway with a long conduction time as the retrograde limb of a circuit. Less often, the mechanism is "atypical" AV node reentry with the "slow"

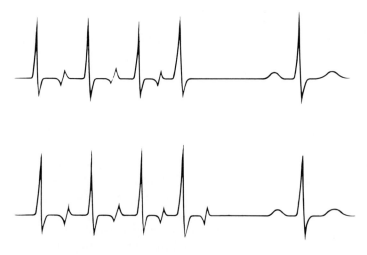

*Figure 12-4*  Value of spontaneous termination in determining mechanism. Termination with the last event being ventricular depolarization (no retrograde P) can occur with either AV node–dependent or independent tachycardia (upper panel). However, consistent termination with the last event being atrial depolarization (lower panel) invariably indicates AV node–dependent tachycardia.

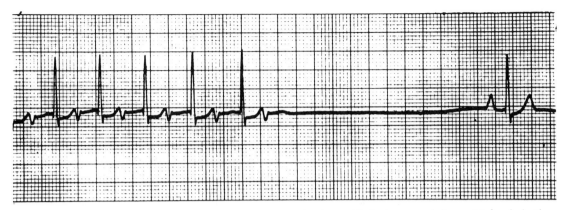

***Figure 12-5***  ECG record in a patient with spontaneous termination, with the last event being atrial depolarization. The mechanism of tachycardia in this patient was AV reentry.

AV nodal pathway serving as the retrograde limb of the circuit (Chap. 6). It is worth emphasizing that the above criteria apply only when AV node–independent tachycardia has been ruled out, since the P wave can obviously be anywhere in the cardiac cycle depending on the PR interval in the latter.

## Acute Management

After reviewing the ECG, the key step at this stage is to classify the tachycardia as AV node–dependent or independent if this is not already apparent. Maneuvers that suddenly depress AV nodal conduction will allow this distinction. Carotid sinus massage or pressure has been used for many years for this purpose.[15,16] Up to 5 s of steady right or left carotid sinus pressure is applied after carotid disease has been excluded historically and by the absence of decreased carotid pulses or bruits. This vagotonic maneuver may be enhanced by pretreating the patient with an anticholinesterase drug such as edrophonium (Tensilon) 5 to 10 mg intravenously. Head-down tilt and the poststrain phase of the Valsalva maneuver are also vagotonic, and beta blockade potentiates the vagal maneuvers. The observation of persistent atrial

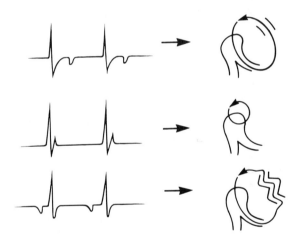

***Figure 12-6***  Value of P wave position within the cardiac cycle. The P wave can be anywhere in the cycle during AV node–independent tachycardia, depending on the PR interval. Consequently, the following guidelines are helpful only if the tachycardia is known to be AV node–dependent (except nonparoxysmal junctional tachycardia). The PR interval is greater than the RP interval with the usual type of AV reentry, with the P wave following the QRS complex (top panel). This relationship is seen far less frequently with AV node reentry. The presence of a P wave within the QRS (middle panel) occurs with AV node reentry. The RP interval is longer than the PR in AV reentry utilizing an unusual accessory pathway with a long conduction time (lower panel) and, less frequently, with the uncommon type of AV node reentry ('fast-slow'). Note that atrial tachycardia with 1:1 AV conduction often has a PR interval shorter than the RP interval.

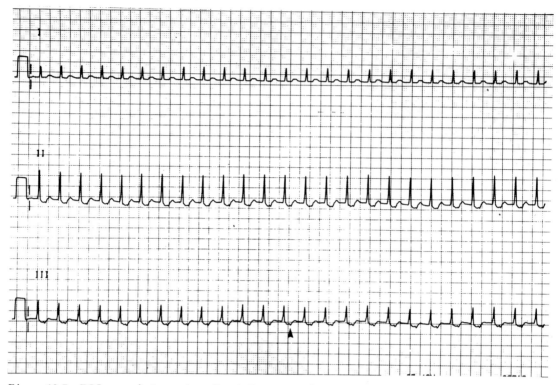

*Figure 12-7*    ECG trace during tachycardia. A P wave can be seen in the ST segment, especially in lead 3 (arrowhead). The PR interval is greater than the RP interval, and this patient had AV reentry utilizing an accessory pathway as the retrograde limb of the circuit.

tachycardia with temporary AV block provides a diagnoses of AV node–independent tachycardia (Fig. 12-8), whereas slowing or abrupt termination of tachycardia indicates AV node–dependent tachycardia.

A transient but intense negative dromotrophic effect can also be readily achieved with the purinergic compounds adenosine or adenosine triphosphate (not available in the United States).[17] One of these compounds will generally expose AV node–independent tachycardia by creating transient AV block and will generally terminate AV node–dependent tachycardia (Fig. 12-9). Some atrial tachycardias will also terminate with adenosine, although this usually occurs after some AV node block has been observed. The calcium antagonist verapamil can be used in a

similar fashion if it is absolutely certain that there is no ventricular tachycardia (Chap. 13).

At this point, the task is simplified. An AV node–dependent tachycardia will have been terminated and an AV node–independent tachycardia will still be present (Table 12-1). Acute treatment strategy for AV node–independent tachycardia of any mechanism involves two steps. The first is slowing of the ventricular response with drugs directed at the AV node (digitalis, calcium antagonists, beta blockers). This step alone will sometimes result in conversion to sinus rhythm, possibly by improving hemodynamics. Once the rate is slowed, therapy with membrane-active medication such as procainamide may be instituted in an attempt to restore sinus rhythm. In general, intravenous medications are used acutely,

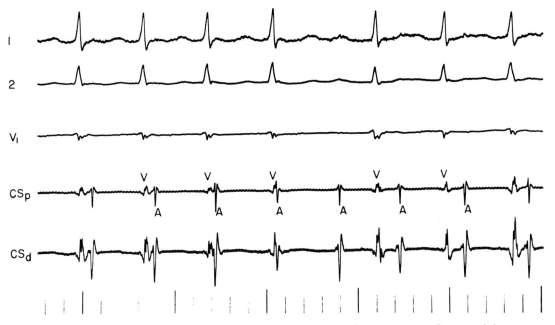

***Figure 12-8***   Use of carotid sinus massage in supraventricular tachycardia. This intracardiac record demonstrates the occurrence of transient AV block during carotid massage without influencing the atrial tachycardia (by definition, AV mode-independent). 1, 2, $V_1$ are ECG leads $CS_p$ and $CS_d$ are proximal and distal coronary sinus electrograms, respectively.

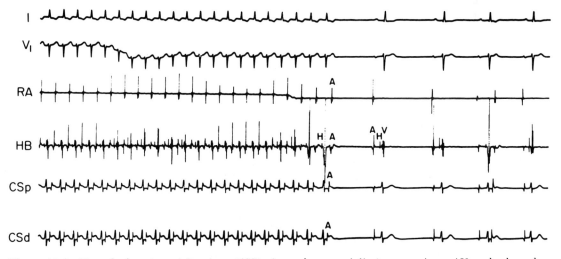

***Figure 12-9***   Use of adenosine triphosphate (ATP, 8 mg by central line) to terminate AV node–dependent tachycardia (AV reentry in this case). Note that tachycardia terminates with an atrial electrogram that blocks in the AV node—i.e., that is not followed by His activation. 1, $V_1$ are ECG leads; $CS_p$ and $CS_d$ are proximal and distal coronary sinus, respectively; HB is His bundle electrogram; and RA is right atrial electrogram.

**Table 12-1    Acute Pharmacological Treatment of Supraventricular Tachycardia**

AV node–independent
  Slow ventricular response (digitalis, beta blockers, calcium antagonists).
  Restore sinus rhythm with membrane-active antiarrhythmic drug such as intravenous procainamide.

AV node–dependent
  In general, direct initial therapy at the AV node (adenosine, calcium antagonists, beta blocker, digitalis).
  Membrane-active drugs (quinidine, procainamide, disopyramide) generally used after failure of initial therapy. Especially useful in nonparoxysmal junctional tachycardia.

Mechanism unknown
  Treat as AV node–independent.

**Table 12-2    Chronic Therapy of Supraventricular Tachycardia**

No therapy
  Indicated in infrequent and well-tolerated tachycardia or when an obvious precipitating course can be identified and eliminated.

Empirical ("trial and error") therapy
  Appropriate for well-tolerated tachycardia.
  Appropriate for frequent tachycardia where results of therapy are more easily assessed.

Therapy guided by electrophysiological testing
  Poorly tolerated tachycardia
  Symptoms of syncope or congestive heart failure with tachycardia.
  Failure of empiric therapy.
  Any circumstance in which it is considered important to identify efficacious therapy expediently.

although oral medication may be considered if the tachycardia is well tolerated. Elective cardioversion is appropriate at any time in the event of serious hemodynamic deterioration or treatment failure. In the latter circumstance, the patient should be adequately "loaded" with antiarrhythmic medication prior to cardioversion to prevent subsequent relapse. Patients with atrial fibrillation lasting longer than 72 h should generally be anticoagulated prior to elective medical or electrical cardioversion (see Chap. 6).

## Approach to Chronic Therapy

The first decision after termination of the acute episode is whether or not chronic therapy is required[18] (Table 12-2). Chronic therapy is not essential if episodes are well tolerated with minor symptoms, if they are infrequent, and if the patient has reasonable access to a medical facility. If a decision is made that further prophylactic therapy is required, the clinician must decide between empiric (trial and error) drug therapy or therapy guided by electrophysiologic

testing. Empirical therapy may be considered if the episodes are not associated with serious symptoms such as syncope or congestive heart failure. It should be considered with reservation in patients with the Wolff-Parkinson-White syndrome, of whom approximately 50 percent have the potential for the occurrence of atrial fibrillation with a rapid ventricular response.[19]

Electrophysiologic testing (Chap. 17) provides the mechanism of tachycardia and, more significantly, provides an expedient, objective measure of the effectiveness of any proposed therapy. It is to be especially recommended in patients with poorly tolerated tachycardia or associated syncope or heart failure. It is useful after repeated empiric drug trials have failed and could be considered under any circumstance where it is desirable to identify efficacious therapy expediently.

## Choice of Chronic Therapy

Antiarrhythmic drugs are the mainstay of therapy for most individuals with AV node–independent tachycardia. Drugs that block the AV node and membrane-active drugs are used in these patients (Chap. 19). When drugs are used for AV node–dependent tachycardia, class 1A or 1C antiarrhythmic drugs (such as quinidine, disopyramide, flecainide, or propafenone) may be considered first, especially in patients with supraventricular tachycardia associated with the Wolff-Parkinson-White syndrome, to provide some protection in the event of atrial fibrillation.

Nonpharmacologic approaches are considered for patients with life-threatening arrhythmias, those who cannot be controlled with a reasonable drug regimen or as first line therapy in certain arrhythmias. Catheter ablation (Chap. 17) is very effective for AV reentry and AV node reentry and can be considered as a matter of preference in patients not wishing to take antiarrhythmic drugs for the long term. Operative therapy (Chap. 20) is considered for patients refractory to medical therapy who cannot be treated by ablation. Catheter ablation of the AV node with pacemaker implantation is also relatively safe and effective (Chap. 17) and is usually considered in patients with drug-refractory AV node–independent arrhythmias such as atrial fibrillation. Permanent antitachycardia pacing devices (Chap. 21) are available for patients with drug-refractory arrhythmias in whom the arrhythmia can be reproducibly terminated by programmed atrial stimulation. Ultimately the choice of nonpharmacologic approach depends on local expertise and individual considerations.

## Commentary

It is not necessary to know the mechanism of supraventricular tachycardia in order to formulate a reasonable treatment strategy. However, the concept of dividing supraventricular tachycardias into AV node–independent versus AV node–dependent types has merit in that the distinction can usually be made without intracardiac recordings or sophisticated equipment and the information is very helpful in formulating a treatment strategy (Table 12-1). This is probably the most important "take-home" message in this section.

## References

1.  Klein GJ et al: Classification of supraventricular tachycardias. *Am J Cardiol* 60:27D–31D, 1987.

2.  Wellens HJJ et al: Second degree block during reciprocal atrioventricular nodal tachycardia. *Circulation* 53:595–599, 1976.

3.  Wu D et al: Clinical, electrocardiographic and electrophysiologic observations in patients with paroxysmal supraventricular tachycardia. *Am J Cardiol* 41:1045–1051, 1978.

4.  Gillette P: The mechanisms of supraventricular tachycardia in children. *Circulation* 54:133–139, 1976.

5.  Gallagher JJ et al: Use of the esophageal lead in the diagnosis of the mechanisms of reciprocating tachycardia. *PACE* 3:440, 1980.

6.  Benditt DG et al: Ventriculoatrial intervals: Diagnostic use in paroxysmal supraventricular tachycardia. *Ann Intern Med* 91:161, 1979.

7.  Prystowsky EN et al: Origin of the atrial electrogram recorded from the esophagus. *Circulation* 61:1017–1023, 1980.

8.  Kuchar DL et al: High frequency analysis of the surface electrocardiograms of patients with supraventricular tachycardia: Accurate identification of atrial activation and determination of the mechanism of tachycardia. *Circulation* 74:1016, 1986.

9.  Riickel A et al: Atrioventricular dissociation detected by suprasternal M-mode echocardiography: A clue to the diagnoses of ventricular tachycardia. *Am J Cardiol* 54:561–563, 1984.

10.  Kuchar DL et al: Surface electrocardiographic manifestations of tachyarrhythmias: Clues to diagnoses and mechanism. *PACE* 11:61–82, 1988.

11.  Bar FW et al: Differential diagnosis of tachycardia with narrow QRS complex (shorter than 0.12 second). *Am J Cardiol* 54:555–560, 1984.

12.  Green M et al: Value of QRS alternation in deter-

mining the site of origin of narrow complex QRS supraventricular tachycardia. *Circulation* 68:368, 1983.

13. Morady F et al: Determinants of QRS alternans during narrow QRS tachycardia. *J Am Coll Cardiol* 9:489, 1987.

14. Kay GN et al: Value of the 12 lead electrocardiogram in discriminating atrioventricular nodal reciprocating tachycardia from circus movement atrioventricular tachycardia utilizing a retrograde accessory pathway. *Am J Cardiol* 59:296–300, 1987.

15. Wald RW et al: Vagal techniques for termination of paroxysmal supraventricular tachycardia. *Am J Cardiol* 46:655–664, 1980.

16. Waxman MB et al: Effects of respiration and posture on paroxysmal supraventricular tachycardia. *Circulation* 62:1011–1020, 1980.

17. DiMarco JP et al: Adenosine: electrophysiologic effects and therapeutic use for terminating paroxysmal supraventricular tachycardia. *Circulation* 68:1254–1263, 1983.

18. Klein GJ et al: An approach to therapy for paroxysmal supraventricular tachycardia. *Am J Cardiol* 61:77A–82A, 1988.

19. Rinne C et al: Relation between clinical presentation and induced arrhythmias in the Wolff-Parkinson-White syndrome. *Am J Cardiol* 60:576–579, 1987.

# Chapter 13

# Wide QRS Tachycardia

Wide QRS tachycardia may be defined as tachycardia having QRS duration of greater than 120 ms, the upper limit of normal QRS duration.[1] Tachycardia fitting this general description may be broadly classified by mechanism into three groups (Fig. 13-1).[2,3] These include ventricular tachycardia (VT), supraventricular tachycardia (SVT) with aberration, and preexcited tachycardia. Supraventricular tachycardia may be defined for this discussion as any tachycardia utilizing the normal atrioventricular (AV) conduction system for ventricular excitation, with the tachycardia either originating in the atria or AV node or requiring one of the latter structures for their perpetuation. These tachycardias include AV node reentrant tachycardia, orthodromic atrioventricular reentrant tachycardia, atrial flutter, atrial fibrillation, sinoatrial node reentrant tachycardia, and atrial tachycardia. Aberration of conduction has been variously defined[2,4] but may be simply defined as "conduction delay or block in the His–Perkinje system during anterograde conduction of impulses over the normal AV conduction system."[2] Conduction block may be fixed or functional. A sudden acceleration of rate, as for the onset of SVT, is a frequent cause of aberration of conduction that may be perpetu-

ated by continuous concealed retrograde conduction into the blocked pathway (see Chap. 3). Although any part of the His–Purkinje system may be involved in this functional block, right bundle branch block and left bundle branch block are by far the most frequent aberration patterns.[2,5–7] The term *preexcited tachycardia* refers to any tachycardia where the ventricles are activated anterogradely over an accessory pathway. The commonest preexcited tachycardia is atrial fibrillation with the ventricular response predominantly a result of anterograde accessory pathway conduction (see Chap. 7). Other preexcited tachycardias include true antidromic tachycardia (anterograde conduction over an accessory AV pathway with retrograde conduction over the normal AV conduction system) and tachycardias utilizing a second accessory pathway as the retrograde limb of a reentrant circuit.

Put more simply, the clinician confronted with a wide QRS tachycardia must decide whether it is VT, SVT with aberrancy (usually functional right or left bundle branch block), or a preexcited tachycardia using an accessory AV pathway to activate the ventricles. The problem is not merely academic, as incorrect diagnosis can lead to inappropriate therapy and potentially lethal consequences.[8,9]

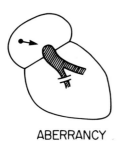 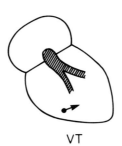 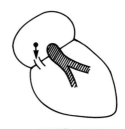

ABERRANCY        VT        PREEXCITATION

*Figure 13-1* Classification of wide QRS tachycardia by mechanism.

## Clinical Assessment

It is especially appropriate to begin with the history, as this may provide the most valuable clue to tachycardia diagnosis before the electrocardiogram (ECG) is even viewed.[5,6] Patients with preexcited tachycardias are considerably younger than patients with VT, the latter usually being in the "coronary prone" age group. Patients with preexcited tachycardia or paroxysmal SVT with aberrancy will more frequently provide a history of long-standing recurrence, often dating back to childhood or early adulthood. A history of heart disease and in particular previous myocardial infarction should lead to a working diagnosis of VT until proved otherwise.

It is most important to appreciate that the hemodynamic status of the patient during tachycardia is not helpful in clarifying the diagnosis. Many practitioners are under the misconception that patients with VT present in dire straits and patients with SVT are not hemodynamically compromised.[10] In fact, patients with VT may present with very little or no evidence of hemodynamic compromise and, conversely, patients with SVT may present with severe hypotension. Determinants of the patient's hemodynamic status are complicated and include the rate of tachycardia, left ventricular function, peripheral vascular tone, and medication; they should not be used to influence the decision regarding diagnosis. Physical examination is nonetheless valuable in elucidating the physical signs of AV dissociation. Atrioventricular dissociation, with rare exceptions, is diagnostic of VT. It is present in 50 percent or more of patients with VT[6,7] and is even more prevalent with advancing age, heart disease, and faster tachycardia rates. The findings are identical to those expected in complete AV block and result from asynchronous activation of the atria and the ventricles. These include intermittent cannon A waves in the jugular venous pulse, variable intensity of the first heart sound, and variability in the magnitude of the systolic blood pressure. These findings are easily overlooked unless the examiner specifically looks for them. Carotid sinus massage with ECG monitoring may also be helpful. With

few exceptions, termination of a tachycardia after this maneuver suggests that the AV node is a critical link in the tachycardia reentrant circuit. Transient AV block may expose atrial flutter or atrial tachycardia. It may even be valuable in exposing ventricular tachycardia with VA conduction if transient retrograde VA block is observed with the maneuver (Fig. 13-2).

## Electrocardiographic Assessment

A careful analysis of the 12-lead ECG and rhythm strips will provide a diagnosis to the experienced observer in the majority of instances.[6,7,11] The following points are important in considering the ECG during tachycardia (see also Chap. 9).

1. A previous 12-lead ECG, if available, should always be examined concurrently. If the tachycardia has a bundle branch block pattern identical to that seen in sinus rhythm, the likely diagnosis is SVT with bundle branch block. On the other hand, if a different wide QRS pattern is present during tachycardia in a patient with fixed bundle branch block, the diagnosis is invariably VT.[5] In a patient with preexcitation, a similar QRS pattern in sinus rhythm tachycardia suggests a preexcited tachycardia.

2. AV dissociation is present in at least half of patients with VT,[7] and its incidence is probably greater in older patients and those with faster VT. On the other hand, AV dissociation in AV nodal reentry or other SVT is exceedingly rate. Thus, the presence of AV dissociation electrocardiographically is a valuable clue to the presence of VT (Fig. 13-3). Atrioventricular dissociation is often best seen in lead $V_1$ but may be seen in any lead in an individual. The rhythm strip should be run using the lead in which P waves appear to be particularly prominent. A "Lewis lead" may be helpful in

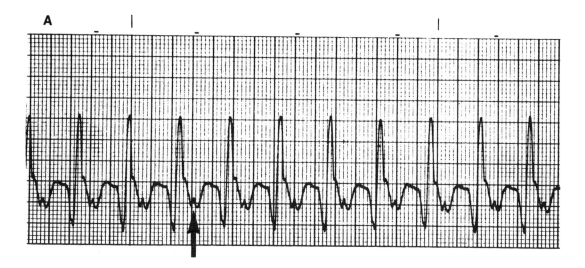

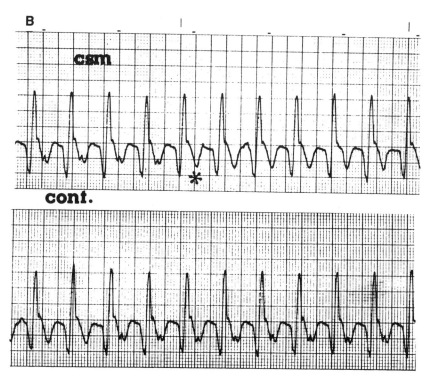

*Figure 13-2*   Carotid massage in wide QRS tachycardia. Panel *A* demonstrates tachycardia with a notch in the ST segment, indicating atrial activity (arrow). The AV relationship is 1 : 1 and the mechanism of tachycardia is not certain. With carotid massage (panel *B*), the P waves are transiently eliminated (asterisk) and the tachycardia is not affected. The latter supports the diagnosis of VT.

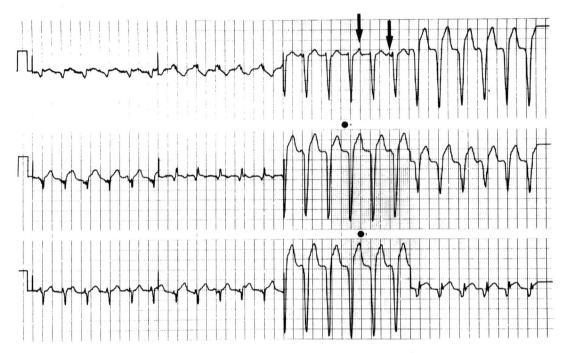

***Figure 13-3***   Wide QRS tachycardia. AV dissociation is evident in V$_1$ *(arrows indicate P waves).*

amplifying P waves. This is a special ECG lead oriented to optimize atrial depolarization. The right-arm electrode is positioned in the right parasternal area near the base of the heart, using a suction electrode. The left-arm electrode is generally in the fourth or fifth interspace, usually in the left parasternal region but it can be moved until an identifiable P wave is observed. The ECG is recorded in the lead 1 position. Although AV dissociation is a valuable finding, it is often difficult to detect electrocardiographically.[5]

3.  Capture beats or fusion beats may be seen in the presence of AV dissociation when a dissociated P wave totally (capture) or partially (fusion) activates the ventricle in advance of the next VT cycle. This results in a "premature" beat during tachycardia that is of supraventricular morphology and usually "narrow" (Fig. 13-4). Factors favoring the observation of fusion beats and capture beats include slower VT rates

with AV dissociation and good anterograde conduction over the AV node. In addition, "pseudonormalization" may occur,[11] resulting in premature complexes of narrower QRS morphology than the dominant wide QRS morphology. For example, a ventricular ectopic from the opposite ventricle could fuse with a VT complex resulting in a narrow QRS. Although frequently cited as "classic" for VT, capture and fusion beats are infrequently seen and difficult to interpret.[5–7]

4.  A QRS width greater than 0.14 s has been observed to occur more frequently in VT than SVT with aberration.[6,7] This is not surprising, since the QRS duration in uncomplicated right bundle branch block and left bundle branch block is usually less than or equal to 0.12 s[12–14] and these are the most common aberration patterns. The QRS in VT secondary to ischemic heart disease is usually wider than that associated with no apparent heart disease.[15] Unfortu-

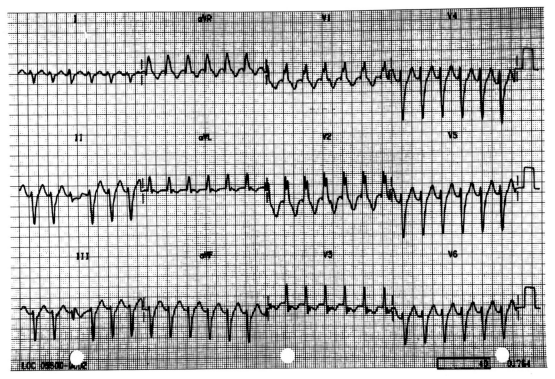

***Figure 13-4***  Wide QRS tachycardia. A capture beat is seen in leads 1, 2, and 3. Atrioventricular dissociation is present in lead V₁.

nately, the QRS can obviously be prolonged greater than 0.14 s during supraventricular rhythm in the presence of heart disease, preexcitation, and/or antiarrhythmic drugs.

5.  It has been observed that a mean QRS axis within the normal range favors a diagnosis of SVT with aberration, while left axis deviation[5] or right axis deviation[5] favors a diagnosis of VT. Certainly, extreme right axis or left axis deviation ("northwest axis") is seldom seen in instances other than VT.

6.  Slight irregularity in tachycardia cycle length may be seen with VT or SVT and is generally not helpful in diagnosis. Of course, striking irregularity should suggest atrial fibrillation and conduction over an accessory pathway should be suspected when the rate in the latter exceeds 200/min.

7.  The rate of tachycardia is of no value in distinguishing VT from SVT.

8.  An abrupt change from one regular wide QRS morphology to another wide QRS morphology is infrequently seen in SVT and suggests VT with multiple morphologies (Fig. 13-5).

9.  Identification of isolated ectopic complexes during sinus rhythm identical to that observed during the wide QRS tachycardia may be helpful in identifying the latter (Fig. 13-6). If an isolated ectopic complex is clearly a PVC, it is likely that wide QRS tachycardia of the same morphology is ventricular. This can be misleading with single-lead recordings.

10. Concordance of QRS complexes in the precordial leads is rarely seen in SVT with aberration and strongly supports a diagnosis of VT.5–7 Positive concordance (QRS predominantly

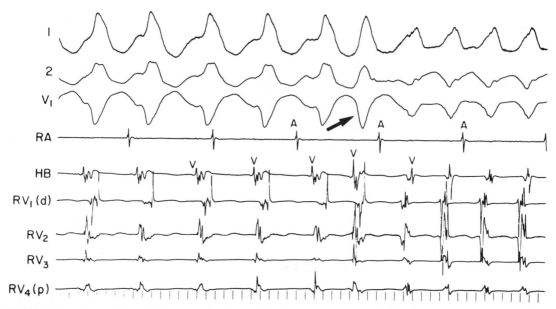

*Figure 13-5*   Abrupt change from one to another wide QRS morphology. The QRS morphology changes abruptly at the arrow. There is also AV dissociation in this patient with VT. HB = His bundle, RA = right atrium, $RV_1$ to $RV_4$ = 4 poles of a quadripolar catheter in the right ventricle.

positive from $V_1$ to $V_6$) suggests a posterobasal origin of VT while negative concordance suggests an anteroapical localization.[6]

11.  In the absence of preexcitation or bundle branch block during sinus rhythm, a number of morphologic features of the QRS complex generally in $V_1$ and $V_6$ have been categorized[6,7,12] and cataloged as to their frequency of occurrence in VT or SVT with aberration (Figs. 13-7 and 13-8). In distinguishing right bundle branch block aberration from VT resembling right bundle branch block, a typical triphasic pattern in $V_1$ favors aberrancy as does a qRs complex in $V_6$ (R greater than s). An rS or a QS complex in $V_6$ favors a diagnosis of VT. To distinguish left bundle branch block aberration from VT resembling left bundle branch block, $V_1$ may be similarly helpful. A typical left bundle branch block pattern in $V_1$ generally has a small initial r wave (less than 30 ms), with a steeply down-sloping S wave. When the initial r is greater than 30 ms in

duration and the down slope of the S wave is broad and notched, a diagnosis of VT is more likely (Fig. 13-8). $V_6$ is less helpful, but a qR or a QS complex favors VT.

### ECG Criteria in Perspective

Are the above criteria an incomprehensible mass of empirical observations to be memorized or can these criteria be logically understood? We have said that the most common types of aberration are due to functional right bundle branch block or left bundle branch block. Thus, it is apparent that right bundle branch block aberration should in general have the characteristics of "typical" right bundle branch block as described in standard textbooks[13,14] (see also Chap. 3). The same obviously holds true for left bundle branch block. Ventricular tachycardia can only be confused with bundle branch block when the activation pattern in VT results in a QRS complex that closely *resembles* right bundle branch block or left bundle branch block. However, when VT mimics

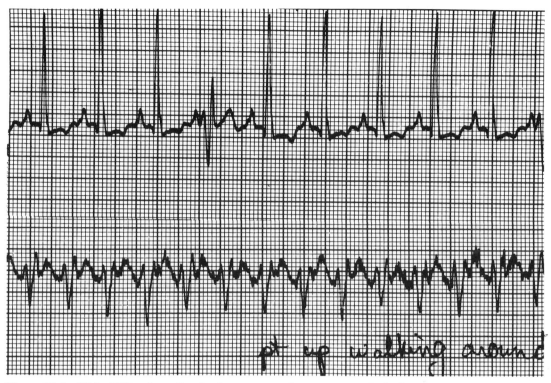

*Figure 13-6*   Wide QRS tachycardia. In the upper panel, a premature QRS (fourth cycle) interrupts the PR segment and (in the known absence of preexcitation) must be a premature ventricular depolarization. This makes it highly probable that the tachycardia in the lower panel (identical to the identified ventricular ectopic) is ventricular.

bundle branch block, the QRS pattern will generally be "atypical" to varying degrees. This is really the unifying concept that brings some order to the criteria listed above. That is, when a wide QRS tachycardia is absolutely typical of a classic right bundle (or left bundle) branch block pattern (Fig. 13-9) it is logical that it is more likely to be a true right bundle (or left bundle) branch pattern. Conversely, the more "atypical" the bundle branch block pattern, the more likely the tachycardia is to be ventricular. *When we use the above QRS criteria, we are essentially saying that a very "typical" bundle branch block pattern is indeed more likely to be SVT with bundle branch block and a very "atypical" one is more likely to be VT masquerading as bundle branch block.* An understanding of this principle immediately makes it possible to appreciate the limitations of these

generally very useful criteria. Antiarrhythmic drugs and organic heart disease can distort the QRS complex and result in "atypical" bundle branch block patterns even in the presence of SVT with aberration. It is thus intuitively obvious that the criteria would be most helpful when the underlying QRS in sinus rhythm is normal. Second, VT originating near the bundle branch system or incorporating the bundle branch system may more closely resemble "typical" bundle branch block patterns and thus be mistaken for SVT with aberration. Finally, preexcited tachycardias involve direct ventricular activation over an accessory AV pathway that bypasses the normal AV conduction system. Ventricular depolarization would then be expected to be identical to VT originating at a site near the distal insertion of the accessory pathway. It is thus obvious that preexcited tachycardia can never

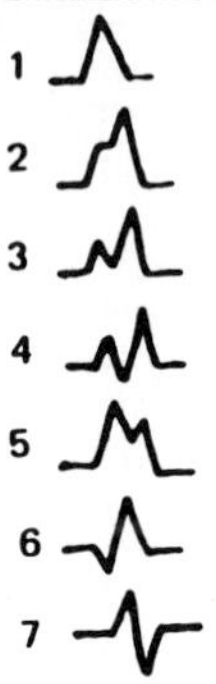

| Type Complex | QRS Configuration in Lead V$_1$ | |
| --- | --- | --- |
| | Aberrant | Ventricular Tachycardia |
| 1 | – | 12 |
| 2 | 7 | 9 |
| 3 | 12 | 2 |
| 4 | 28 | 2 |
| 5 | – | 4 |
| 6 | 1 | 12 |
| 7 | – | 4 |
| | 48 | 45 |

A

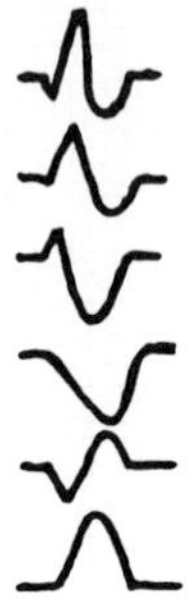

| Type Complex | Aberrant | Ventricular Tachycardia |
| --- | --- | --- |
| 1 | 31 | 2 |
| 2 | 15 | 10 |
| 3 | 2 | 18 |
| 4 | – | 11 |
| 5 | – | 3 |
| 6 | – | 1 |
| | 48 | 45 |

B

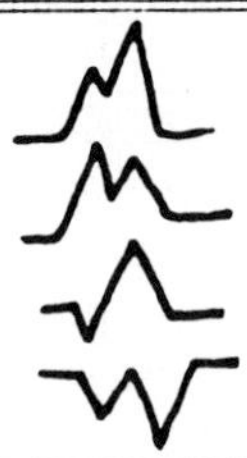

| Type Complex | Aberrant | Ventricular Tachycardia |
| --- | --- | --- |
| 1 | 10 | 11 |
| 2 | 12 | 10 |
| 3 | – | 3 |
| 4 | – | 1 |
| | 22 | 25 |

C

*Figure 13-7*   QRS morphology in aberration and VT. The relative frequency of VT and SVT with aberration is documented in panels *A, B,* and *C* in a manuscript from Wellens et al.[7] *(From Wellens HJJ:* Am J Med 64:27, 1978. *Reproduced by permission.)*

be distinguished from VT by morphological criteria unless one is an expert at pattern recognition or knows that the patient has the Wolff-Parkinson-White syndrome.

## Ancillary Investigations

Although the history, physical examination, and 12-lead ECG should provide a diagnosis in the majority of instances, it is worth remembering a few points that could be helpful in difficult cases. The presence of AV dissociation results in a beat by beat variability of chamber size, ejection times, and hemodynamics. Consequently, the presence or absence of AV dissociation is readily evident on an M mode echocardiogram.[16,17] The variation in mitral valve opening time in particular is usually striking in the presence of AV dissociation (Fig. 13-10). Esophageal electrocardiography can be done with routinely available equipment including an ECG cart, alligator connectors, and a pacing lead[18] (see Chap. 18). A bipolar permanent pacing lead is especially suitable for this purpose and can be advanced through the nares into

# V₁ AND V₂

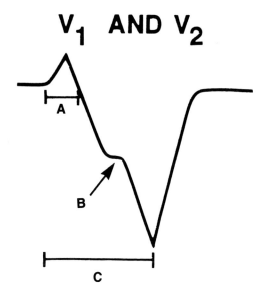

*Figure 13-8* Distinction of VT from aberrancy with left bundle branch block in $V_1$. With left bundle branch block morphology, features favoring VT in lead $V_1$ include initial r greater than 30 ms *(A)*, a notch in the down slope of the s wave *(B)*, and the interval from the QRS onset to the nadir *(C)* greater than 70 ms. *(From Wellens HJJ, Brugada P: Cardiology Clinics. Saunders, Philadelphia, 1987. Reproduced by permission.)*

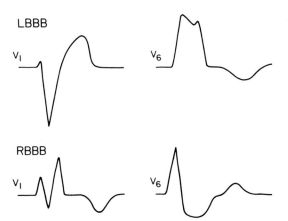

*Figure 13-9* Typical right bundle branch block (RBBB) and left bundle branch block (LBBB). In LBBB, $V_1$ has a small r and a deep S with a rapid down slope. In RBBB, $V_1$ typically is triphasic, with the initial R of lesser amplitude than the subsequent $R_1$. $V_6$ has a terminal s that is widened and of less amplitude than the initial R.

the esophagus as far as it will go. The bipolar leads are then connected to the right- and left-arm leads of the ECG, respectively, and lead 1 is monitored. The pacing lead is then withdrawn slowly until an adequate atrial deflection is visualized. Electrophysiologic testing using intracardiac recording and programmed stimulation should rarely be required for the initial diagnosis, although ultimately it is the most accurate and predictable way of determining the mechanism of tachycardia.

A pharmacologic test that would readily distinguish VT from SVT with aberration would be very useful in the emergency setting. The ideal pharmacologic agent would have to be safe regardless of the mechanism of tachycardia and specific for one mechanism. Verapamil is generally very specific for prolonging AV nodal conduction and refractoriness and terminating paroxysmal SVT while generally being ineffective in VT. Unfortunately, verapamil is a peripheral vasodilator and has negative inotropic properties which create a dangerous situation in many patients with VT.[8,9] Adenosine or adenosine triphosphate may prove to be useful for this purpose. When administered intravenously by rapid bolus, adenosine results in a marked transient increase in AV nodal conduction time and refractoriness. The effect of this agent is too transient (seconds) to have any serious adverse consequences, but it generally serves to terminate paroxysmal SVT, utilizing the AV node as a critical link, or at least to cause transient AV block in cases of atrial tachycardia or flutter with aberrant QRS conduction (Fig. 13-11).[19] Therefore adenosine may well become a useful "diagnostic test" for VT versus SVT, although it must be remembered that some types of VT can be adenosine-sensitive.

## Acute Therapy

It is evident that therapy for wide QRS tachycardia depends on the specific arrhythmia diagnosis if this is known with some degree of confidence. When tachycardia is associated with cardiovascular collapse

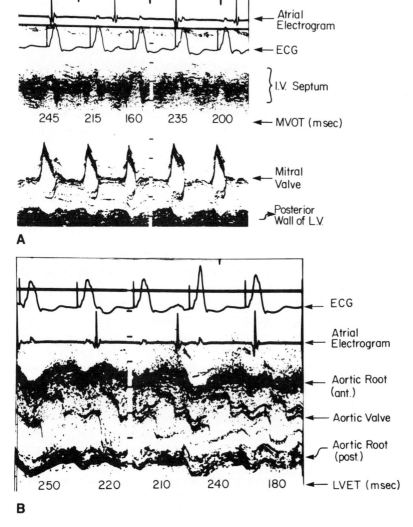

Atrial
Electrogram

ECG

} I.V. Septum

245   215   160   235   200   ← MVOT (msec)

Mitral
Valve

Posterior
Wall of L.V.

**A**

ECG

Atrial
Electrogram

Aortic Root
(ant.)

Aortic Valve

Aortic Root
(post.)

250   220   210   240   180   ← LVET (msec)

**B**

*Figure 13-10*   M-mode echo-cardiography with AV dissocia-tion. In this example of AV dissociation with ventricular pacing, there is a striking vari-ability of mitral valve opening time (MVOT) *(A)* and ejection time (LVET) *(B)*. MVOT is the time from mitral opening to mitral closure while LVET is the time from aortic valve opening to closure. The vari-ability in MVOT and LVET reflects variability of stroke vol-ume with AV dissociation.

or severe hemodynamic compromise, cardioversion is always appropriate and does not require knowledge of the mechanism of tachycardia. A 12-lead ECG should be done, if possible, before cardioversion. Situations will arise, however, where the physician is confronted with a hemodynamically stable wide QRS tachycardia in the emergency setting but is unsure of the mechanism of tachycardia. Certainly, verapamil is not to be used in this setting unless ventricular tachycardia (with rare exceptions[20]) has been ruled out. In this setting, a class 1 agent such as procainamide is a reasonable choice, as it would have efficacy for both VT and SVT. A reasonable sequence of interventions in an unknown tachycardia might include adenosine, procainamide, lidocaine, and cardioversion.

**A**

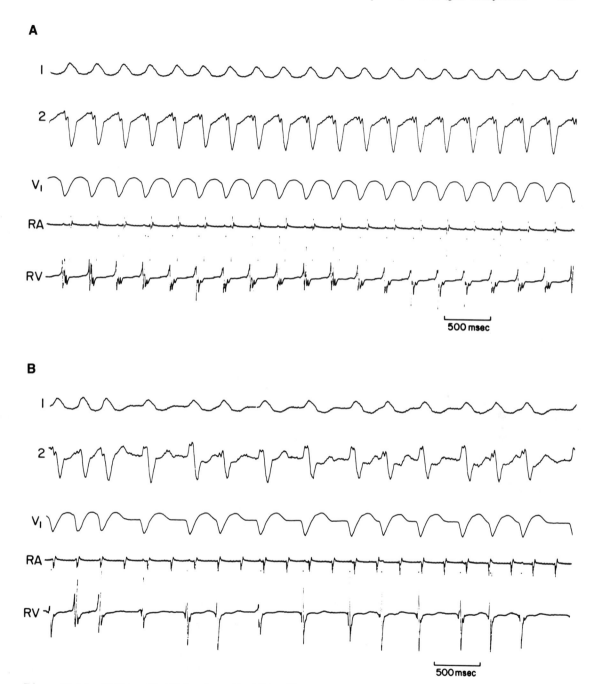

**B**

*Figure 13-11*   ATP in wide QRS tachycardia. This wide QRS tachycardia has a 1 : 1 AV relationship (panel *A*). An intravenous bolus of ATP, 20 mg, results in continuation of atrial tachycardia in the presence of AV block (panels *B* and *C*) and establishes the diagnosis.

**C**

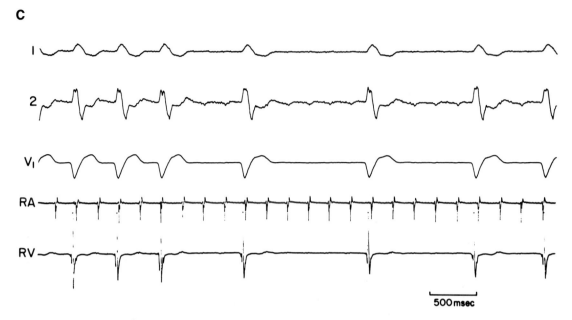

*Figure 13-11 (Continued)*

## Illustrative Cases (Fig. 13-12–13-17)

**EXAMPLE 1 (FIG. 13-12):** The patient is a 43-year-old man presenting with tachycardia 3 weeks after myocardial infarction. There is a suggestion of "capture-fusion" beats (lead $V_5$, arrow), but p waves are clearly not seen. The QRS morphology resembles RBBB but is atypical (see $V_1$, $V_6$). The diagnosis is VT.

**EXAMPLE 2 (FIG. 13-13):** The patient is a 35-year-old woman with a history of recurrent paroxysmal tachycardia since childhood. A typical LBBB morphology is observed. A working diagnosis of SVT with aberration is indicated and was confirmed at electrophysiologic study.

**EXAMPLE 3 (FIG. 13-14):** The patient is a 63-year-old man who presented with tachycardia 3 years after uncomplicated myocardial infarction. AV dissocia-

tion is not clearly evident. The QRS resembles RBBB but is quite "atypical" (Fig. 13-9). A working diagnosis of VT is appropriate and was confirmed at electrophysiology study.

**EXAMPLE 4 (FIG. 13-15):** The patient is a 54-year-old woman with cardiomyopathy. The QRS resembles LBBB but the QRS duration is 160 ms. AV dissociation is not evident. Nonetheless, a working diagnosis of VT should be made on the basis of history.

**EXAMPLE 5 (FIG. 13-16):** The patient is a 38-year-old man with cardiomyopathy. AV dissociation is evident in $V_1$ (arrows indicate P waves). The QRS morphology resembles LBBB but is atypical (Fig. 13-8). Some variability of the QRS is probably related to fusion complexes. The diagnosis of ventricular tachycardia was confirmed at electrophysiology study.

**EXAMPLE 6 (FIG. 13-17):** The patient is a 21-year-old man with recurrent paroxysmal tachycardia and no history of cardiac disease. The tachycardia recorded

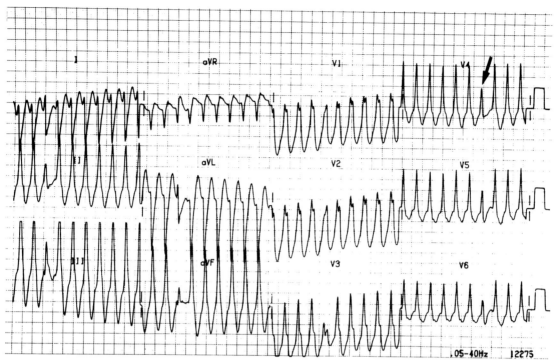

*Figure 13-12*

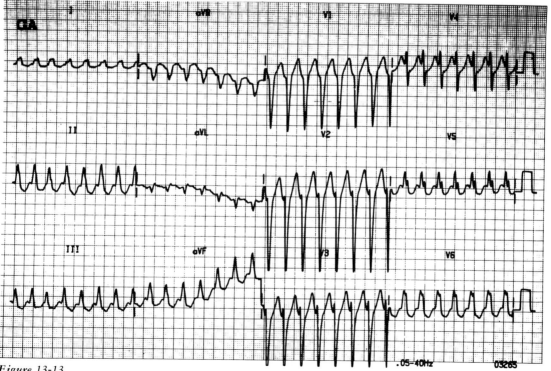

*Figure 13-13*

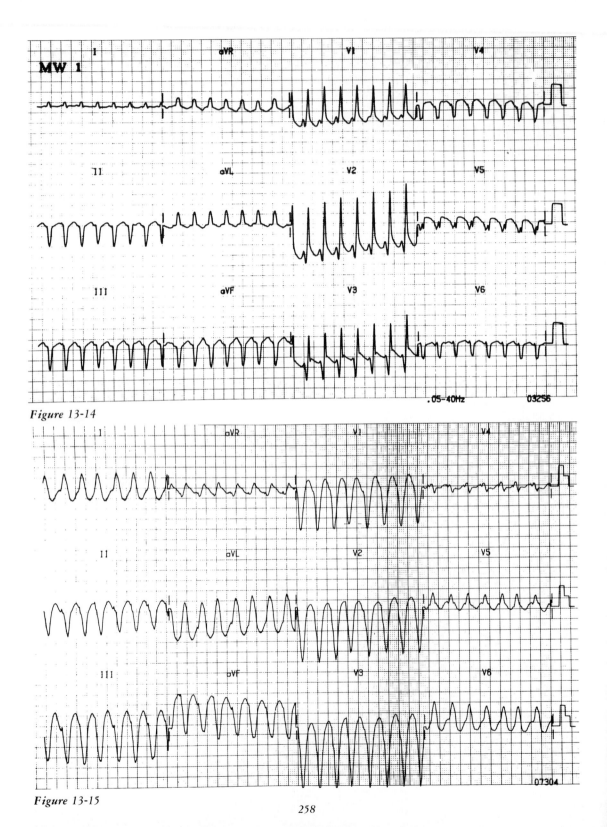

MW 1

.05=40Hz    03256

Figure 13-14

07304

Figure 13-15

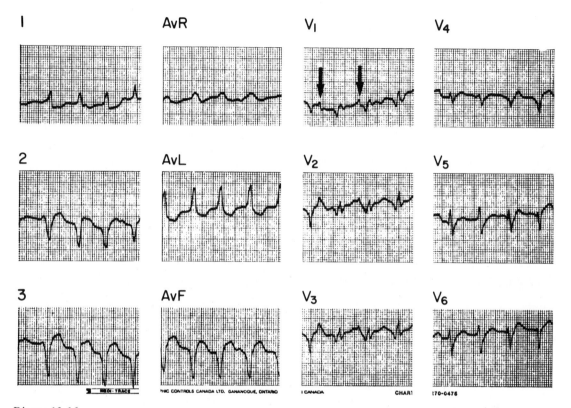

I    AvR    V₁    V₄

2    AvL    V₂    V₅

3    AvF    V₃    V₆

*Figure 13-16*

in panel A may be VT or preexcited tachycardia. The resting ECG shows a short PR interval (panel B), but preexcitation is only clearly evident with coronary sinus pacing (panel C). The similarity of panels *A* and *C* supports the diagnosis of preexcited tachycardia, which was shown to be antidromic at electrophysiological testing.

## Commentary

In the majority of instances, a diagnosis in wide QRS tachycardia should be made on the basis of history, physical examination, and ECG analysis (Table 13-1). If the physician is uncertain of the

*Table 13-1   Acute Assessment of Wide QRS Tachycardia*

- History . . . age, previous myocardial infarct

- Examination . . . evidence for AV dissociation

- ECG . . . AV dissociation, "typical" or "atypical" bundle branch block pattern

- Echocardiogram . . . variable mitral or aortic valve opening time

- Esophageal recording

- When in doubt, the working diagnosis is ventricular tachycardia!

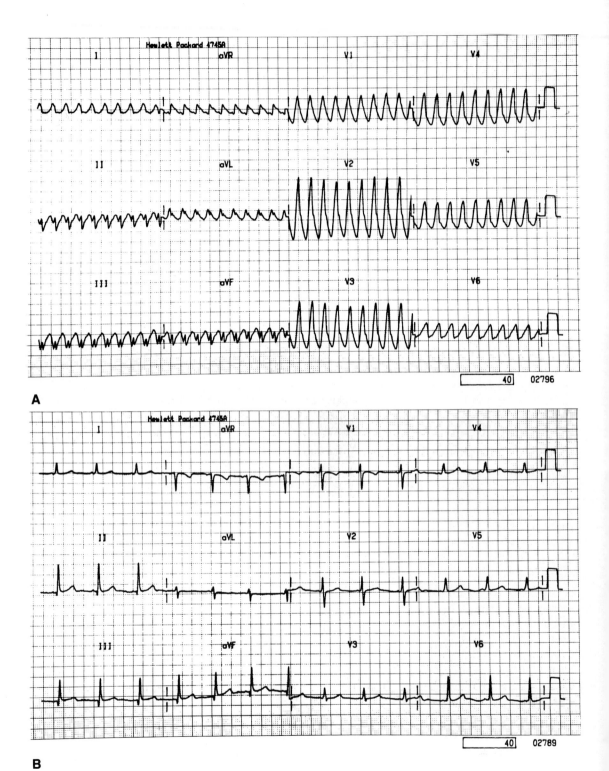

**A**

**B**

*Figure* 13-17

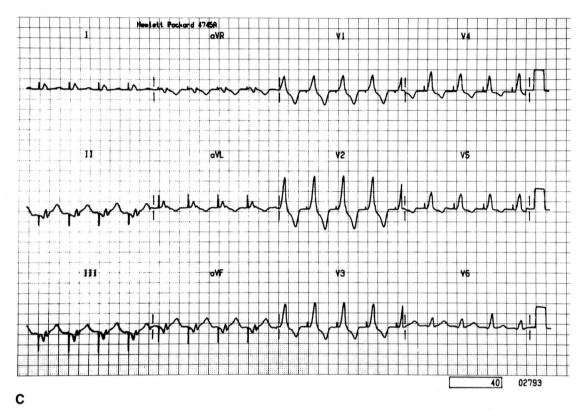

**C**

*Figure 13-17 (Continued)*

diagnosis after this, it is imperative that the working diagnosis be VT until proved otherwise. This is reasonable in that the great majority of adult patients presenting with wide QRS tachycardia are ultimately shown to have VT,[5,6] and therapy directed at VT is in most cases also appropriate for SVT. The converse is not always true, especially in the case of verapamil. The most common pitfall in diagnosis is to make a mistaken diagnosis of SVT with aberration instead of VT when the arrhythmia is "too well tolerated for VT" or the "QRS is not wide or bizarre enough for VT."

## References

1. Goldman MJ: Definitions of electrocardiographic configurations, in *Principles of Clinical Electrocardiography*. Lange, Los Altos, California, 1973.

2. Akhtar M: Electrophysiolgic bases for wide QRS complex tachycardia. *PACE* 6:81, 1983.

3. Miles WM et al: Evaluation of the patient with wide QRS tachycardia. *Med Clin North Am* 68:1015, 1984.

4. Watanabe Y: Terminology and electrophysiologic concepts in cardiac arrhythmias: I. Aberrant conduction. *PACE* 1:231, 1978.

5. Akhtar M et al: Role of electrophysiologic studies in supraventricular tachycardia, in Brugada P, Wellens HJJ (eds): *Cardiac Arrhythmias: Where to Go from Here*. Futura Publishing, Mount Kisco, New York, 1987, pp 233–242.

6. Wellens HJJ, Brugada P: Diagnosis of ventricular tachycardia from the 12-lead electrocardiogram, in Barold SS (ed): *Cardiology Clinics,* vol 5, no 3, *12-Lead Electrocardiography.* Saunders, Philadelphia, 1987, pp 511–525.

7. Wellens HJJ et al: The value of the electrocardiogram in the differential diagnosis of a tachycardia with a widened QRS complex. *Am J Med* 64:27, 1978.

8. Stewart RB et al: Wide complex tachycardia: Misdiagnosis and outcome after emergent therapy. *Ann Intern Med* 104:766, 1986.

9. Buxton AE et al: Hazards of intravenous verapamil for sustained ventricular tachycardia. *Am J Cardiol* 59:1107, 1987.

10. Morady F et al: A prevalent misconception regarding wide-complex tachycardias. *JAMA* 254:2790, 1985.

11. Schamroth L, Agathangelou N: QRS normalization by ventricular fusion. *PACE* 4:448, 1981.

12. Sandler JA, Marriott HJL: The differential morphology of anomalous ventricular complexes of RBBB-type in lead V1. *Circulation* 31:551, 1965.

13. Goldman MJ: Intraventricular conduction defects, in *Principles of Clinical Electrocardiography.* Lange, Los Altos, California, 1973.

14. Cooksey JD et al: *Clinical Vectorcardiography and Electrocardiography,* ed 2. Year Book, Chicago, 1977.

15. Coumel P: Diagnostic Significance of the QRS waveform in patients with ventricular tachycardia, in Bardol SS (ed): *Cardiology Clinics* Volume 5 #3 *12-Lead Electrocardiography.* Saunders, Philadelphia, 1987, pp 527–540.

16. Manyari DE et al: A simple echocardiographic method to detect atrioventricular dissociation: A useful aid in the differential diagnosis of regular tachycardia with wide QRS complexes. *Chest* 81:67, 1982.

17. Drinkovic N: Subcostal M-mode echocardiography of the right atrial wall for differentiation of supraventricular tachycardias with aberration from ventricular tachycardia. *Am Heart J* 107:326, 1984.

18. Hammill SC, Pritchett ELC: Simplified esophageal electrocardiography using bipolar recording leads. *Ann Intern Med* 95:14, 1981.

19. Sharma AD et al: ATP in wide QRS tachycardia (in preparation).

20. Klein GJ et al: Recurrent ventricular tachycardia responsive to verapamil. *PACE* 7:938, 1984.

# Chapter 14

# Undiagnosed Syncope, Dizzy Spells, Palpitations

## Transient Loss of Consciousness

The term *syncope* refers to a transient loss of consciousness due to temporary impairment of cerebral perfusion.[1] The differential diagnosis of transient loss of consciousness is very extensive and covers a broad spectrum of associated cardiac and noncardiac conditions.[1-3] The more common forms of syncope are listed in Table 14-1. Fortunately, the differential diagnosis can usually be narrowed considerably by a careful history and physical examination and some simple laboratory assessment.[4,5]

The broad goals of assessment in a patient presenting with syncope are threefold. The key goal,

### Table 14-1 Major Categories of Loss of Consciousness

A. Neurological
  i. Seizure
B. Cardiogenic/vascular
  i. Arrhythmic (bradycardia or tachycardia)
  ii. Hemodynamic, such as LV outflow obstruction, left atrial myxoma, pulmonary embolus, ischemia (rare), exertion with fixed cardiac output, pulmonary hypertension
  iii. Reflex peripheral vascular, such as vasovagal (most common), carotid hypersensitivity, micturition, cough and swallow syncope, orthostatis, vasodilating medications.
C. Miscellaneous
  i. Includes hysteria, hyperventilation, hypoglycemia

but often the most elusive, is the documentation of etiology during a spontaneous spell. Under ideal circumstances, the spell is witnessed by a physician, who documents physical findings, blood pressure, electrocardiogram (ECG), and perhaps even an electroencephalogram (EEG) during the episode. Failure to monitor or witness the episode is the fundamental difficulty in such patients and results in diagnosis by inference, with all its attendant vagaries. A secondary goal is the documentation of associated medical and, in particular, cardiac disease. This can considerably narrow the diagnostic possibilities. Finally, the third goal is to identify by laboratory testing abnormalities that suggest a potential diagnosis. Reproduction of symptoms by provocative maneuvers improves the degree of confidence of the implied diagnosis. In the absence of actual data during syncope, identification of abnormalities may provide the basis for a "therapeutic trial."

### Assessment

A careful history is perhaps the single most productive part of the diagnostic workup.[4] Obviously, the patient may be the least helpful person in providing this history, and every effort should be made to obtain the history from one or more reliable witnesses if these are available. The observations of ambulance attendants, who may be the first medical personnel to see the patient, may also be valuable. Syncope due to an arrhythmia is typically associated with a slight prodrome of light-headedness or no prodrome.

The period of loss of consciousness is relatively brief (a few minutes or less) and the patient generally awakes without any impairment of consciousness. A history of rapid heartbeat prior to syncope may suggest a rapid tachycardia as the cause, but patients with rapid tachycardia may have syncope without any awareness of a racing heart.

A thorough general physical examination with emphasis on the cardiovascular and neurologic systems is aimed at diagnosing conditions potentially associated with syncope. This examination should include assessment of blood pressure, both supine and upright, and carotid sinus massage.[6] This should be performed with ECG monitoring and caution when there is evidence for cerebrovascular disease. Initially, gentle massage is performed one side at a time on the right and left carotid sinus areas in the neck. This is followed by more aggressive pressure if no response is noted. Asystole longer than 3 s is suggestive of cardioinhibitory carotid sinus syndrome, while a marked fall in blood pressure even after the heart rate resumes suggests the vasodepressor variety. If initially negative, it is useful to repeat this maneuver on other occasions. Unfortunately, pauses of 3 s and longer can occur in the aged without a history of symptoms. Thus, a positive result without reproduction of symptoms must be interpreted with caution.

## Laboratory Assessment

Because syncope is sporadic and may be due to a wide range of disorders, it is difficult to recommend a list of laboratory investigations on a "cookbook" basis. Specific laboratory investigations must be guided by clues provided during the history and physical examination. It is intuitively obvious that no single test will be terribly rewarding or "cost-effective" if the etiology is not evident by the history and physical examination.[4,5,7,8] If seizures are not witnessed during syncope, it is rare to uncover a neurologic cause. In this situation extensive neurologic tests will usually not be productive. In the overtly normal patient with syncope, a broad laboratory search for medical disease is frequently pursued, with particular emphasis on cardiac and autonomic

reflex mechanisms. The most frequently used investigations include the following:

- The EEG
- The 12-lead ECG
- The graded treadmill exercise test
- The echocardiogram
- Ambulatory monitoring or transtelephonic monitoring
- Cardiac electrophysiologic assessment using intracardiac recording and programmed stimulation
- Upright tilt testing

### The Electroencephalogram

The EEG is frequently used but rarely helpful. It is probably unnecessary in a patient with a reliable history typical of cardiac syncope or where expert neurologic opinion deems it unlikely to be productive. It is reasonable to do an EEG where the history is vague and a seizure disorder cannot be ruled out with confidence.

### The 12-Lead Electrocardiogram

The 12-lead ECG is very valuable and may reveal preexcitation, conduction defects, myocardial infarction, or other abnormalities suggesting a possible cause of syncope. The ST segment and QT interval should be carefully examined for abnormalities suggesting the long QT syndrome. The arrhythmia associated with the latter, namely torsade de pointes ventricular tachycardia (VT), frequently presents as syncope or "seizure," and often the only diagnostic clue short of recording the ECG during an episode is the finding of a long QT interval on the standard ECG. Polymorphic VT unrelated to the QT syndrome can mimic torsade de pointes (Fig. 14-1).

### The Graded Treadmill Exercise Test

A graded treadmill exercise test is especially useful when syncope is associated with exercise. Its standard use is otherwise debatable, as syncope due to intermittent atrioventricular (AV) block or

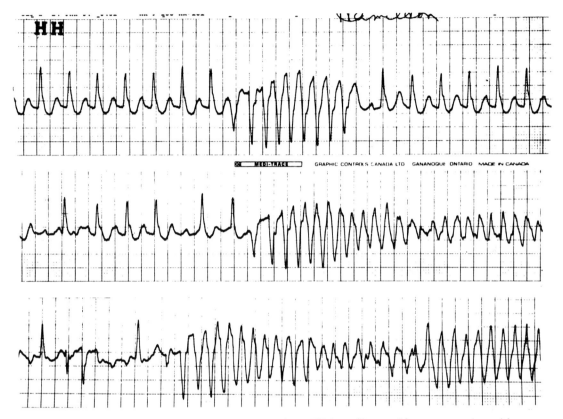

*Figure 14-1*  Documentation of spontaneous polymorphous VT in a 40-year-old man presenting with syncope. The arrhythmia occurs in a background of atrial flutter, raising the possibility of an alternative diagnosis of flutter with 1:1 AV conduction. The QT interval in this particular patient was normal.

tachycardia will rarely be exposed by this test. Treadmill testing is certainly indicated when silent myocardial ischemia is a consideration (Fig. 14-2), although ischemia per se is not a usual cause of syncope. In our view, this test is sufficiently inexpensive and noninvasive to justify its use if a cardiac cause of syncope is suspected.

### The Echocardiogram

The two-dimensional echocardiogram will again not be "cost-effective" when applied to a large population of patients with undiagnosed syncope. Nonetheless, it is an excellent test for detecting associated cardiac disease—such as left atrial myxoma, asymmetric septal hypertrophy, or early cardio-

myopathy—that may elude physical examination. The echocardiogram and ECG provide key data relating to presence or absence of cardiac disease which affects prognosis and subsequent evaluation (Ref. 9; Fig. 14-3). Electrophysiologic testing becomes an early consideration in patients with heart disease, while noninvasive tests are done initially in others (Fig. 14-3).

### Ambulatory Monitoring or Transtelephonic Monitoring

Ambulatory (Holter) monitoring is of most value in patients with frequent symptoms (several per week), since the probability is high that aggressive ambulatory monitoring will be successful in provid-

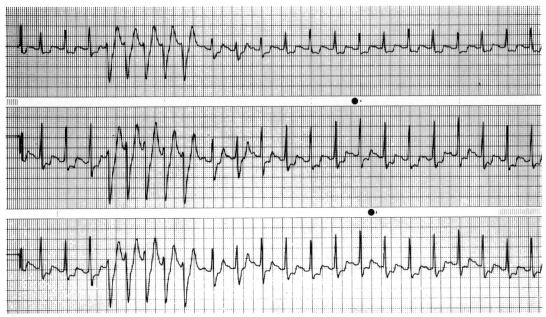

***Figure 14-2***  Ventricular tachycardia induced by ischemia during exercise testing in a diabetic man with syncope. The patient was presyncopal with longer runs of VT. During exercise, the ST segments became abnormal but the patient did not experience chest pain. At angiography, he had severe coronary heart disease. Leads $V_5$, $V_2$, and AVF are shown.

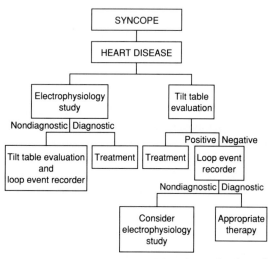

***Figure 14-3***  Suggested algorithm for evaluation of patients with syncope. (*Reproduced with permission from Prystowsky EN et al: Diagnostic evaluation and treatment strategies for patients at risk of serious cardiac arrhythmias: Part I. Syncope of unknown origin. Mod Concepts Cardiovasc Dis 60:49, 1991.*)

ing an ECG during a spell. Ambulatory monitoring for periods of 24 to 48 h is considerably less helpful in patients with infrequent episodes of syncope, since it is unlikely that the recording will be obtained during a spell. Nonetheless, arrhythmias and conduction abnormalities may be detected even during asymptomatic periods, and these can provide clues to the etiology of syncope.[10] One must be cautious in ascribing the cause of syncope to asymptomatic abnormalities, especially those that are frequently observed in populations without syncope. It is reasonable to assume that the more "serious" the abnormality, the more likely it is to be related to the cause of syncope, although this has not been proved; and any abnormality occurring in the absence of symptoms must be interpreted with caution. The optimal recording time has not been established. In general, the yield for recording longer than 24 h improves only slightly for patients with infrequent symptoms.[11,12] Patient-activated devices or transtelephonic monitors may be very useful in patients with infrequent episodes of syncope if the syncope is preceded by a prodrome sufficiently long to allow activation of the device. Even without a prodrome, such devices may be useful in the hands of a close companion or spouse who can be instructed on the use of the device in the event of syncope. Ambulatory loop ECG recorders are capable of storing the previous several minutes of ECG when activated by the patient and are generally more useful than hand-held devices in patients with syncope.[13] Clearly, none of these devices is practical in patients with episodes of syncope separated by months or years.

*Electrophysiologic Testing (Chap. 17)*

The techniques of intracardiac recording and programmed stimulation have proved very useful in the management of patients with paroxysmal tachycardia and these techniques have been utilized in the assessment of patients with loss of consciousness of unknown etiology. A typical protocol[14] would include the following:

1.  The recording of basic intervals, that is the (PA), atrio-His (AH), and His-ventricle (HV) intervals.
2.  Assessment of sinus node function, including determining the sinus node recovery time and the sinoatrial conduction time.
3.  Incremental atrial pacing (to induce arrhythmias and assess potential block below the His bundle) and incremental ventricular pacing.
4.  Atrial and ventricular extrastimulus testing at multiple sites and multiple cycle lengths to induce arrhythmias. It must be appreciated that the sensitivity of induced ventricular arrhythmias increases with the aggressiveness of the protocol, but specificity deteriorates (Fig. 14-4). In general, a ventricular arrhythmia induced with three or more extrastimuli is less likely to be related to reality than one induced with more conservative techniques unless the arrhythmia induced is sustained monomorphic VT, an arrhythmia rarely seen in normals.[15]

5.  Tests directed at assessing the integrity of the autonomic nervous system at electrophysiologic study.[16-18] For example, reversal of severe bradycardia or conduction abnormality with atropine suggests hypervagotonia,[18] while atrioventricular node conduction and refractoriness are highly dependent on autonomic tone.[17]

Electrophysiologic testing is a sensitive means of detecting abnormalities of AV conduction and inducing arrhythmias, but the yield is less with undiagnosed sick sinus syndrome.[19] Abnormalities are detected far more frequently than with ambulatory monitoring applied to the same patient.[20] Generally, the yield of abnormalities is lowest in patients without any evidence of heart disease[21] and highest in patients with organic heart disease,[7,20] forming the basis of the syncope workup proposed in Fig. 14-3. Predictors of a positive electrophysiologic study include an ejection fraction less than 40, left bundle branch block on the ECG, the presence of coronary artery disease, previous myocardial infarction, male gender, and injury sustained during syncope.[22] In addition, the inducibility of VT is much higher if late potentials can be recorded using signal-averaging techniques.[23] Of note, the presence of late potentials with a QRS duration $<110$ ms in a patient with no ventricular dysfunction is less specific. Most investigators have found a lower recurrence rate of syncope when treatment is based on the results of electrophysiologic testing (2 to 27 percent) than when no electrophysiologic abnormalities are detected or no efficacious therapy can be found at such testing (18 to 80 percent recurrence).[7,8,19,24] One large study, however, found absolutely no difference in recurrence rate of syncope when the results were guided by electrophysiologic testing.[20] Although data generally support the efficacy of electrophysiologic testing, the superiority of electrophysiologically guided versus empirical therapy has not been rigorously demonstrated. This would require a large study with randomization of patients to electrophysiologically guided and nonelectrophysiologically guided groups.

Currently, electrophysiologic testing is recom-

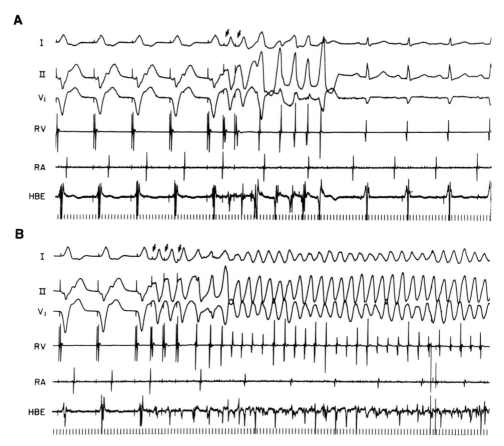

***Figure 14-4*** Induction of sustained polymorphous VT during electrophysiologic testing for syncope in a 54-year-old woman without heart disease. The significance of this arrhythmia is not clear, but it is generally thought to be nonspecific. The patient had no further syncope over 2 years of follow-up without treatment. Arrows indicate ventricular extrastimuli after a standard drive of 8 cycles.

mended in any patient with recurrent syncope when the diagnosis is not evident after noninvasive assessment and attempts to document the causes during syncope electrocardiographically. It should be used earlier in the evaluation of patients with heart disease. Because of the high spontaneous remission rate, electrophysiologic assessment is generally not recommended after a single syncopal spell in a patient without heart disease. Electrophysiologic testing is justified after a first episode of the patient has sustained a significant injury during the episode or if severe organic heart disease with a potential for a life-threatening arrhythmia is present.[7] The presence

of heart disease and inducible monomorphic VT in a patient with undiagnosed syncope carries a particularly unfavorable prognosis.[25] Syncope associated with advanced congestive heart failure carries an ominous prognosis regardless of etiology or results of electrophysiologic testing.[26]

Intuitively, the results of electrophysiologic testing would be expected to be most reliable when an abnormality is reproduced that exactly reproduces the patient's spontaneous symptoms. Otherwise, the results of electrophysiologic testing are merely inferential and, in effect, a therapeutic trial is embarked upon based on this inference. In theory, the more "severe" and specific the abnormality, the more likely it is to be related to the cause of syncope. It has been suggested[7,22] that these severe abnormalities include sinus node recovery time greater than 3 s, HV interval greater than 100 ms,[27] block below the His bundle during spontaneous or atrial paced rhythm when this cannot be explained by an Ashman phenomenon, unimorphic sustained VT and supraventricular tachycardia when it is secondary to AV nodal reentry or AV reentry.[14,21,28] A thorough electrophysiologic evaluation should be done since unexpected arrhythmic causes of syncope may be found—for example, VT in patients with ventricular preexcitation.[29] Atrial flutter or fibrillation may be considered as potentially causative of syncope if it is sustained and reproduces the patient's spontaneous symptoms.

Unfortunately, patients with severe organic heart disease may exhibit several abnormalities[7,8,19] possibly suggesting both tachycardia and bradycardia. Patients with electrocardiographic left bundle branch block in particular may have both severe infra-His conduction abnormalities and inducible VT.[19,30] With multiple potential etiologies, it would appear reasonable to direct treatment at all abnormalities considered to be severe and specific based on the above criteria. Finally, the significance of a negative study is not clear. It certainly does not rule out a paroxysmal bradycardia (Fig. 14-5).[30]

### Upright Tilt Testing (Chap. 18)

Clinically, the classic "vasovagal" episode has been diagnosed by a history suggesting a typical precipitating event, prodrome, and sequelae.[32] More recently, it has been recognized that the classic presentation may be less frequent than a presentation with sudden and apparently unprecipitated loss of consciousness, especially in the younger patient without organic heart disease.[33] The tendency to "vasovagal" or "vasodepressor" syncope can be exposed by a relatively simple test—namely, upright tilt testing[33-35] as described in Chap. 18. Although the mechanism for an abnormal response is not definitively established, it is thought to be a reflex related to venous pooling, which leads to more aggressive left

ventricular contractility in a chamber with decreased volume.[36] Tilt testing can be used not only diagnostically but as an end point to assess therapy, with some suggestion that disopyramide[37] and beta blockade[34] may be useful to prevent or attenuate the response. The latter concept has recently been challenged in placebo-controlled trials which have failed to demonstrate efficacy for these agents.[38,39] Many issues remain to be resolved with upright tilt testing, such as standardization of protocols, reproducibility, sensitivity, and specificity, and use as an end point for drug therapy, but there is little doubt that it is a clinically useful test to expose the vasodepressor tendency in the patient with syncope of undetermined etiology. Tilt testing should precede electrophysiologic testing in the workup of patients, especially in younger patients without heart disease.

### Commentary

In spite of many scholarly publications on syncope, many clinicians still feel uneasy with our current management of these patients. Many facts conspire to make recurrent syncope a frustrating problem. The patient may relate a poor history or no witness may be available to describe the spell. Infrequent occurrences of syncope frustrate attempts to document the disorder electrocardiographically. The patient is frequently elderly, with chronic medical diseases and multiple potential etiologies for syncope.[40] The diagnostic workup may suggest no abnormalities or multiple abnormalities of unclear specificity. In the absence of ECG documentation during a spell, our therapy is essentially inferential, with variable degrees of confidence in the inference. Ultimately, what is really required is improved technology in the area of long-term physiologic recording in order to achieve our primary goal: the monitoring of physiologic parameters during an episode.[41]

Several points can be kept in mind even if a diagnosis has not been reached after extensive evaluation:

1.   The prognosis in patients with syncope is highly variable and depends on the prognosis

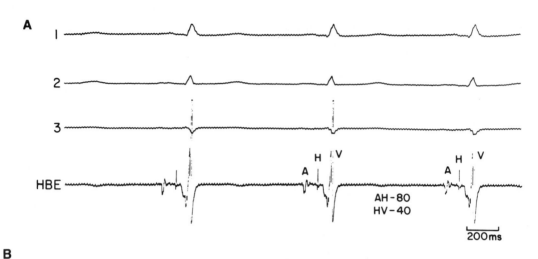

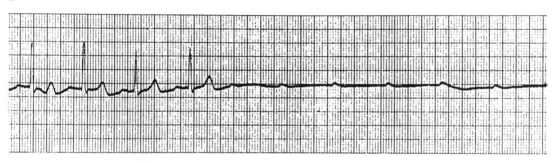

*Figure 14-5*    Panel *A* shows normal conduction intervals in a 55-year-old male with recurrent syncope. The anterograde Wenckebach cycle length was 380 ms. Panel *B* shows transient complete heart block, as subsequently recorded during spontaneous syncope.

of the pathologic process causing syncope.[4] A great deal of anxiety can be relieved by telling healthy patients without demonstrated medical disease that their prognosis is essentially good.

2. Recurrence of syncope is highly variable and spontaneous remission is frequent, especially after single episodes or clusters of episodes.[7,14,19,20]

3. Close companions or relatives can often be trained to take the pulse, listen to the chest for the heartbeat, or apply a transtelephonic monitor. Some patients do not find it difficult to adopt a "cautious" lifestyle until the prognosis is clear or until a diagnosis is made. This

would include refraining from driving and other situations where a loss of consciousness might cause serious injury to the patient or others.

Can an empirical trial of therapy without any corroborating data ever be considered? Empirical cardiac pacing in patients with a "typical" history of Stokes-Adams disease has met with some success,[21,42] although the number of patients has been limited and the high spontaneous remission rate makes this difficult to prove. Nonetheless, great pressure can be exerted in cases where syncope is recurrent, injury has occurred, and the workup is negative. In our opinion, a therapeutic trial of pacing may be advocated in selected instances; it has been advocated by others as a reasonable medical decision.[43]

## Undiagnosed Dizzy Spells and Palpitations

Symptoms of light-headedness, "dizzy spells," and palpitations occur very commonly and frequently do not have an arrhythmic basis when assessed with ambulatory monitoring.[10] A potential arrhythmic etiology can be assessed with routine ambulatory monitoring if the spells are sufficiently frequent or with a patient-activated monitor[12,44] if they are less frequent. At times, it may suffice to teach patients to take their own pulse during symptoms and report the result to the physician. More detailed investigation and, in particular, electrophysiologic testing are rarely indicated in these patients, as the essential diagnostic information should be obtainable by monitoring techniques. It may even be argued that episodes that are too brief or too infrequent to be assessed by patient-activated monitors are not worth investigating further. An exception may be the occurrence of presyncopal spells in a patient with heart disease. Electrophysiologic testing is justifiable if one is suspicious of VT in such a patient.

## References

1. Sobel BE, Roberts R: Hypotension and syncope, in Braunwald E (ed): *Heart Disease: A Textbook of Cardiovascular Medicine.* Saunders, Philadelphia, 1984, p 932.

2. Thomas JE, Hammill SC: Syncopal disorders, in Brandenburg RO, Fuster V, Giuliani ER, et al (eds): *Cardiology—Fundamentals and Practice.* Year Book, Chicago, 1987, p 689.

3. Weissler AM, Warren JV: Syncope: Pathophysiology and differential diagnosis, in Hurst JW, Logue RB, Rackley CE, et al (eds): *The Heart: Arteries and Veins.* McGraw-Hill, New York, 1986, p 507.

4. Kapoor W et al: A prospective evaluation and follow up of patients with syncope. *N Engl J Med* 308:197, 1983.

5. Day SC et al: Evaluation and outcome of emergency room patients with transient loss of consciousness. *Am J Med* 73:15, 1982.

6. Davies AB et al: Carotid sinus hypersensitivity in patients presenting with syncope. *Br Heart J* 42:583, 1979.

7. Morady F: The evaluation of syncope with electrophysiologic studies. *Cardiol Clin* 4:515, 1986.

8. Olshanksky B et al: Significance of inducible tachycardia in patients with syncope of unknown origin: A long term follow up. *J Am Coll Cardiol* 5:216, 1985.

9. Prystowsky EN et al: Diagnostic evaluation and treatment strategies for patients at risk of serious cardiac arrhythmias: Part I. Syncope of unknown origin. *Mod Concepts Cardiovasc Dis* 60:49, 1991.

10. Gibson TC, Heitzman MR: Diagnostic efficacy of 24 hour electrocardiographic monitoring for syncope. *J Am Coll Cardiol* 53:1013, 1984.

11. Hertzeanu H et al: Holter monitoring in dizziness and syncope. *Acta Cardiol* 34:775, 1979.

12. Lewis RP et al: Arrhythmic syncope: What to do when ambulatory monitoring is non-diagnostic. *Trans Am Clin Climatol Assoc* 96:131, 1984.

13. Linzer M et al: Incremental diagnostic yield of loop electrocardiographic recorders in unexplained syncope. *Am J Cardiol* 66:214, 1990.

14. Bachinsky WB et al: Usefulness of clinical characteristics in predicting the outcome of electrophysiologic studies in unexplained syncope. *Am J Cardiol* 69:1044, 1992.

15. Brugada P et al: Results of a ventricular stimulation protocol using a maximum of 4 premature stimuli in patients without documented or suspected ventricular arrhythmias. *Am J Cardiol* 52:1214, 1983.

16. Jordan JL et al: Studies on the mechanism of sinus node dysfunction in the sick sinus syndrome. *Circulation* 57:217, 1978.

17. Mann DE et al: Effects of upright posture on anterograde and retrograde atrioventricular conduction in patients with coronary artery disease, mitral valve prolapse or no structural heart disease. *Am J Cardiol* 60:625, 1987.

18. McLaran CJ et al: Increased vagal tone as an isolated finding in patients undergoing electrophysiological testing for recurrent syncope: Response to long term anticholinergic agents. *Br Heart J* 55:53, 1986.

19. Teichman SL et al: The value of electrophysiologic studies in syncope of undetermined origin: Report of 150 cases. *Am Heart J* 110:469, 1985.

20. Doherty JU et al: Electrophysiologic evaluation and follow-up characteristics of patients with recurrent unexplained syncope and presyncope. *Am J Cardiol* 55:703, 1985.

21. Gulamhusein S et al: Value and limitations of clinical electrophysiologic study in assessment of patients with unexplained syncope. *Am J Med* 73:700, 1982.

22. Krol RB et al: Electrophysiologic testing in patients with unexplained syncope: Clinical and noninvasive predictors of outcome. *J Am Coll Cardiol* 10:358, 1987.

23. Gang ES et al: Detection of late potentials on the surface electrocardiogram in unexplained syncope. *Am J Cardiol* 58:1014, 1986.

24. Olshansky B et al: Significance of inducible tachycardia in patients with syncope of unknown origin: A long-term follow-up. *J Am Coll Cardiol* 5(2 pt 1):216, 1985.

25. Bass EB et al: Long-term prognosis of patients undergoing electrophysiologic studies for syncope of undetermined origin. *Am J Cardiol* 62:1186, 1988.

26. Middlekauff HR et al: Syncope in advanced heart failure: High risk of sudden death regardless of origin of syncope. *J Am Coll Cardiol* 21:110, 1993.

27. Scheinman MM et al: Value of the HQ interval in patients with bundle branch block and the role of prophylactic permanent pacing. *Am J Cardiol* 50:1316, 1982.

28. Yee R, Klein GJ: Syncope in the Wolff-Parkinson-White syndrome: Incidence and electrophysiologic correlates. *PACE* 7(3 pt 1):381, 1984.

29. Lloyd EA et al: Syncope and ventricular tachycardia in patients with ventricular preexcitation. *Am J Cardiol* 52:79, 1983.

30. Ezri M et al: Electrophysiologic evaluation of syncope in patients with bifascicular block. *Am Heart J* 106:693, 1983.

31. Fujimura O et al: The diagnostic sensitivity of electrophysiologic testing in patients with syncope caused by transient bradycardia. *N Engl J Med* 321:1703, 1989.

32. Weissler AM, Warren JV: Vasodepressor syncope. *Am Heart J* 57:786, 1959.

33. Almquist A et al: Provocation of bradycardia and hypotension by isoproterenol and upright posture in patients with unexplained syncope. *N Engl J Med* 320:346, 1989.

34. Waxman AM et al: Isoproterenol induction of vasodepressor-type reaction in vasodepressor-prone persons. *Am J Cardiol* 63:58, 1989.

35. Fitzpatrick AP et al: Methodology of head-up tilt testing in patients with unexplained syncope. *J Am Coll Cardiol* 17:125, 1991.

36. Rea AF: Neurally mediated hypotension and bradycardia: Which nerves? How mediated? *J Am Coll Cardiol* 14:1633, 1989.

37. Milstein S et al: Usefulness of disopyramide for prevention of upright tilt-induced hypotension-bradycardia. *Am J Cardiol* 65:1339, 1990.

38. Brignole M et al: A controlled trial of acute and long-term medical therapy in tilt-induced neurally mediated syncope. *Am J Cardiol* 70:339, 1992.

39. Morillo CA et al: A placebo controlled trial of intravenous and oral disopyramide for prevention of neurally mediated syncope induced by head-up tilt. *J Am Coll Cardiol* (in press) 1993.

40. Lipsitz LA: Syncope in the elderly. *Ann Intern Med* 99:92, 1983.

41. Murdock CJ et al: Feasibility of long-term electrocardiographic monitoring with an implanted device for syncope diagnosis. *PACE* 13:1374, 1990.

42. Klein GJ, Gulamhusein S: Arrhythmias as a cause of syncope (editorial). *Stroke* 13:746, 1982.

43. Kwoh CK et al: Repeated syncope with negative diagnostic evaluation: To pace or not to pace. *Med Decis Making* 4:351, 1984.

44. Fogel RI et al: Are event recorders useful and cost effective in the diagnosis of palpitations, presyncope and syncope? *Circulation* 21:358A, 1933.

# Chapter 15

# *Cardiac Arrest*

Sudden cardiac death is a major epidemiologic problem in the United States; it is estimated that a patient dies from this disorder once every minute.[1] The prevalence of sudden cardiac death varies with the population studied, but it remains the most common cause of mortality in adults below age 65.[2] Cardiac arrest as a cause of sudden death is usually due to ventricular fibrillation (Fig. 15-1) or rapid sustained ventricular tachycardia, but it may be due to bradyarrhythmias in a smaller percentage of patients.[3-7] The usual victim of cardiac arrest is an individual with heart disease, most frequently coronary artery disease, with substantial left ventricular dysfunction. Thus, the workup of a patient who has been resuscitated from cardiac arrest requires a thorough history, physical examination, and laboratory evaluation to identify any reversible predisposing factors for recurrent cardiac arrest. Although not yet proven, efforts to identify and prophylactically treat patients at high risk for cardiac arrest may result in a decrease in the incidence of sudden death.

## History and Physical Examination

### History

The history is a critical part of the workup of the cardiac arrest victim. Diverse etiologies can lead to the common pathway of sudden cardiac death due to ventricular fibrillation, although most patients have some form of heart disease (Table 15-1). Coronary artery disease is the most common cardiac abnormality associated with sudden cardiac death.[8-11] Coronary angiography performed on 79 survivors of out-of-hospital cardiac arrest demonstrated that 64 (81 percent) patients had coronary artery disease, with approximately two-thirds having significant obstruction of two or three coronary arteries.[11] It is interesting to note that severe obstruction of the left main coronary artery was relatively rare in this series. In another study, Perper et al.[12] showed that a 75 percent or greater stenosis in three or four major coronary artery vessels was present in 61 percent of hearts identified at autopsy, and two vessels were involved in another 15 percent. Thus, significant coronary artery disease, whether identified at cardiac catheterization in survivors of cardiac arrest or from postmortem studies, is the most frequently associated heart disease in cardiac arrest patients in the industrialized world. For this reason it is critically important to obtain a complete and thorough history for angina pectoris, risk factors for coronary artery disease such as cigarette smoking, and a family history for atherosclerotic disease.

*Table 15-1    Common Conditions Associated with Sudden Cardiac Death*

Coronary artery disease
Cardiomyopathy
   Chronic
      Hypertrophic
      Dilated
   Acute myocarditis
Congenital heart disease
Electrophysiologic abnormalities
   Wolff-Parkinson-White syndrome
   Idiopathic ventricular tachycardia/fibrillation
   Long QT syndrome
Miscellaneous
   Proarrhythmia with drugs
   Electrolyte abnormalities

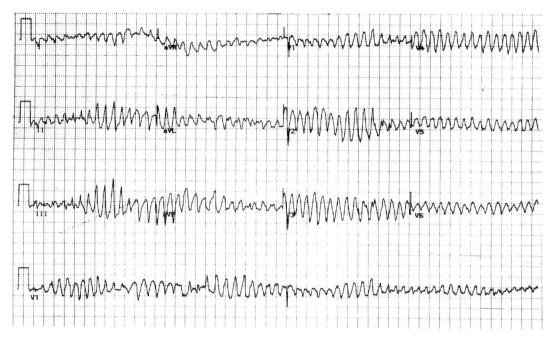

*Figure 15-1*    Twelve-lead ECG of ventricular fibrillation obtained at electrophysiologic study.

It is very important to determine whether cardiac arrest in a patient with coronary artery disease was related to an acute reversible cause such as acute myocardial infarction or Prinzmetal's angina. Proof that acute reversible ischemia without myocardial infarction initiated ventricular fibrillation will be very difficult in most patients unless they were undergoing electrocardiographic (ECG) monitoring at the time of the event or a witness was present to verify that the patient had symptoms of severe chest pain prior to collapse. The patient with cardiac arrest who undergoes resuscitative efforts almost always has recent memory loss and will not be able to recall the moments preceding loss of consciousness. Thus, the history from the patient regarding chest pain prior to cardiac arrest will be unreliable. Since myocardial damage does not occur due to the reversible ischemia, there will be no biochemical or electrocardiographic evidence of acute myocardial infarction. Practically then, reversible severe ischemia as the initiating factor for ventricular fibrillation will be very difficult to confirm in most instances by history alone.

Evidence of acute myocardial infarction is extremely important for prognostic purposes. Cobb and associates[13] evaluated 424 survivors of ventricular fibrillation and noted that the 1-year mortality was 2 percent in patients who had had an acute myocardial infarction and 22 percent in patients without evidence of acute infarction. Thus, it is important to evaluate carefully the history and other laboratory data necessary to diagnose acute myocardial infarction as the cause of cardiac arrest (Fig. 15-2A and B). It is interesting that the majority of patients successfully resuscitated from cardiac arrest have no evidence of acute myocardial infarction,[14] although the data from pathology studies are not as definitive.[15–17]

A history of congestive heart failure regardless of etiology is significant, and these individuals are at increased risk for sudden cardiac death.[18] It is particularly important to determine whether there is a familial history of sudden cardiac death for two reasons. First, this may be the initial clue to identification of a pathophysiologic abnormality such as hypertrophic or dilated cardiomyopathy or to the

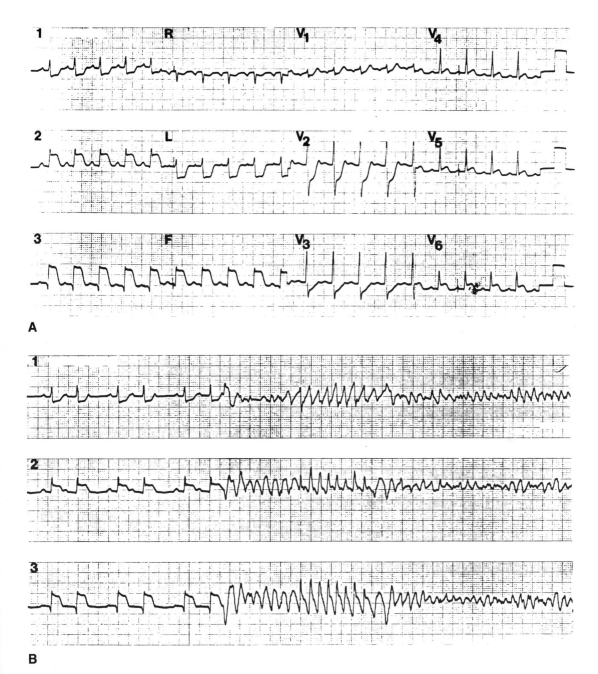

*Figure 15-2* Ventricular fibrillation as a consequence of acute myocardial infarction. *A.* Twelve-lead ECG demonstrating acute ischemic changes represented by ST elevation in leads II, III, aVF, and $V_4$–$V_6$, with reciprocal changes in other leads, in a patient who suffered an inferior-wall myocardial infarction. *B.* A continuous rhythm strip of ECG leads I, II, and III demonstrates both Wenckebach second-degree AV block on the left-hand side of the figure followed by ventricular fibrillation.

long-QT syndrome.[19-24] Second, recognition of a familial pattern of sudden cardiac death may enable the clinician to evaluate other family members at possible risk for ventricular fibrillation.

The history should include current medications the patient is taking, especially antiarrhythmic drugs or other agents known to prolong the QT interval; diuretics that have a propensity for lowering serum potassium levels; any nonprescription drugs—for example, decongestants; or illicit agents such as cocaine. These agents may by themselves or in combination with other factors lead to the development of life-threatening ventricular arrhythmias. Drugs that prolong the QT interval, especially in the presence of hypokalemia, can lead to torsade de pointes ventricular tachycardia that can degenerate into ventricular fibrillation. This arrhythmia tends to occur in patients treated with antiarrhythmic agents such as quinidine and is more likely to occur in the presence of bradycardia and hypokalemia. Proarrhythmic events with other drugs can also occur[25] (Fig. 15-3). It is very important to differenti-

ate a true tachyarrhythmia from artifact noted during ECG monitoring, which can lead to the wrong diagnosis (Fig. 15-4).

Other clues to etiologic factors may be a history of a recent viral illness that could cause myocarditis; a history of palpitations, presyncope, or syncope that suggests a tachyarrhythmia; or the association of exercise prior to onset of cardiac arrest. The latter might signify a causative role for enhanced sympathetic tone, underlying ischemia, or valvular dysfunction. Some generalized disorders—for example, systemic lupus erythematosus, scleroderma, or sarcoidosis—affect the heart, and their presence should be ascertained. Finally, it is often difficult to identify psychologic factors predisposing to ventricular fibrillation, although they are certainly operative in some individuals.

### Physical Examination

Physical examination may reveal the presence of cardiac disease or systemic manifestations of other

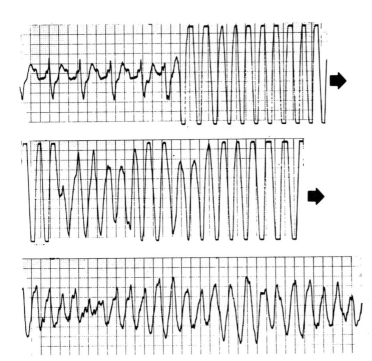

*Figure 15-3* Proarrhythmic effect during continuous telemetry monitoring in a patient receiving propafenone at 225 mg three times daily. The top ECG strip demonstrates sinus rhythm on the left followed by sustained rapid ventricular tachycardia that later degenerated into ventricular fibrillation. This patient was being treated for monomorphic sustained ventricular tachycardia and never previously experienced a polymorphic sustained ventricular arrhythmia.

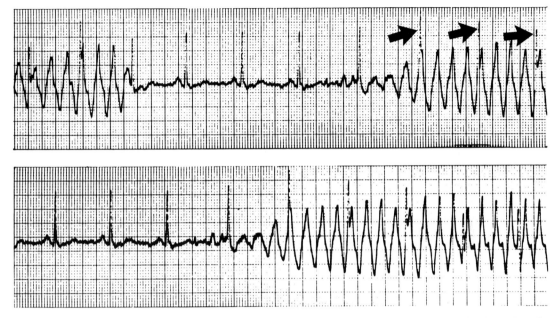

*Figure 15-4*  Artifact resembling malignant ventricular tachycardia during telemetry ECG monitoring. Note that the arrows point to continuous regular ventricular depolarizations throughout the apparent ventricular tachycardia that is actually artifact. One should always evaluate such rhythm strips by identifying regular QRS complexes with a pair of calipers and then "march" the calipers through the apparent ventricular tachycardia to determine whether regular ECG complexes are present. This will aid substantially in confirming the diagnosis of artifact.

diseases that could aggravate an underlying cardiac problem or by themselves be implicated in cardiac arrest. The cardiac exam may reveal an S3 or S4 gallop, suggestive of systolic and diastolic dysfunction, respectively. Cardiac murmurs may be detected, most importantly those of aortic outflow tract obstruction. Mitral valve prolapse with a click or murmur is a relatively common finding, but the incidence of sudden cardiac death in isolated mitral valve prolapse is relatively rare. Possible exceptions are patients with a family history of sudden cardiac death, prolongation of the QT interval, or substantial mitral regurgitation with redundant mitral valve leaflets. Evidence for atherosclerosis may be detected by findings of peripheral vascular disease such as decreased arterial pulses and the presence of xanthomas or xanthelasma. The neck should be palpated carefully to detect any thyromegaly, and peripheral signs of thyrotoxicosis should be sought. Many systemic

diseases, such as vasculitides and infiltrative disorders, can affect the heart. Thus, peripheral findings of disorders such as systemic lupus erythematosus, sarcoidosis, and other systemic disorders need to be investigated. Even with the most thorough physical examination, most patients have few findings suggestive of anything other than cardiac disease.

## Laboratory Evaluation

It is essential to perform serial cardiac enzymes and ECGs in patients resuscitated from cardiac arrest so as to determine whether an acute myocardial infarction has occurred. The ECG is also valuable to uncover conditions such as the long-QT syndrome, evidence of previous myocardial infarction, nonspecific findings suggestive of cardiomyopathy, and the presence of ventricular preexcitation. It is well documented that patients with Wolff-Parkinson-White syndrome can experience sudden cardiac death that is thought to occur by a rapid ventricular preexcited response during atrial fibrillation, degenerating into ventricular fibrillation.[26,27] Serum electrolytes may detect the presence of a predisposing condition such as marked hypokalemia, but the chemistry screen is usually unrevealing. A chest radiograph is important to evaluate cardiac as well as pulmonary abnormalities. Determination of left ventricular function is critically important, and we often use echocardiography for this purpose. Echocardiography yields data on ventricular function, ventricular size and wall thickness, and valvular function. In our estimation, it is the single most important noninvasive test to identify multiple forms of cardiac pathology. A 24-h ECG recording is minimally useful in a patient who has had cardiac arrest. However, continuous in-hospital ECG monitoring

may detect spontaneous ventricular fibrillation on rare occasions (Fig. 15-5). Thus, for both diagnostic and safety reasons, all patients hospitalized for evaluation of cardiac arrest should have continuous ECG monitoring.

Patients without an obvious precipitating cause for cardiac arrest should routinely have a treadmill exercise test, hemodynamic cardiac catheterization with cineangiography, and electrophysiologic evaluation. In our experience, it is relatively rare for a sustained ventricular tachyarrhythmia to emerge during exercise testing in survivors of cardiac arrest.[28] However, one such example of exercise-induced ventricular fibrillation in a patient resuscitated from cardiac arrest is shown in Fig. 15-6. In this patient, ventricular fibrillation occurred in the first few minutes after the end of the exercise test, a time not unusual for ventricular tachycardia or fibrillation to occur.[29] Cardiac catheterization is especially important to document the presence and severity of coronary artery disease and, as noted later, it is

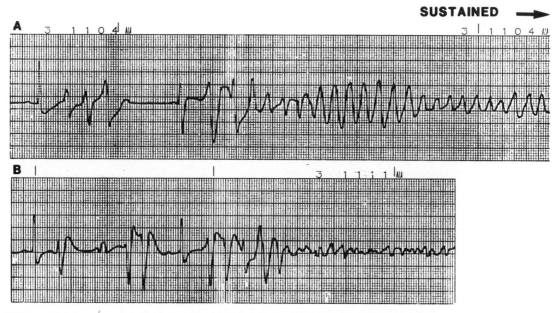

*Figure* 15-5   Ventricular fibrillation occurring spontaneously during in-hospital continuous ECG telemetry monitoring at 11:04 A.M. that was successfully defibrillated (A). At 11:11 A.M. VF recurred and again DC shock restored sinus rhythm (B).

SUSTAINED ➞

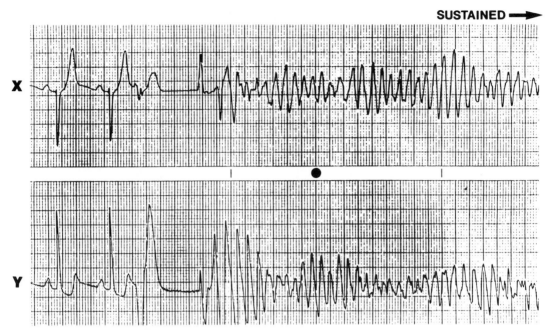

*Figure 15-6*   Ventricular fibrillation occurring in the first 3 min after termination of treadmill exercise testing in a patient with a history of cardiac arrest.

important to evaluate and treat all significant patho-physiologic disorders in survivors of cardiac arrest. Thus, patients with significant coronary artery disease may require specific antiarrhythmic therapy as well as anti-ischemic treatment.

A complete electrophysiologic evaluation should be performed unless an unequivocal precipitating cause for cardiac arrest is identified—for example, acute ischemia. This includes incremental atrial and ventricular pacing as well as programmed atrial and ventricular stimulation. In patients with ventricular preexcitation, induction of atrial fibrillation is a critical part of the study; in some patients, atrial fibrillation with a rapid preexcited ventricular response will degenerate into ventricular fibrillation (Fig. 15-7). This is a relatively rare cause of sudden cardiac death.[30,31] More common is the induction of sustained ventricular tachycardia or ventricular fibrillation at electrophysiologic study in a patient with underlying cardiac dysfunction.[32,33] Induction

of a sustained ventricular tachyarrhythmia depends on the type of heart disease and is more commonly seen in patients with coronary artery disease.[34] In a review of 1233 survivors of cardiac arrest undergoing electrophysiologic evaluation, 42 percent of patients had inducible sustained monomorphic ventricular tachycardia, while sustained polymorphic ventricular tachycardia or ventricular fibrillation was initiated in 16 percent of patients.[32] Thus, 42 percent of patients had either nonsustained ventricular tachycardia or no ventricular tachycardia initiated. Sustained monomorphic ventricular tachycardia induced at elec-trophysiologic study is considered a relatively specific arrhythmia identifying patients at risk for the sponta-neous occurrence of the same or similar tachycardia. In contrast, ventricular fibrillation initiated at electro-physiologic study may be a nonspecific finding in certain patients. We feel it is important to consider both the method of induction of ventricular fibrilla-tion as well as the patient in whom it is induced

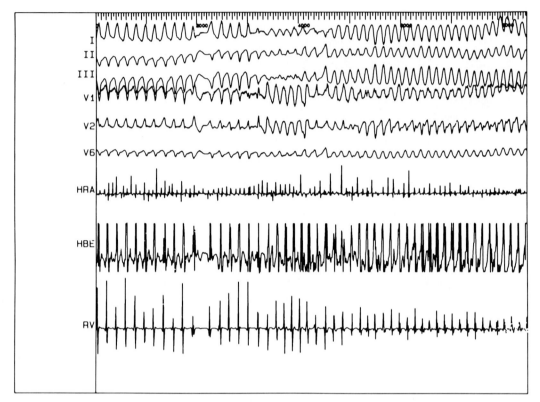

*Figure 15-7*    Atrial fibrillation degenerating into ventricular fibrillation in a patient with ventricular preexcitation. Atrial fibrillation is documented by the grossly irregular and rapid atrial arrhythmia noted on the high right atrial (HRA) endocardial recording. The left-hand portion of the figure demonstrates a rapid ventricular rate due to conduction over an accessory pathway; the right-hand portion shows the degeneration of this rhythm into ventricular fibrillation that required DC shock. This was recorded during electrophysiologic testing.

prior to making a judgment regarding its specificity. For example, in our opinion, initiation of rapid sustained monomorphic ventricular tachycardia that subsequently degenerates into ventricular fibrillation using one ventricular extrastimulus or polymorphic ventricular tachycardia using two ventricular extrastimuli has relatively more specificity than initiation of ventricular fibrillation using close-coupled triple extrastimuli (Figs. 15-8 and 15-9). Although decidedly uncommon, triple ventricular extrastimuli at close-coupled intervals can initiate ventricular fibrillation in patients with normal ventricular function, as noted in Fig. 15-10 in a patient with Wolff-Parkinson-White syndrome without a history of

cardiac arrest. As with all tests in medicine, the electrophysiologic results must be integrated into the total patient evaluation prior to making any clinical judgment regarding specificity.

## General Approach to Therapy

The initial approach to therapy is to identify any potential reversible causes of cardiac arrest and correct them. Most patients who have a cardiac arrest have multiple problems but no clearly identifiable cause-

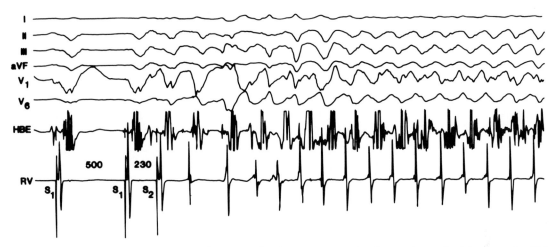

**Figure 15-8**   Rapid ventricular tachycardia initiated using one extra stimulus at electrophysiologic study. This rhythm quickly degenerated into ventricular fibrillation. (*From Knilans TK, Prystowsky EN: Antiarrhythmic drug therapy in the management of cardiac arrest survivors. Circulation 85(suppl I):I-118, 1992. Reproduced with permission from the American Heart Association.*)

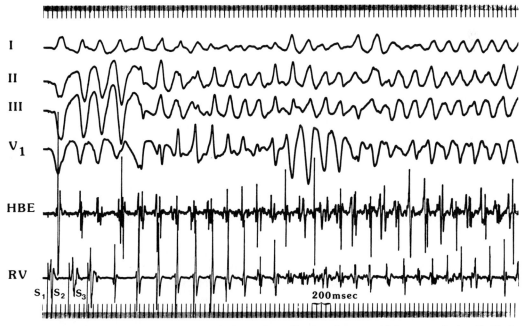

**Figure 15-9**   Initiation of polymorphic ventricular tachycardia that degenerated into ventricular fibrillation at electrophysiologic study using two extrastimuli ($S_2$ and $S_3$).

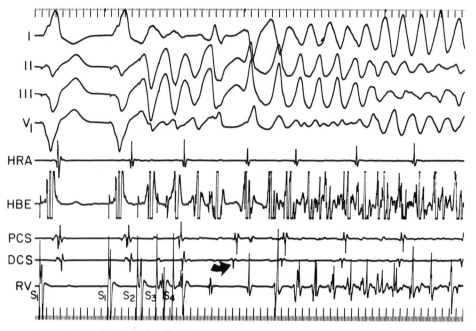

***Figure 15-10*** Initiation of ventricular fibrillation in a patient with a normal ventricle and Wolff-Parkinson-White syndrome. Three close-coupled extrastimuli ($S_2$, $S_3$, $S_4$) initiated a nonclinical arrhythmia in this patient. Note that retrograde conduction to the atrium occurs over a left-sided free-wall accessory pathway confirmed by the eccentric atrial activation pattern with distal coronary sinus as the earliest ventriculoatrial interval (*arrow*).

and-effect relationship of any specific factor to the malignant ventricular arrhythmia. Exceptions may be acute myocardial infarction or severe hypokalemia—for example, serum potassium levels below 2.0 meq/L. We do not recommend further workup of the patient who has ventricular fibrillation in the first 48 h of an acute myocardial infarction, as these individuals have a very low recurrence rate after hospital discharge.[13] For the majority of patients who have no identifiable reversible cause of the cardiac arrest, we offer the following approach, as noted in Fig. 15-11.

Therapy initially is directed at optimizing treatment for coexistent heart failure or ischemia. Empiric antiarrhythmic drug therapy for survivors of out-of-hospital cardiac arrest is not useful and may even be harmful;[35,36] we suggest serial electrophysiologic-pharmacologic testing to judge drug efficacy.[32] Most data in this area have been obtained from patients who have coronary artery disease, and it is not clear

whether similar results can be obtained from patients without coronary artery disease. In fact, it is reasonable to select an implantable cardioverter defibrillator as the first treatment option in a patient who has a cardiomyopathy and cardiac arrest.

At electrophysiologic study, nearly 40 percent of patients surviving a cardiac arrest will have no inducible sustained ventricular tachyarrhythmias.[32] We currently think that patients without inducible sustained ventricular tachycardia or ventricular fibrillation should receive an implantable cardioverter defibrillator (Fig. 15-11). Several studies have shown that these individuals are at significant risk for recurrent cardiac arrest if left untreated.[33,37,38] Further work is necessary to determine whether this group can be subdivided into relatively high- and low-risk segments. Implantable defibrillators in this group of patients appear to decrease subsequent sudden death, although no good control studies are available for analysis at present.[38]

*Figure 15-11* Treatment strategy for cardiac arrest survivors. (Key: VT = ventricular tachycardia; VF = ventricular fibrillation; LVEF = left ventricular ejection fraction; CAR = coronary artery revascularization (+, yes; −, no); ICD = implantable cardioverter defibrillator; PREV = previous; MI = myocardial infarction; LV func = left ventricular function; Rx = treatment.) (*From Knilans TK, Prystowsky EN: Antiarrhythmic drug therapy in the management of cardiac arrest survivors. Circulation 85(suppl I):I-118, 1992. Reproduced with permission from the American Heart Association.*)

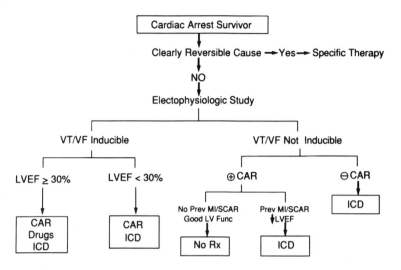

It is important to evaluate carefully the necessity for revascularization in patients with coronary artery disease. As noted in Fig. 15-11, in patients without inducible sustained ventricular tachycardia or ventricular fibrillation, an implantable defibrillator as sole therapy is given to those who require no coronary artery revascularization. Further, it is our current bias to withhold defibrillator therapy in that very small group of patients who have relatively normal ventricular function in association with severe coronary artery disease in whom we think the initiating cause for ventricular fibrillation was an acute ischemic event that did not lead to myocardial infarction and in whom satisfactory revascularization is given. Antiarrhythmic drug therapy in patients without inducible ventricular tachyarrhythmias is administered primarily to suppress secondary arrhythmias such as atrial fibrillation or nonsustained ventricular tachycardia that may be symptomatic or cause the defibrillator to be activated. In some individuals, antiarrhythmic drug therapy may slow the ventricular tachycardia rate enough to prevent syncope prior to defibrillator discharge and restoration of sinus rhythm. In essence, drugs are given more as secondary therapy in this group of patients, since their efficacy for the prevention of ventricular fibrillation cannot be judged by electrophysiologic testing.

Induction of sustained ventricular tachyarrhythmia allows the option for serial electrophysiologic-pharmacologic testing (Fig. 15-11). Although any such patient is theoretically a candidate for serial drug testing, it is our current practice to reserve this approach for patients with a left ventricular ejection fraction of 30 percent or greater. We have chosen this approach because recent data suggest that recurrence is unacceptably high in patients with suppressible ventricular tachycardia or fibrillation during drug therapy who have left ventricular ejection fraction below 30 percent.[32,33] It is not unreasonable to prescribe antiarrhythmic drugs to these patients for secondary reasons in addition to defibrillator treatment. For those individuals who have ejection fraction 30% or more, we recommend serial electrophysiologic-pharmacologic testing. Coronary artery revascularization should be performed for all patients if deemed necessary. As noted by several investigators,[32] excellent long-term results can be achieved in individuals with higher ejection fractions who have suppressible sustained ventricular tachycardia or fibrillation. There is no single superior drug for these patients in our experience. Several drugs can be used for initial therapy—such as sotalol, quinidine, disopyramide, and propafenone—assuming that contraindications are not present. If initial drug treatment is ineffective, subsequent combination therapy with quinidine or disopyramide with mexiletine might be chosen, although amiodarone is also a reasonable selection. The number of drug trials that should be attempted is an unanswered question and depends upon patient and physician preference. However, if two drug trials fail to yield nonsuppressibility of sustained ventricular tachyarrhythmias, the likelihood of subsequent trials proving successful markedly diminishes.[32] Thus, one could try two drug trials and then progress to a defibrillator; although several additional trials may be warranted in some patients who prefer a pharmacologic approach.

## Risk Stratification

Few patients with out-of-hospital cardiac arrest will undergo sufficiently early resuscitative efforts to allow survival to the hospital and discharge in a relatively well state.[39] Thus, it is extremely important to develop more efficient emergency medical services systems to provide prompt electrical defibrillation for these individuals.[40,41] Along with this approach should go an effort to identify individuals at high risk for sudden cardiac death so that an attempt to prevent the first event can be made. This approach involves risk stratification, as noted in Fig. 15-12.[42,43]

Three specific subgroups for patients at potential risk for sudden cardiac death are noted in Fig. 15-12. Individuals at minimal risk are those who have premature ventricular complexes or even nonsustained ventricular tachycardia but who have no heart disease or left ventricular dysfunction. Data suggest that these individuals require no specific antiarrhythmic therapy unless their arrhythmias are symptomatic. The right-hand column in Fig. 15-12 represents the highest risk for sudden cardiac death and contains patients who have a history of sustained ventricular tachycardia or ventricular fibrillation. Most commonly these individuals have heart disease and substantial left ventricular dysfunction, with nearly two-thirds having a left ventricular ejection fraction below 40 percent. These individuals require antiarrhythmic therapy. Patients who have heart disease of variable severity with nonsustained ventricular arrhythmias

| Arrhythmia | PVCs; VT-NS | PVCs / VT-N | VT-S; VF |
|---|---|---|---|
| Heart Disease | Absent | Present | Present |
| LV Dysfunction | Absent | Absent / Present | Present |
| Potential Risks for SCD | Minimal | Intermediate | High |

*Figure 15-12*   Risk stratification for patients with ventricular arrhythmias. In the intermediate column, there are shades of gray. As the gray color darkens, patients are at increased risk for cardiac arrest as they approximate the characteristics noted in patients who have already demonstrated sustained ventricular tachycardia or ventricular fibrillation. In essence, these are individuals with substantial left ventricular dysfunction who have nonsustained ventricular tachycardia. (*From Prystowsky EN: Antiarrhythmic therapy for asymptomatic ventricular arrhythmias. Am J Cardiol 61:102A, 1988. Reproduced by permission.*)

causing minimal symptoms are at intermediate risk for sudden cardiac death and present the clinician with the most difficult therapeutic decisions. It is easy, at present, to be a therapeutic nihilist with these patients, since no prospective data are available demonstrating that any form of antiarrhythmic therapy will prevent sudden cardiac death in this group. In fact, information has been published to suggest that there was an increase in sudden cardiac death among survivors of myocardial infarction who were given antiarrhythmic drug therapy.[44] Nevertheless, it is not unreasonable to engage in risk stratification of these individuals and to provide therapy guided by electrophysiologic testing for those individuals at apparent highest risk for sudden death.[42,43] This approach is controversial and will have to be verified by ongoing prospective multicenter studies.

## *Commentary*

Survivors of out-of-hospital cardiac arrest are the fortunate minority of this common cause of death in adults. Aggressive workup is necessary to identify and correct any obvious precipitating factors. Most patients will need some form of specific long-term antiarrhythmic treatment. Methods to judge efficacy of therapy are recommended, and empiric drug treatment is discouraged until confirmatory data supporting this approach are published. The overwhelming majority of patients do not survive their cardiac arrest. Thus, methods (risk stratification) to identify patients at high risk for sudden death and subsequent treatment of these individuals to prevent cardiac arrest appear reasonable although not yet proven.

## *References*

1. Gillum FR: Sudden coronary death in the United States, 1980–1985. *Circulation* 79:756, 1989.
2. Cupples LA et al: Long- and short-term risk of sudden coronary death. *Circulation* 85:I-11, 1992.
3. Prystowsky EN et al: The recognition and treatment of patients at risk for sudden death, in Eliot RS, Saenz A, Forker AD (eds): *Cardiac Emergencies*. Mount Kisco, New York, Futura, 1982, p 353.
4. Cobb LA, et al: Sudden cardiac death: I. A decade's experience with out-of-hospital resuscitation. *Mod Concepts Cardiovasc Dis* 49:31, 1980.
5. Liberthson RR, et al: Pre-hospital ventricular defibrillation: Prognosis and follow-up course. *N Engl J Med* 291:317, 1974.
6. Myerburg RJ et al: Clinical, electrophysiologic and hemodynamic profile of patients resuscitated from pre-hospital cardiac arrest. *Am J Med* 68:568, 1980.
7. Luu M et al: Diverse mechanisms of unexpected cardiac arrest in advanced heart failure. *Circulation* 80:1675, 1989.
8. Kuller L et al: Epidemiologic study of sudden and unexpected deaths due to arteriosclerotic heart disease. *Circulation* 34:1056, 1966.
9. Liberthson RR et al: Pathophysiologic observations in pre-hospital ventricular fibrillation and sudden cardiac death. *Circulation* 49:790, 1974.
10. Reichenbach DD et al: Pathology of the heart in sudden cardiac death. *Am J Cardiol* 39:865, 1977.
11. Weaver WD et al: Angiographic findings and prognostic indicators in patients resuscitated from sudden cardiac death. *Circulation* 54:895, 1976.
12. Perper JA et al: Arteriosclerosis of coronary arteries in sudden, unexpected deaths. *Circulation* 52(suppl III):III-27, 1975.
13. Cobb LA et al: Sudden cardiac death: II. Outcome of resuscitation; management, and future directions. *Mod Concepts Cardiovasc Dis* 49:37, 1980.
14. Baum RS et al: Survival after resuscitation from out-of-hospital ventricular fibrillation. *Circulation* 50:1231, 1974.
15. Spain DM, Bradess VA: The relationship of coronary thrombosis to coronary atherosclerosis and ischemic heart disease. (A necropsy study covering a period of 25 years.) *Am J Med Sci* 240:701, 1960.
16. Roberts WC, Buja LM: The frequency and significance of coronary arterial thrombi and other observations in fatal acute myocardial infarction: A study of 107 necropsy patients. *Am J Med* 52:425, 1972.
17. Davies MJ: Anatomic features in victims of sudden coronary death. *Circulation* 85:I-19, 1992.
18. Packer M: Sudden unexpected death in patients with

congestive heart failure: A second frontier. *Circulation* 72:681, 1985.

19. Maron BJ et al: Sudden death in hypertropic cardio-myopathy: A profile of 78 patients. *Circulation* 65:1388, 1982.

20. Nava A et al: Familial occurrence of right ventricular dysplasia: A study involving nine families. *J Am Coll Cardiol* 12:1222, 1988.

21. Jervell A, Lange-Nielsen F: Congenital deaf-mutism, functional heart disease with prolongation of the Q-T interval, and sudden death. *Am Heart J* 54:59, 1957.

22. Romano C et al: Aritimie cardiache rare dell'eta pediatrica. *Clin Pediatr (Bologna)* 45:656, 1963.

23. Ward O: A new familial cardiac syndrome in children. *J Irish Med Assoc* 54:103, 1964.

24. Moss AJ, Robinson J: Clinical features of the idiopathic long QT syndrome. *Circulation* 85(suppl I): I-140, 1992.

25. Minardo JD et al: Clinical characteristics of patients with ventricular fibrillation during antiarrhythmic drug therapy. *N Engl J Med* 319:257, 1988.

26. Klein GJ et al: Ventricular fibrillation in the Wolff-Parkinson-White syndrome. *N Engl J Med* 301:1080, 1979.

27. Fananapazir L et al: Procainamide infusion test: Inability to identify patients with Wolff-Parkinson-White syndrome potentially at risk of sudden death. *Circulation* 77:1291, 1988.

28. Evans JJ et al: Comparison of ventricular tachycardia induction between exercise and electrophysiologic testing in patients with ventricular tachycardia. *Circulation* 70(II):II-423, 1984.

29. Dimsdale JE et al: Post-exercise peril. *JAMA* 251:630, 1984.

30. Prystowsky EN et al: Wolff-Parkinson-White syndrome and sudden cardiac death. *Cardiology* 74(suppl 2):67, 1987.

31. Klein GJ et al: Asymptomatic Wolff-Parkinson-White: Should we intervene? *Circulation* 80:1902, 1989.

32. Knilans TK, Prystowsky EN: Antiarrhythmic drug therapy in the management of cardiac arrest survivors. *Circulation* 85(suppl I):I-118, 1992.

33. Wilbur DJ et al: Out-of-hospital cardiac arrest: Use of electrophysiologic testing in the prediction of long-term outcome. *N Engl J Med* 318:19, 1988.

34. Prystowsky EN et al: Induction of ventricular tachycardia during programmed electrical stimulation: Analysis of pacing methods. *Circulation* 73(suppl II):II-32, 1986.

35. Moosvi AR et al: Effect of empiric antiarrhythmic therapy in resuscitated out-of-hospital cardiac arrest victims with coronary artery disease. *Am J Cardiol* 65:1192, 1990.

36. Hallstrom AP et al: An antiarrhythmic drug experience in 941 patients resuscitated from an initial cardiac arrest between 1970 and 1985. *Am J Cardiol* 68:1025, 1991.

37. Roy D et al: Clinical characteristics and long-term follow-up in 119 survivors of cardiac arrest: Relation to inducibility at electrophysiologic testing. *Am J Cardiol* 52:969, 1983.

38. Fogoros RN et al: Long-term outcome of survivors of cardiac arrest whose therapy is guided by electrophysiologic testing. *J Am Coll Cardiol* 19:780, 1992.

39. Cobb LA et al: Community-based interventions for sudden cardiac death: Impact, limitations, and changes. *Circulation* 85(suppl I):I-98, 1992.

40. Cummins RO et al: Improving survival from sudden cardiac arrest: The "chain of survival" concept. *Circulation* 83:1832, 1991.

41. Haynes BE et al: A statewide early defibrillation initiative including laypersons and outcome reporting. *JAMA* 266:545, 1991.

42. Prystowsky EN: Antiarrhythmic therapy for asymptomatic ventricular arrhythmias. *Am J Cardiol* 61:102A, 1988.

43. Prystowsky EN et al: Diagnostic evaluation and treatment strategies for patients at risk for serious cardiac arrhythmias, Part 2: Ventricular tachyarrhythmias and Wolff-Parkinson-White syndrome. *Mod Concepts Cardiovasc Dis* 60:55, 1991.

44. The Cardiac Arrhythmia Suppression Trial (CAST) Investigators: Preliminary report: Effect of encainide and flecainide on mortality in a randomized trial of arrhythmia suppression after myocardial infarction. *N Engl J Med* 321:406, 1989.

# Chapter 16

# Arrhythmias during Acute Myocardial Infarction

Arrhythmias associated with acute myocardial infarction are generally related to myocardial ischemia or necrosis variably complicated by left ventricular dysfunction, metabolic and electrolyte abnormalities, and therapeutic interventions. The contribution to prognosis of any arrhythmia is difficult to assess, although it is clear that the independent contribution of any arrhythmia is usually small relative to the degree of myocardial damage. The general principles relating to assessment and management of arrhythmias as detailed elsewhere are applicable, and only issues related to acute infarction are highlighted in this section.

## Bradycardia and Conduction Defects

### Sinus Node Dysfunction

Sinus node dysfunction is observed in 4 to 5 percent of patients with acute infarction and is more prevalent with inferior infarction.[1] The presentation may be sinus bradycardia or bradycardia alternating with supraventricular tachycardia. Bradycardia is usually caused by enhanced vagal tone, ischemia or necrosis of the sinus node or medication. Treatment is considered if bradycardia is compromising cardiac output or is felt to be contributing to ventricular arrhythmia.[2] Intravenous atropine given cautiously in 0.5 mg aliquots (total dose up to 2.5 mg over

$2^{1}/_{2}$ h) may be attempted,[2] with temporary atrial or ventricular pacing used if necessary. Doses less than 0.4 mg should be avoided since they may worsen bradycardia. Temporary pacing should be considered when antiarrhythmic medication is used to treat associated tachycardia. Atrial pacing is preferable to ventricular pacing with "bradycardia-hypotension" syndrome or with right ventricular infarction. Sinus node dysfunction resolves spontaneously in the majority of patients, although patients with the bradycardia-tachycardia syndrome may need permanent pacing[2,3] if the problem is persistent.

### Bundle Branch Block

The presence of bundle branch block or intraventricular conduction disturbance may be associated with a two- or threefold increase of in-hospital mortality,[4-6] with this excess mortality largely accounted for by associated left ventricular dysfunction.[6] Approximately 12 percent of patients with acute infarction will have bundle branch block or bifascicular block. The challenge to the clinician is to select the patient who is destined to develop sudden complete heart block with an inadequate escape rhythm and to institute prophylactic temporary pacing. Temporary pacing may not influence mortality[5] but can prevent the turbulence and potential morbidity associated with emergency temporary pacemaker insertion. In contrast to the 6 percent incidence of complete heart block in the patient without intraventricular conduction disturbance, the patient with conduction disturbance may have a 13 to 70 percent incidence.[6]

Many studies have attempted to define the risk of complete heart block with specific single and combinations of intraventricular conduction disturbances.[4–10] These studies are limited by inadequate patient numbers, inability to distinguish new from previous conduction block, and variable interventions. Not surprisingly, they fail to provide consistent guidelines to predict complete heart block. A unifying concept was proposed by Lamas et al.[11] in a study where individual conduction defects were assigned a value of 1 [first-degree atrioventricular (AV) block, Mobitz type I or II AV block, left anterior fascicular block, left posterior fascicular block, right or left bundle branch block] and the subsequent total point score related to the risk of complete heart block (Fig. 16-1). A score of 3 or more was found to carry a risk of 36 percent for the development of AV block, and an analysis of published data by the authors provided a similar hierarchy of risk. This study fails to weigh risk factors individu-

ally and has other limitations, but it is intuitively reasonable and easy to apply pending the availability of further data.

Some investigators have recommended measuring the His–ventricle (HV) interval directly to assess His-Purkinje conduction and have proposed that a prolonged HV interval may be predictive of complete heart block.[6,9] We do not recommend catheter measurement of the HV interval to decide who will need temporary pacing. Noninvasive measurement of the HV interval by signal averaging techniques may prove useful in the future. In addition, improvements in external chest wall pacing[12] may allow consistent ventricular capture and tolerability and obviate many of our concerns regarding the consequences of sudden complete heart block.

### Indications for Pacing

Available data do not permit "cookbook" guidelines regarding temporary pacing with acute infarction; individual clinical judgment and available facilities will continue to be important. Nonetheless, we can recommend temporary pacing with the occurrence of alternating bundle branch block, Mobitz type II second-degree AV block with bundle branch block,[6,8] or conduction disturbance with a score of 3 or more.[11] When the decision is borderline, it may be remembered that the risk of complete heart block is lower with a first infarct if the patient is in Killip class 1 or 2.[8] The decision to institute permanent pacing is even more difficult. There does not appear to be a benefit from permanent pacing with bifascicular block (right bundle branch block plus left anterior or posterior fascicular block), with mortality generally ascribed to ventricular fibrillation in this group.[10] Permanent pacing should be considered after Mobitz type II second-degree or complete heart block with bundle branch block even if the former resolve prior to discharge.[6] Of note, indications for pacing may require revision in patients who undergo acute coronary revascularization with thrombolytic therapy or angioplasty.

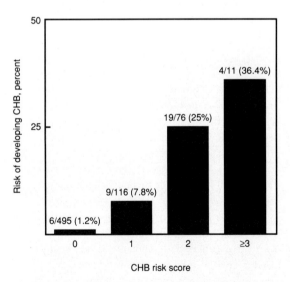

*Figure 16-1*    Risk of developing complete heart block as a function of risk score. In this scheme, each individual conduction defect (see text) is assigned an unweighted value of 1. *(Reproduced with permission from Lamas GA et al: Am J Cardiol 57:1213, 1986.)*

### Complete AV Block

Two patterns of complete AV block have been identified with acute infarction, each with distinct characteristics and therapeutic implications[13]:

1. *Atrioventricular block without bundle branch block* is generally associated with inferior myocardial infarction, occurs at the level of the AV node, and is felt to be related largely to edema and, to a lesser extent, ischemia and hypervagotonia. It occurs within 2 weeks of infarction (peak, 2 days) and frequently displays a progression from first-degree to second-degree (usually Mobitz type I) to third-degree AV block. The escape rhythm during the latter is "junctional," with a narrow QRS, and the rate is 40/min or greater in over 50 percent of cases.[14,15] Heart block may be atropine-responsive in up to 50 percent of cases[15] and temporary pacing is indicated only if bradycardia impairs hemodynamics. Pacing may also be considered if the escape QRS becomes wider (lower escape focus), if there has been previous remote infarction, and if there is a need for antiarrhythmic medication that may depress the escape rhythm.[13] Permanent pacing is rarely required as AV block invariably resolves even though it may occasionally take several weeks.

2. *Atrioventricular block with bundle branch block* is generally associated with anterior myocardial infarction and is largely related to necrosis of the conducting system involved in extensive infarction. The onset is often abrupt with a slow (generally less than 40/min), wide QRS escape rhythm and accompanying hemodynamic deterioration or collapse. Atrioventricular block is rarely atropine-sensitive and isoproterenol may temporarily enhance the escape rate. Patients generally are older, more likely to have or develop congestive heart failure, and have a high mortality (30 percent for patients in Killip class 1 and 2 and 60 to 100 percent in Killip class 3 and 4).[8,9] Permanent pacing has been recommended even if AV block resolves, due to the possibility of subsequent recurrences,[4,16] although improved survival may be difficult to demonstrate[17]

because death is usually related to heart failure or ventricular arrhythmia.

## Supraventricular Arrhythmias

Although the pathophysiology of supraventricular arrhythmias is complex, the management of these arrhythmias is essentially similar to that for supraventricular arrhythmias in other contexts except for a few unique considerations.

### Sinus Tachycardia

Sinus tachycardia is usually an appropriate physiologic response to a primary problem, and its therapy involves a search for and correction of these factors where possible. These include pain and anxiety, hypovolemia, left ventricular failure, and pericarditis. Even sinus tachycardia as an apparent isolated problem correlates with larger infarction, more ischemia, and a higher prevalence of pericarditis and other complications[18] and may be an independent predictor of subsequent mortality. Sinus tachycardia may reflect a "hyperdynamic" circulation and be associated with a high cardiac output and enhanced oxygen demand. In such instances, beta-blocker therapy has been advocated, but only after careful consideration and exclusion of other primary causes.[19,20]

### Atrial Ectopy

Atrial ectopy is also multifactorial and often related to another primary problem such as atrial distention due to ventricular dysfunction or pericarditis. Antiarrhythmic therapy is generally not recommended, although frequent atrial ectopy may rarely have adverse effects on cardiac output or may be a harbinger of atrial fibrillation.

### Paroxysmal Supraventricular Tachycardia

Paroxysmal supraventricular tachycardia is said to occur in 2 to 5 percent of patients with acute infarction. In contrast to the ambulatory, usually younger patient with recurrent supraventricular tachycardia ("PAT"), the mechanism of tachycardia is usually *not* AV nodal reentry or atrioventricular reentry, which terminates abruptly with carotid massage or AV nodal blocking drugs. Rather, the mechanism is usually focal atrial tachycardia related to intraatrial reentry or abnormal automaticity. Focal atrial tachycardia is managed in a way similar to atrial flutter or fibrillation. Initial treatment is directed at slowing the ventricular response by enhancing AV block during tachycardia (digitalis, verapamil, diltiazem, beta blockers). A membrane-active drug (quinidine, procainamide, etc.) is then given in an attempt to restore sinus rhythm. Accelerated junctional rhythm (>60/min) or junctional tachycardia (>120/min) may or may not be AV-dissociated. These rhythms are probably related to AV junctional ischemia or edema (if digitalis toxicity is ruled out) and may be treated, if necessary, with membrane-active antiarrhythmic drugs.

### Atrial Flutter and Fibrillation

Atrial flutter frequently presents with a 2:1 AV response and consequently a regular ventricular rate of 150/min. If flutter waves are not clearly discernible on the resting electrocardiogram (ECG), they can be unmasked with judicious carotid sinus massage, creating higher-grade temporary AV block. Medical management involves initial rate control with AV nodal blocking drugs followed by membrane-active drugs (quinidine type). Atrial flutter can frequently be terminated with atrial pacing techniques, transvenous or esophageal (Chap. 18). Alternatively, continuous atrial pacing at a rate exceeding the flutter rate may slow the ventricular response where flutter cannot be terminated. Cardioversion at relatively low energies (50 joules or less) may be appropriate in selected individuals where the procedure outlined above is not successful.

Atrial fibrillation is considerably more common than flutter, occurring in up to 10 percent of patients.[20] Early cardioversion can be considered if loss of atrial contractility or excessive rate is seriously compromising cardiac output. Otherwise, medical management again involves rate control followed by a membrane-active drug. Newer intravenous agents under investigation such as the class 1C (flecainide, propafenone) or class 3 (amiodarone) drugs have negative dromotropic effects on the AV node in addition to membrane-active properties and may prove useful as single agents.

## Ventricular Arrhythmias

### Ventricular Ectopy

The major goal in the treatment of ventricular ectopy is the prevention of ventricular tachycardia (VT) and fibrillation. Lown[21] originally proposed that complex (multiform, couplets or greater, R-on-T phenomenon) and frequent (>5/min) ventricular ectopy heralded ventricular fibrillation (VF) and should be treated to prevent this.[22] There would be no controversy surrounding this recommendation if the "warning" arrhythmias did indeed precede VF and therapy were safe and effective. However, other investigators have subsequently pointed out that VF frequently (up to 83 percent) occurs in the absence of ventricular ectopy and ventricular ectopy is common in the absence of VF.[23–25] That is, ventricular ectopy is neither sensitive nor specific for predicting VF. Trials aimed at assessing the efficacy of antiarrhythmic drugs (generally lidocaine but also quinidine, disopyramide, procainamide, and beta blockers) have demonstrated reduction of premature ventricular complexes (PVCs).[26] Lidocaine has been most extensively studied with some[27,28] but not all[29] studies showing a decrease in the incidence of VF in addition to PVC reduction. This potential benefit must be weighed against the cost and toxicity of lidocaine or other drugs selected.

Available data do not allow a clear recommendation for the use of antiarrhythmic drugs prophylactically, whether or not ventricular ectopy is present. Three approaches are generally followed: (1) Some do not treat patients prophylactically in the presence or absence of ectopy. The rationale is that therapy is not of proven efficacy and rapid treatment of primary ventricular fibrillation does not have permanent adverse consequences. (2) Others recommend the treatment of "warning" arrhythmias as advocated by Lown, an approach that many find intuitively attractive even in the absence of clear demonstration of efficacy. (3) Finally, some advocate lidocaine prophylaxis in all patients or at least in those considered to be at "high" risk for primary ventricular fibrillation (age less than 50 years, no previous history of congestive heart failure or myocardial infarction, within 6 h of acute infarction),[20] and some endorse this with considerable enthusiasm.[30] If lidocaine is used in this manner, it should be started as soon as possible, either in the emergency room or at initial contact with the patient, since the greatest risk for VF is within the first 6 h of chest pain. The dose should be carefully monitored and levels obtained in selected patients such as those with congestive failure who may have impaired drug metabolism or clearance. Antiarrhythmics should be used with caution in the presence of conduction disturbances, since they may aggravate the latter or suppress subsidiary pacemakers in the event of complete heart block. Lidocaine should be stopped at 36 h,[31] with further monitoring (especially in patients with conduction disturbance and congestive heart failure) to assess the need for chronic therapy.

Immediate defibrillation in the critical care unit is the rule, and lidocaine prophylaxis will not decrease mortality. Thus, the primary use of this agent is to prevent the psychological consequences of being resuscitated. This is a reasonable goal, but it is also important to monitor closely for adverse effects of lidocaine toxicity.

### Ventricular Tachycardia and Fibrillation

#### Ventricular Fibrillation

Ventricular fibrillation occurs in 4 to 18 percent of patients with acute infarction[20] and is more frequently seen with Q-wave infarction. An important distinction is made between unexpected or "primary"

VF and "secondary" VF in the context of severe left ventricular (LV) failure. The majority of primary VF occurs early, with 60 percent occurring within the first 4 to 6 h and 80 percent by 12 h. Late VF (1 to 6 weeks) occurs more commonly with larger transmural infarcts often accompanied by arrhythmias and conduction defects. Primary VF has been said not to affect prognosis when rapidly treated, although some investigators[32] have suggested a worse prognosis after this event.

#### Ventricular Tachycardia

Accelerated idioventricular rhythm or "slow" VT (rate 60 to 120/min) is observed in 20 percent of patients with both anterior and inferior infarction. It may be paroxysmal or nonparoxysmal and is felt to be due to abnormal automaticity of ischemic Purkinje fibers. Treatment is generally not required, although lidocaine may be used if hemodynamic impairment is present. "Slow" VT may be a harbinger of more rapid VT if the rate exceeds 75/min in anterior myocardial infarction.[33]

Ventricular tachycardia is generally defined as three or more successive ventricular ectopic depolarizations at a rate of 100 to 120/min or greater. It may be self-terminating or sustained. New wide QRS tachycardia in the context of acute myocardial infarction should be considered to be VT unless proved otherwise (Chap. 13). Treatment of VT is directed at correcting potential aggravating factors and using membrane-active antiarrhythmic drugs. Lidocaine is the most commonly used initial drug, with procainamide as an alternative. Other drugs—both approved and currently investigational (bretylium, amiodarone, propafenone, flecainide, and others)—are used for resistant VT. Ventricular tachycardia occurring in the early stages of infarction (first 48 h) does not correlate with late VT, and acute therapy is generally discontinued after this time frame under continuous monitoring to assess the need for further interventions and therapy. Although it is controversial, some consider chronic therapy for most patients with sustained monomorphic VT that occurs early. Ventricular tachycardia occurring in the later stages of infarction (10 days or later) in the absence of an obvious inciting factor requires further investigation, with consideration of subsequent long-term prophylaxis. The precise point when "early" becomes "late" and VT can no longer be directly attributed to the acute effects of infarction is not known and requires further study.

### Recurrent Ventricular Tachycardia or Fibrillation

Recurrent primary VT or VF in the course of acute infarction remains a challenging and emotionally draining problem for all involved. Patients are frequently lucid and may be hemodynamically stable between episodes and must endure frequent cardioversions and defibrillations. Under the pressure of the situation, multiple antiarrhythmic drugs are often used, and it soon becomes unclear whether these are aggravating or ameliorating the situation. Although this problem will never be simple, it is important to have an orderly approach with a vigorous effort to correct reversible factors such as electrolyte imbalance, oxygenation, and volume status. Drugs should initially be given one at a time, and a drug should not be discarded until it is clear that efficacy is not present at an adequate dose (and preferably, an adequate blood level). Drugs with significant negative inotropic effects (such as disopyramide and some class 1C agents) should be avoided. Lidocaine, procainamide, and bretylium are commonly used, and "rapid" intravenous loading with amiodarone may be helpful.[34] Insertion of a pacing lead may be helpful if the patient has a relatively more stable VT that may be terminated by pacing techniques, and investigational specialized catheters capable of lower-energy countershock or defibrillation may prove useful in the future.[35]

We consider it important to proceed with early cardiac catheterization when it becomes apparent that one is dealing with recurrent primary VT or VF. This identifies potentially correctable factors such as coronary stenosis or ventricular aneurysm and, at the very least, makes it clear when there is very severe LV dysfunction that greatly influences further therapeutic options (Figs. 16-2 and 16-3).

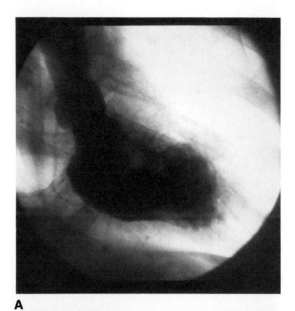

**A**

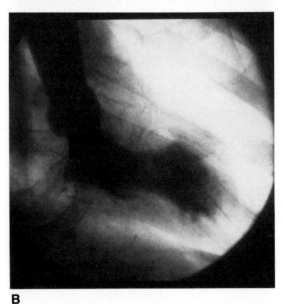

**B**

*Figure 16-2*  End-diastolic (*A*) and end-systolic (*B*) frames from a patient with recurrent drug refractory VT after acute myocardial infarction. This patient had an occluded left anterior descending artery with otherwise normal coronary arteries. There is a discrete anteroapical aneurysm with otherwise good ventricular function. Aneurysmectomy guided by myocardial mapping prevented further VT.

Cardiac transplantation can be considered in selected individuals. Implantable defibrillating devices can be considered, but generally the frequency of VT or VF is prohibitive for the rational use of such a device in this setting. A difficult decision not to resuscitate may also be considered by all involved in selected cases, although the legal and ethical considerations surrounding this decision remain to be established in most countries.

## Commentary

Many of the issues presented in this chapter remain controversial because of insufficient controlled data and the difficulty of extrapolating from published data to a given patient. Clinical judgment and individual considerations allow for variable approaches, and what may be right for one institution may not be right for another. Consider a clinician confronted with a patient developing bifascicular block in the course of acute infarction. At a well-staffed urban hospital with rapidly available expertise in temporary transvenous pacing or chest wall pacing, the clinician may decide that the morbidity of prophylactic temporary pacing is not justified by the risk of complete AV block. The same clinician in a more sparsely staffed rural hospital, given the same patient, may make the exactly opposite decision. The issue of prophylactic lidocaine for all patients with acute infarction can be viewed similarly. Even if lidocaine were unequivocally efficacious in reducing the incidence of primary VF, many clinicians could reasonably argue that the cost and potential morbidity of lidocaine in all patients may not be justified by preventing a few episodes of primary ventricular fibrillation in a setting where defibrillation is prompt. Under different circumstances, the opposite conclusion could be reached. Last, the widespread use of thrombolytic drugs may alter the natural history of acute events and change our approach to these problems.

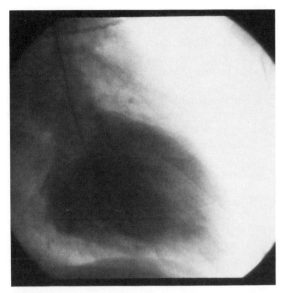

**A**

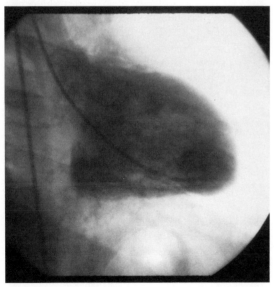

**B**

*Figure 16-3* End-diastolic (*A*) and end-systolic (*B*) frames in another patient with recurrent VF after acute myocardial infarction. There was diffuse inoperable coronary disease and the end-systolic and diastolic frames are virtually identical. This patient does not have a surgical option and his prognosis is very poor. A cardiac transplant may be considered if feasible.

# *References*

1. Parameswaran R et al: Sinus node dysfunction in acute myocardial infarction. *Br Heart J* 38:93, 1976.
2. Scheinman MM et al: Use of atropine in patients with acute myocardial infarction and sinus bradycardia. *Circulation* 52:627, 1975.
3. Rokseth R, Hatle L: Sinus arrest in acute myocardial infarction. *Br Heart J* 33:639, 1971.
4. Atkins JM et al: Ventricular conduction blocks and sudden death in acute myocardial infarction: Potential indications for pacing. *N Engl J Med* 288:281, 1973.
5. Nimetz AA et al: The significance of bundle branch block during acute myocardial infarction. *Am Heart J* 90:439, 1975.
6. Klein RC et al: Intraventricular conduction defects in acute myocardial infarction: Incidence prognosis therapy. *Am Heart J* 108:1007, 1984.
7. Pine MB et al: Excess mortality and morbidity associated with right bundle branch block and left anterior fascicular block. *J Am Coll Cardiol* 1207:1212, 1983.
8. Hindman MC et al: The clinical significance of bundle branch block complicating acute myocardial infarction: Incidence for temporary and permanent pacemaker insertion. *Circulation* 58:689, 1978.
9. Roos JC, Dunning AJ: Bundle branch block in acute myocardial infarction. *Eur J Cardiol* 6:403, 1978.
10. Watson RDS et al: The Birmingham trial of permanent pacing in patients with intraventricular conduction disorders after acute myocardial infarction. *Am Heart J* 108:496, 1984.
11. Lamas GA et al: A simplified method to predict occurrence of complete heart block during acute myocardial infarction. *Am J Cardiol* 57:1213, 1986.
12. Zoll PM et al: External noninvasive temporary cardiac pacing and clinical trials. *Circulation* 71:937, 1985.
13. Norris RM: Heart block in posterior and anterior myocardial infarction. *Br Heart J* 31:352, 1969.
14. Tans AC et al: Clinical setting and prognostic significance of high degree atrioventricular block in acute inferior myocardial infarction. *Am Heart J* 99:4, 1980.
15. Feigl D et al: Early and late atrioventricular block in acute myocardial infarction. *J Am Coll Cardiol* 4:35, 1984.
16. Ritter WS et al: Permanent pacing in patients with transient trifascicular block during acute myocardial infarction. *Am J Cardiol* 38:205, 1976.
17. Ginks WR et al: Long term prognosis after acute anterior infarction with atrioventricular block. *Br Heart J* 39:186, 1977.
18. Crimm A et al: Prognostic significance of isolated sinus tachycardia during the first three days of acute myocardial infarction. *Am J Med* 76:983, 1984.
19. Nelson WP: Supraventricular arrhythmias: Diagnosis treatment and prognosis, in Karliner JS, Gregoratos G (eds): *Coronary Care*. Churchill Livingstone, New York, 1981, p 339.
20. Pasternak RC et al: Arrhythmias in acute myocardial infarction, in Braunwald E (eds): *Heart Disease: A Textbook of Cardiovascular Medicine*. Saunders, Philadelphia, 1988, p 1262.
21. Lown B et al: The coronary care unit. New perspectives and directions. *JAMA* 199:188, 1967.
22. Campbell RWF et al: Relation of ventricular arrhythmias to ventricular fibrillation. *Br Heart J* 43:109, 1980.
23. Lie KJ et al: Observations on patients with primary ventricular fibrillation complicating acute myocardial infarction. *Circulation* 52:755, 1975.
24. El-Sherif N et al: Electrocardiographic antecedents of primary ventricular fibrillation: Value of the R on T phenomenon in myocardial infarction. *Br Heart J* 38:415, 1976.
25. Lawrie DM et al: Ventricular fibrillation complicating acute myocardial infarction. *Lancet* 2:523, 1968.
26. Josephson ME: Treatment of ventricular arrhythmias after myocardial infarction. *Circulation* 74:653, 1986.
27. Koster RW, Dunning J: Intramuscular lidocaine for prevention of lethal arrhythmias in the prehospitalization phase of acute myocardial infarction. *N Engl J Med* 313:1105, 1985.
28. Lie KJ et al: Lidocaine in the prevention of primary ventricular fibrillation: A double blind randomized study of 212 consecutive patients. *N Engl J Med* 291:1324, 1974.
29. Dunn HM et al: Prophylactic lidocaine in the early phase of suspected myocardial infarction. *Am Heart J* 110:353, 1985.
30. Lie KJ: Lidocaine and prevention of ventricular fibrillation complicating acute myocardial infarction. *Int J Cardiol* 7:321, 1985.
31. Wagner GS: Arrhythmias in acute myocardial infarction. *Med Clin North Am* 68:1001, 1984.
32. Thompson P, Sloman G: Sudden death in hospital

after discharge from coronary care unit. *Br Heart J* 4:136, 1971.

33.  deSoyza N et al: Association of accelerated idioventricular rhythm and paroxysmal ventricular tachycardia in acute myocardial infarction. *Am J Cardiol* 34:667, 1974.

34.  Installe E et al: Intravenous amiodarone in the treatment of various arrhythmias following cardiac operations. *J Thorac Cardiovasc Surg. 81:302, 1981.*

35.  Yee R et al: Low energy countershock using an intravascular catheter in an acute cardiac care setting. *Am J Cardiol* 50:1124, 1982.

# Part IV

## Methods and Therapy

# Chapter 17

# *Techniques in Electrophysiologic Testing*

Programmed electrical stimulation of the heart was introduced by Durrer and colleagues[1] as a technique to study the mechanisms of cardiac arrhythmias in humans. A critical adjunct to this earlier work was the development of a catheter method to record His bundle potentials in humans.[2] Through the use of these techniques, it is possible to diagnose with certainty various forms of supraventricular and ventricular tachycardia as well as to identify the site of atrioventricular (AV) block. Over the past two decades, clinical electrophysiology has undergone transformation from an esoteric subspeciality of cardiology, concerned primarily with diagnosing various cardiac arrhythmias and investigating electrophysiologic properties of the heart, to an area vital to the management of patients with arrhythmias, including the ability to cure patients by endocardial catheter ablation. This chapter describes the techniques and applications of electrophysiologic testing.

## Electrophysiologic Testing Methods

### Electrical Equipment

Electrophysiologic procedures are specialized cardiac catheterizations that involve the recording of intracardiac electrograms and programmed electrical stimulation of the heart.[3] Requisite equipment includes a fluoroscope with multiple view capability, at least one defibrillator, a variety of electrode catheters, a junction box isolated from the patient, a recording apparatus with an oscilloscope and the ability to provide a hard copy of the records, a method to store data for retrieval (e.g., tape recorder, optical disk), and a programmed electrical stimulator. Computerized recording systems are becoming standard equipment for many laboratories. After catheters are in position in the heart, they are connected to the electrical junction box, which transmits electrical signals from within the heart to the recording equipment and allows pacing stimuli from the programmed stimulator to be directed to various cardiac chambers.

An example of the recording and stimulation apparatus is noted in Fig. 17-1, which consists of two racks of equipment. In the left-hand rack, from top to bottom, there is a monitor for blood pressure recordings, a 16-channel oscilloscope, two sets of switches that allow electrocardiographic or intracardiac signals to be positioned at any one of the 16 channels on the oscilloscope and strip recorder, respectively, and a strip recorder. The electrical signals are filtered and amplified as needed. In this particular system, the monitor on the top of the right-hand rack shows a computerized listing of each data channel that can be changed by a keyboard noted above the tape recorder on the bottom of the rack. Underneath the top screen is a storage oscilloscope that enables detailed on-line analysis of electrical events. The middle portion of the right-hand rack contains the programmed electrical stimulator and its controls (Fig. 17-2).

The custom-designed programmed electrical stimulator shown in Fig. 17-2 is quite complex;

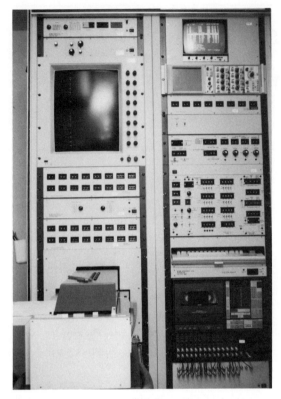

*Figure* 17-1    Electrophysiologic equipment. *(See text for details.)*

many simpler devices exist. Certain requisite features for any stimulator include capability for incremental and programmed stimulation, external and intracardiac sensing, multiple extrastimuli, and variable pulse width and amplitude of stimuli.

### Catheter Insertion and Manipulation Techniques

Insertion of catheters is almost always performed using the percutaneous technique, and cut downs are rarely needed. The three most common catheterization sites are the groin, the subclavian area, and the antecubital fossa. The route chosen for catheter insertion depends primarily on the accessibility of the venous or arterial system and the intracardiac catheter position required for study. Prior to catheter insertion, each area is prepped and draped in a sterile

manner and local anesthesia is administered with a 21- or 23-gauge needle. Some antecubital veins are hard to feel. In such instances it is better to acquire venous access before giving local anesthesia, which can obscure the venous landmarks. While administering anesthesia to deeper tissues, it is useful to confirm venous access prior to removing the needle. After an area has been appropriately anesthetized, an 18-gauge thin-wall needle is inserted into the vessel. When free-flowing blood is confirmed through the needle, a flexible-tip guide wire is placed into the vessel through the needle and the needle is removed. An introducer and sheath are placed over the wire into the artery or vein, the guide wire is removed, and the electrode catheter is inserted through this sheath. We prefer a right femoral artery approach when a catheter is positioned in the left ventricle. Recordings of the His bundle electrogram are obtained most easily with a catheter advanced from the femoral vein, which allows the catheter position to be kept stable throughout the study—a difficult task when the His bundle catheter is introduced through an antecubital, subclavian, or internal jugular vein.[4] These latter approaches are often used when a catheter is inserted into the coronary sinus or during repeat electrophysiologic testing to determine efficacy of therapy using a single catheter. The antecubital approach is especially desirable for repeat electrophysiologic studies because it is associated with very low risk and the patient can be ambulated immediately after catheter removal—a substantial psychological benefit. Placement of the catheter in the right atrium or right ventricle can be accomplished easily from any venous route. After catheters are in place, heparin anticoagulation may be given intravenously, although its use is variable among electrophysiology laboratories. An absolute benefit of anticoagulation has not been proved for decreasing thrombophlebitis during catheterization of veins, but it is required in any patient in whom arterial catheterization is performed.

No specific electrode catheter can be used for all studies; rather, several types are necessary to attain certain intracardiac positions in individuals. Figure 17-3A demonstrates three quadripolar electrode catheters with separate curves. The top two

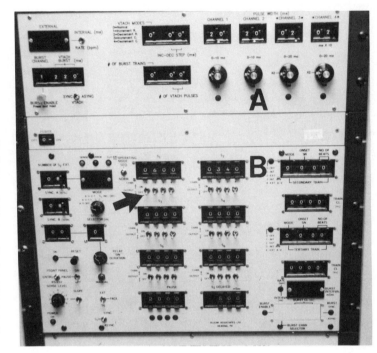

*Figure* 17-2   Programmed electrical stimulator. *A*. Controls to regulate current (mA) and pulse duration (ms) output to each of four pacing channels. Other features include a digital readout of heart rate, a setup for rapid burst pacing, and various pacing modalities to terminate tachycardia. *B*. This custom-built stimulator has many features not essential for routine studies. In the center are selectors for the pacing drive train interval ($S_1$) and choice of up to five extrastimuli ($S_2$ to $S_6$). Each stimulus can be directed to any one of four output channels (*arrow*).

catheters have somewhat gentle bends; the primary difference between them is the interelectrode spacing, which is 5 mm on the top catheter and 10 mm on the middle catheter. A quadripolar catheter is used when simultaneous bipolar pacing and recording are performed. Newer systems using digital acquisition allow pacing and recording from the same electrode pair. Special catheters are also available to record monophasic action potentials (MAP) from atrial or ventricular endocardium (Fig. 17-4).[5] MAP recordings may prove useful to help diagnose arrhythmias caused by afterdepolarizations.

There are advantages and disadvantages for each catheter. For example, when a femoral approach is used to attain a site in the high right atrium, use of the 5-mm interelectrode spacing enables one to pace the high right atrium and record from this area (Fig. 17-5A). However, the close spacing of the electrode poles often obscures distinct atrial electrograms during pacing. In comparison, use of a quadripolar catheter with 10-mm interelectrode spacing, with

the distal electrode pair positioned in the high right atrium, allows for excellent separation of the pacing artifact and atrial recording, but the proximal recording poles are actually situated in the mid to low right atrium, depending on the atrial size (Fig. 17-5B). A catheter with an acute bend (Fig. 17-3A, bottom) is very useful to position in the right ventricular apex when a femoral vein approach is used. In some instances it is important to have a catheter with a flexible distal tip that can be manipulated into various shapes once the catheter is situated in the heart (Fig. 17-3B). This type of catheter is especially useful for delivery of radiofrequency energy, as noted below. In summary, catheters are available in several diameters (French sizes), electrode arrays, and curvature; selection of a particular catheter will depend on the objectives of the study.

Recordings can be either unipolar or bipolar as demonstrated in Fig. 17-6. In this example, a quadripolar catheter was situated with its tip at the right ventricular apex. Proximal and distal bipolar

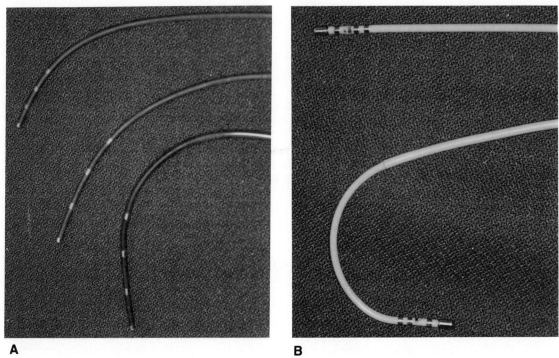

**A**                    **B**

*Figure 17-3*   Types of electrode catheters. *A.* Three quadripolar catheters are shown, the top two with gentle curves and the bottom one with an acute curve. *B.* Flexible-tip catheter in its straight and curved configurations. (*See text for details.*)

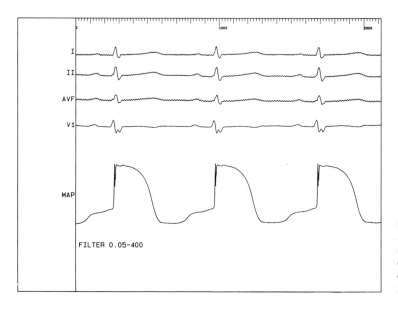

*Figure 17-4* Monophasic action potential (MAP) recording. The MAP was recorded using a catheter with a contact electrode positioned at the right ventricular apex. The MAP resembles a transmembrane action potential recorded with a microelectrode in vitro. The duration of the MAP closely approximates local ventricular refractoriness.

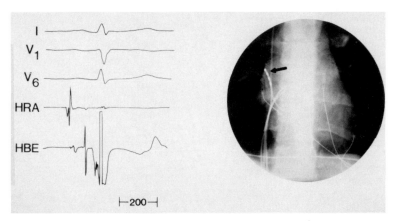

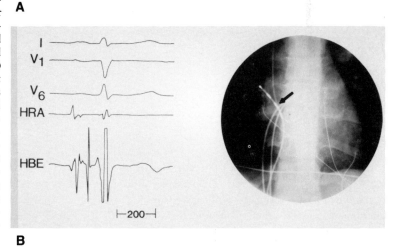

*Figure 17-5*   Right atrial catheterization site. *A.* A quadripolar electrode catheter with 5-mm interelectrode spacing was inserted from the right femoral vein, and the distal electrode pair (*arrow*) was positioned in the high right atrium (*right*). The proximal poles are near the high right atrium and record primarily an atrial deflection on the high right atrial electrogram (HRA) (*left*). *B.* The proximal poles (*arrow*) on a catheter with 10-mm electrode spacing between poles in the same patient record from lower atrial tissue as reflected by a substantial ventricular deflection on the HRA recording (*left*).

electrograms were recorded as well as unipolar electrograms from each pole of the catheter. An electrical field is present during activation of cardiac muscle. In a unipolar lead, the rapid or intrinsic deflection represents activation of the myocardium directly underneath the electrode.[6] Thus, only one rapid component will be present. The electrogram configuration in a bipolar lead may contain several relatively rapid deflections. The bipolar electrogram is the algebraic sum of the two unipolar leads.[6] The closer the bipolar spacing, the sharper the electrogram (Fig. 17-5A). Unipolar and bipolar electrograms require different filter settings, which vary depending on the

equipment used. Typically, unipolar electrograms are more unfiltered—for example, 0.05 to 400 Hz. Common bipolar settings range from 30–40 to 400–500 Hz.

Local activation in healthy tissue is easier to determine with a unipolar tracing that demonstrates a single rapid deflection when the electrical wavefront arrives at the electrode and is useful for precise mapping purposes. A closely coupled bipolar electrode pair may yield better results in infarcted tissue. Under routine circumstances, bipolar recordings are used because of their stability and greater resistance to motion artifact and changes in amplitude under

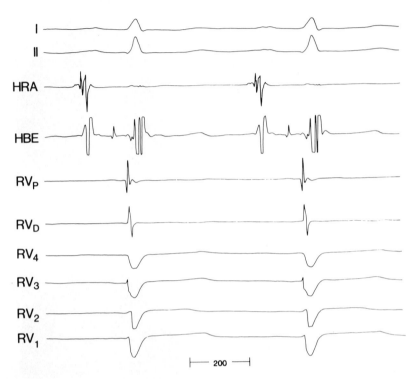

*Figure 17-6* Bipolar and unipolar electrograms. Simultaneous recordings from electrocardiogram (ECG) leads I and II and bipolar intracardiac electrograms from the high right atrium (HRA), His bundle area (HBE), and right ventricular proximal $(RV_p)$ and distal $(RV_D)$ electrode pair. Unipolar RV electrograms are recorded using each of the four poles from the most proximal $(RV_4)$ to the most distal $(RV_1)$. (*See text for details.*)

various conditions throughout the study. Further, close-spaced bipolar electrodes—for example, 1 to 2 mm interelectrode distance—enable excellent identification of local activation and are preferred in many instances over unipolar electrograms.

The His bundle area is surprisingly easy to locate in the vast majority of patients. Using the femoral approach, the catheter is initially manipulated to a site where the recording bipolar pair overlies the middle of the spine during fluoroscopy

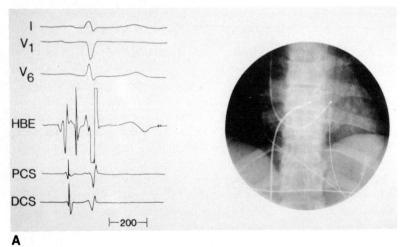

**A**

*Figure 17-7* His bundle recording site. *A*. Ideal catheter position with large-amplitude atrial and His bundle electrograms. *B*. Catheter moved more into the ventricle reduces the amplitude of both the atrial and His bundle electrogram. *C*. Catheter positioned more proximally produces a large atrial but small His potential. Simultaneous ECG leads I, $V_1$, $V_6$ recorded with intracardiac HBE and coronary sinus electrograms.

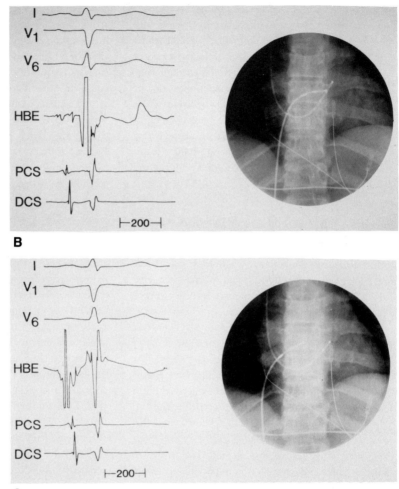

*Figure* 17-7 *(Continued)*     **C**

in the posterior-anterior view (Fig. 17-7*A*). The goal is to record a large His deflection with a relatively large atrial deflection at the same time, which is accomplished in this instance. One should fine-tune the catheter position to obtain such a recording. However, note that slight movements of the catheter to a more distal position (Fig. 17-7*B*) result in a decrease in the atrial potential and His deflection amplitude and that a more proximal recording site increases the atrial amplitude but diminishes that of the His bundle electrogram (Fig. 17-7*C*).

## Programmed Electrical Stimulation

Programmed electrical stimulation encompasses two basic modes of pacing. To assess conduction over the atrioventricular conduction system or an accessory pathway, incremental atrial or ventricular pacing is used. The heart is paced starting at a relatively slow rate, and progressively faster rates are used until block occurs over the tissue being evaluated. To evaluate refractoriness, a drive train at a constant paced cycle length or during sinus rhythm is selected and extrastimuli are introduced late in diastole and then at progressively more premature intervals until either block occurs in the tissue evaluated or local refractoriness at the site of stimulation is encountered. Both incremental pacing and introduction of one or more extrastimuli are used to initiate supraventricular and ventricular tachycardia; at times bursts of a rapid constant cycle length are necessary to achieve this aim. In most situations we recommend pacing stimuli of twice diastolic threshold current strength and 2-ms pulse width.

### Electrophysiologic Evaluation of the Sinus Node

Two atrial stimulation techniques are typically used to test sinus nodal function.[7-9] The most useful test to uncover sinus nodal dysfunction is atrial overdrive pacing to determine the sinus node recovery time.[8] This test is based on a normal electrophysiologic property of pacemaker cells known as overdrive suppression of spontaneous depolarization.[10] After atrial overdrive pacing is terminated, the pacemaker cells in the sinus node remain quiescent for a period of time and then resume spontaneous activity. If a marked depression of automaticity occurs at the end of pacing, a prolonged pause will be noted, and this presumably identifies sinus node dysfunction. In our experience, this test is specific but insensitive to diagnose sinus node dysfunction in patients in whom the diagnosis has not been confirmed by routine electrocardiography.

Sinus node testing is performed by pacing the high right atrium after the patient is in a quiet, restful state. Before pacing, the mean spontaneous sinus rate is calculated using approximately 10 intervals. It is important to use multiple pacing cycle lengths to obtain the maximal sinus node recovery time.[11] We use cycle lengths of 800 to 350 ms in 50-ms decrements as the paced cycle lengths for testing, and we pace for 30 s with a 30-s rest between pacing runs. In patients with slower spontaneous rates, we prefer to test the slowest atrial paced rate that can capture the sinus node without interference. Measurement of the sinus node recovery

time is taken as the interval from the high right atrial depolarization of the last paced beat to the high right atrial depolarization of the first return sinus beat, and this is considered the primary pause.[8] In some patients there may be an excessively long pause after the first sinus return beat; this is classified as a secondary pause.[12] Figure 17-8 is an example from a patient with both a primary and secondary pause, the latter of which was excessively long. Because the sinus node recovery time is influenced by the underlying basic sinus rate, a variety of methods have been proposed to obtain the corrected sinus node recovery time (CSNRT).[7] We prefer the method of subtraction of the mean sinus cycle length from the primary pause to obtain the CSNRT. The maximal CSNRT is taken after evaluation of all paced cycle lengths. We prospectively evaluated 131 patients in a drug-free state and noted a 95 percent confidence interval for the upper value for maximal CSNRT of 500 ms, which was independent of age or gender.[11] It should be remembered that an abnormal maximal CSNRT suggests sinus node dysfunction but is not in itself an indication for implantation of a permanent pacemaker.

Determination of the sinoatrial conduction time (SACT) is another test of sinus node function.[9] The SACT is based on the principles of reset of an automatic focus, described in Chap. 2. During sinus rhythm, the cardiac cycle is scanned by a premature atrial stimulus every eighth cycle. Atrial stimuli are introduced at the sinus node region beginning with an $A_1A_2$ interval approximately 10 ms less than sinus cycle length and decrementing by 10 to 20 ms until the stimulus fails to capture the atrium. A stylized sequence is illustrated in Fig. 17-9. Initially, the atrial extrastimulus ($A_1A_2$) at late coupling intervals fails to alter the return cycle ($A_2A_3$) (panel A, Fig. 17-9), indicating that the extrastimulus did not reset the sinus node (zone of compensation or collision). At earlier coupling intervals, the return cycle is advanced (noncompensatory pause), indicating that the sinus node has been depolarized and reset (panel B, Fig. 17-9). The $A_2A_3$ interval is then plotted as a function of $A_1A_2$ (Fig. 17-10). At the reset zone, the sinoatrial conduction time is calculated as

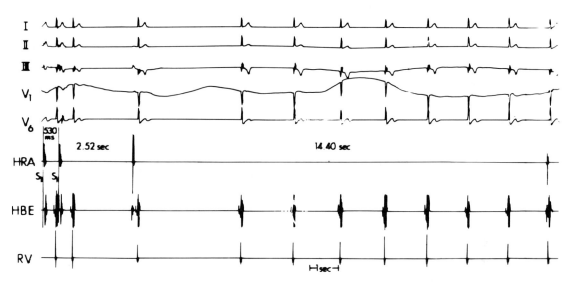

*Figure 17-8*   Abnormal sinus node recovery time. There is a 2.52-s primary pause, which yielded a markedly abnormal CSNRT. More impressive is the 14.40-s secondary pause before resumption of sinus node activity. A junctional escape rhythm prevented total asystole (note the His deflection before each ventricular electrogram on the HBE lead) in this patient. The patient had a history of recurrent syncope that did not recur after a permanent pacemaker was implanted. The presumption was that a stable junctional rhythm did not always occur with prolonged sinus pauses. (*From Prystowsky EN, Noble RJ: Electrophysiologic studies: Who to refer. Heart Dis Stroke 1:188, 1992. Reproduced by permission.*)

SACT = $A_2A_3$ − SCL/2, where $A_2A_3$ is the interval from $A_2$ to the return sinus cycle $A_3$ and SCL is the sinus cycle length. It is assumed that the atrial impulse enters the sinus node retrogradely and resets the node, and the sinus impulse exits anterogradely to initiate the return cycle. The SACT is then represented by the total interval $A_2A_3$ minus the sinus cycle length—divided by two since the interval includes both conduction time into and out of the sinus node. At still earlier coupling intervals (panel C, Fig. 17-9), the extrastimulus may be more or less interpolated, indicating that the premature atrial

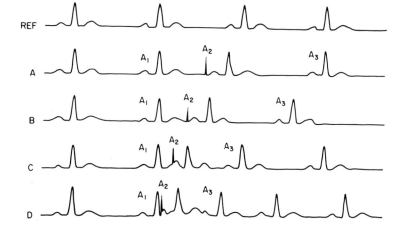

*Figure 17-9*   Schematic illustration of the results of the atrial extrastimulus technique. $A_1A_2$ is the coupling interval between the last sensed high right atrial electrogram and the atrial electrogram following the extrastimulus. $A_2A_3$ is the returned atrial cycle. *A* represents the zone of compensation, *B* zone of reset, *C* zone of interpolation, and *D* zone of reentry. In this "ideal" representation, there is no sinus arrhythmia. REF = reference ECG lead.

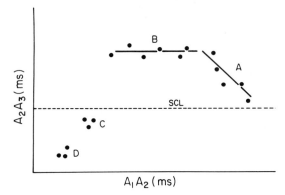

*Figure 17-10*   Schematic curve illustrating atrial extrastimulus testing for calculation of sinoatrial conduction time. Four classic zones are depicted, including the zone of compensation (A), the zone of reset (B), the zone of interpolation (C), and the zone of reentry (D), as discussed in the text. SCL = sinus cycle length.

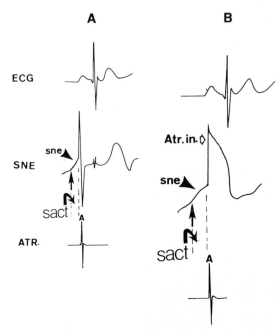

*Figure 17-11*   Direct calculation of sinoatrial conduction time. The slow upstroke of the sinus node potential is labeled SNE and the sinoatrial conduction time is calculated from the onset of this potential to the onset of rapid atrial depolarization, as depicted. Atr. in. = atrial injury pattern. (*From Ref. 14. Reproduced by permission.*)

stimulus failed to alter sinus node automaticity, presumably because it encountered refractoriness in the sinus node region (sinus node refractory period). Still earlier atrial extrastimuli can initiate sinus node reentrant responses (panel *D*, Fig. 17-9).

An alternative method of calculating SACT involves pacing the sinus node region for 8 to 16 cycles just faster than baseline sinus rate.[13] By similar reasoning to the longer method, SACT = $A_2A_3$ − SCL/2, where $A_2A_3$ is the interval from the last paced atrial cycle to the first return cycle. These techniques for SACT are subject to substantial experimental error and are very difficult to use in patients with sinus arrhythmia. Normal values for SACT range from <100 to <170 ms. More recently, direct methods to measure sinoatrial conduction time through endocardial catheter recordings have been developed[14–16] (Fig. 17-11). Evaluation of the sinus node effective refractory period (SNERP) is another test of sinus node function.[17,18] The SNERP is determined during atrial pacing, using the atrial extrastimulus technique. The SNERP is defined as the longest premature atrial interval that results in interpolation (Fig. 17-12). The normal range for SNERP at an atrial paced cycle length of 600 ms is 250 to 380 ms (mean $325 \pm 39$ ms) and is prolonged

with sinus node dysfunction.[18] Overall, we think that overdrive atrial pacing yields the most useful clinical assessment of sinus node function.

## Electrophysiologic Evaluation of Atrioventricular and Ventriculoatrial Conduction System

Incremental atrial and ventricular pacing is used to ascertain anterograde block in the AV node and His-Purkinje system and retrograde block in the ventriculoatrial system, respectively. (See also Chap. 1.) Incremental atrial pacing is started at the longest pacing cycle length that can consistently capture the atrium without interference from the underlying

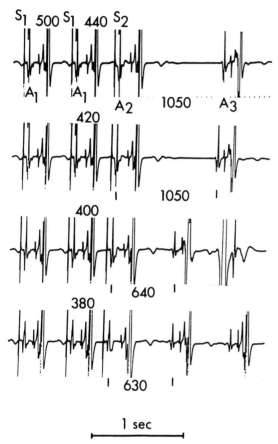

S₁ 500 S₁ 440 S₂

A₁  A₁  A₂  1050  A₃
420

1050
400

640
380

630

| 1 sec

*Figure 17-12* Illustration of the measurement of sinus node effective refractory period (SNERP). An atrial extrastimulus is made progressively premature using a drive cycle of 500 ms. At a critical prematurity of the extrastimulus (400 ms), there is an abrupt shortening of the cycle length of the return atrial cycle, indicating failure of conduction to the sinus node region. This interval is the SNERP.

sinus rate. The cycle length is progressively shortened in 10-ms decrements until AV nodal block occurs or the patient develops symptoms due to hypotension. In patients with abnormal His-Purkinje conduction, block below the His bundle depolarization may occur during atrial pacing, as noted in Fig. 17-13.[19] Atrial pacing should be continued until AV node block occurs, so that both the AV node as well as the His-Purkinje system can be evaluated.

We stress that, for accurate determination of His–Purkinje conduction, *incremental* atrial pacing should be used—not the sudden onset of atrial pacing at various rates. The latter technique can result in a sudden shortening of the atrial cycle length in a patient with a relatively slow heart rate and subsequent block below the recorded His potential. Block below the His in this context is a physiologic event, as previously reported.[20] Block below the His recording can also occur in situations in which there is sudden loss of atrial capture during an incremental atrial pacing run (Fig. 17-14). In this patient, without interruption of the atrial drive train, Wenckebach block occurred in the AV node during incremental pacing, but no block below the His depolarization was noted. However, in Fig. 17-14, note that the second atrial stimulus fails to result in an atrial depolarization, yielding a relatively long cycle length, and the third captured complex demonstrates block below the His depolarization. Infra-His block here is physiologic and not pathologic.

Incremental ventricular pacing to the point at which ventriculoatrial (VA) block occurs should also be performed. In some patients without accessory pathways, there is minimal increase in the VA conduction time until a paced cycle length 20 to 40 ms prior to block. This is a normal finding and does not imply the presence of an accessory pathway.[21] Other patients demonstrate a progressive increase in the VA interval until block occurs, and still other patterns of conduction—such as intermittent VA conduction—can occur (Fig. 17-15). In some patients there is complete VA block during all paced cycle lengths, as noted in Fig. 17-16, taken from a 15-year-old girl after successful radiofrequency endocardial catheter ablation of a left free-wall accessory pathway. Ventriculoatrial block at all paced cycle lengths has no clinical relevance to anterograde conduction over the AV conduction system and frequently occurs in patients with otherwise normal anterograde AV conduction.[22]

Programmed atrial stimulation is used to characterize AV node and His-Purkinje refractoriness. Similarly, programmed ventricular stimulation is used to evaluate refractoriness of the VA conduction

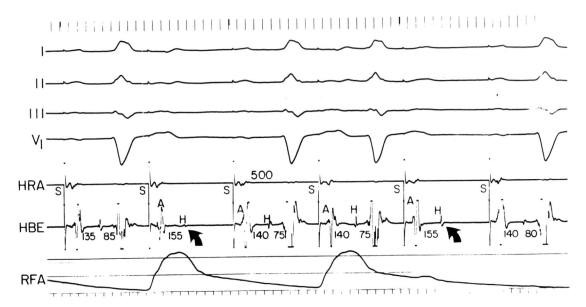

*Figure 17-13*  Mobitz type II second-degree AV block. Atrial pacing at 500 ms results in block below the recorded His deflection (*arrow*), and variable His-Purkinje conduction times from 75 to 85 ms are noted. There is also some slight variability in the AH interval, possibly due to changes in autonomic tone depending on the timing of the arterial pulse pressure before AV node activation. RFA = right femoral artery pressure.

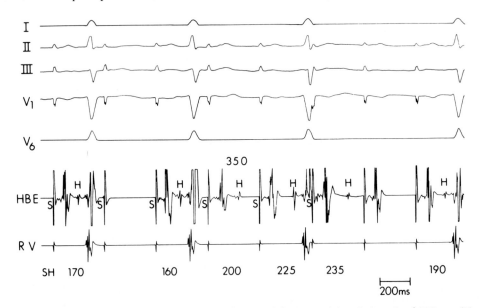

*Figure 17-14*  Infra-His block due to long-short paced interval during atrial cycle length of 350 ms. The second atrial paced stimulus (S) fails to capture the atrium, allowing a sudden long interval to occur, closed by the third stimulus, which causes atrial depolarization and conduction to the ventricles. The fourth stimulus results in block below the His deflection—not a pathologic finding in this situation. Recurrence of block below the His can occur in subsequent beats (sixth stimulus) and is also not abnormal. Note that AV node Wenckebach block also occurs at this cycle length, as evidenced by a progressive increase in the AH interval, measured here for simplicity from the stimulus artifact to the His depolarization (SH).

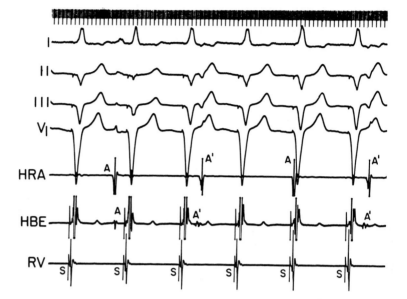

*Figure    17-15    Intermittent ventriculoatrial    conduction.* Note that the first paced ventricular complex does not conduct to the atria, and this is followed by a ventricular fusion beat due to partial activation of the ventricles by a sinus-conducted complex. The third and sixth placed beats conduct retrograde to the atria (A′) as noted by the low-to-high atrial activation sequence (His bundle A′ before HRA A′).

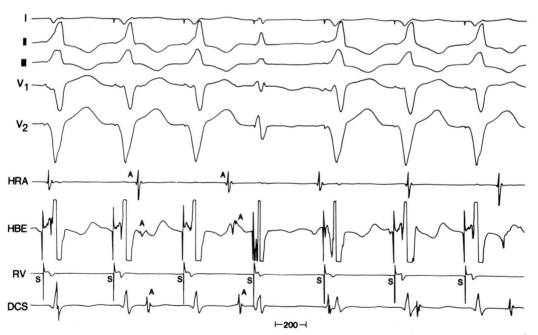

*Figure 17-16*    Complete ventriculoatrial block. During ventricular pacing at a constant cycle length shorter than the sinus cycle length, VA dissociation is present and the fourth QRS complex is a fusion beat. There is a persistent high-to-low atrial activation sequence throughout.

system. We recommend testing refractoriness during sinus rhythm as well as during at least one paced cycle length. After eight either sensed or paced atrial cycles, a premature atrial complex is introduced, beginning in late diastole, and shortened progressively until atrial refractoriness is achieved. In our experience, approximately one-third of patients will demonstrate AV node refractoriness at relatively slow (e.g., 800 ms) atrial cycle lengths, and AV node block will occur in another 30 to 40 percent at faster atrial paced rates. This is due to an increase in the AV node effective refractory period in the normal adult AV node during faster atrial rates. However, approximately 20 to 30 percent of patients will not demonstrate AV node block at atrial pacing cycle lengths of 400 ms or greater, because AV node refractoriness is less than atrial refractoriness at these rates. An example of AV node refractoriness is demonstrated in Fig. 17-17 in a patient who had dual AV node physiology without initiation of tachycardia because of poor VA conduction. Refractoriness of the VA conduction system is tested during ventricular pacing at a constant cycle length, with the introduction of progressively shorter premature ventricular complexes until ventricular refractoriness is achieved.

### Initiation of Tachycardia

Various pacing techniques can be used to initiate supraventricular and ventricular tachycardias (VT). In some patients, especially those with atrioventricular reentry, incremental atrial or ventricular pacing will initiate supraventricular tachycardia. Bursts of atrial pacing at rapid fixed cycle lengths are also useful to initiate AV and AV node reentry and certain types

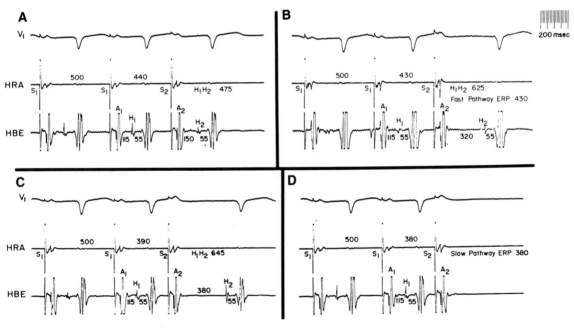

*Figure 17-17*  Determination of refractoriness of the fast and slow AV node conduction pathways. The right atrium was paced at 500 ms and a premature atrial complex of 440 ms conducted over the AV node with a $H_1H_2$ of 475 ms (*A*). An $A_1A_2$ of 430 ms blocked in the fast AV node pathway, as noted by a sudden increase in $H_1H_2$ to 625 ms (*B*). Conduction occurred over the slow AV node pathway at $A_1A_2$ 390 ms (*C*), but block was present at $A_1A_2$ 380 ms (*D*). The effective refractory period (ERP) of the fast and slow AV node pathways are 430 and 380 ms, respectively.

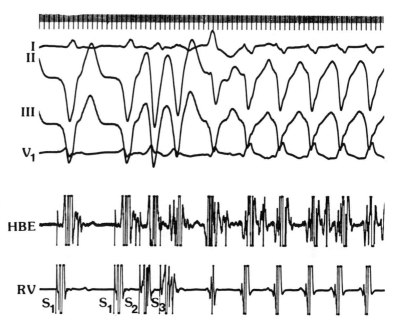

*Figure 17-18*   Induction of sustained monomorphic ventricular tachycardia during ventricular pacing and double extrastimuli ($S_2S_3$). There is variable VA conduction and a His depolarization is not noted before each ventricular electrogram on the HBE tracing.

of atrial tachycardia. Ventricular pacing techniques often initiate AV reentry but are much less successful in inducing AV node reentry. (see Chap. 7). Incremental and burst pacing do not often initiate sustained monomorphic VT, which usually requires pacing of the ventricle with introduction of one to three extrastimuli (Fig. 17-18)[23] (see Chap. 9). Illustrated in Fig. 17-19 is the initiation of AV node reentry with the introduction of only one premature atrial complex during sinus rhythm. In contrast, the patient shown in Fig. 17-20 required two atrial extrastimuli to cause block in the fast AV node pathway and initiate AV node reentry.

## Endocardial Catheter Mapping

Mapping to determine the site of origin of supraventricular tachycardia employs several catheters located at various areas in the right and left atria. The His bundle catheter is left in place and the right atrium

is mapped in one of several ways. A modified Brockenbrough technique developed by Gallagher et al.[24] can be used to map the tricuspid annulus. A luminal bipolar electrode catheter is inserted into the right atrium and a thin flexible stylus with a directional pointer at its end is inserted into the catheter. The electrode is then positioned at various points around the tricuspid annulus. The base of the left atrium is mapped using a catheter that is positioned within and along the length of the coronary sinus to map various points. This is useful primarily in AV reentry but cannot be used to map other points in the left atrium, which might require the introduction of a flexible-tipped catheter into the left atrium by a transseptal technique or retrogradely via the aorta. Right atrial sites can also be mapped with a tip-deflecting catheter. Figure 17-21 is an example of a map of the base of the left atrium in a patient with AV reentry.

During VT, catheters are inserted into the right and left ventricles to map the site of origin of tachycardia. Various criteria have been used by different investigators to localize tissue at or near the

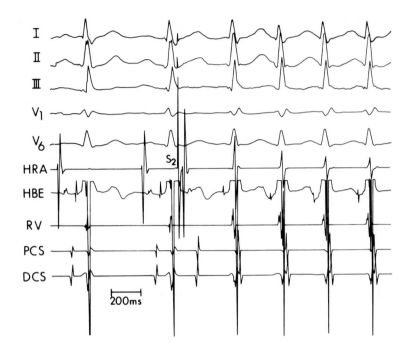

*Figure 17-19*   Initiation of AV node reentry with one atrial extrastimulus (S₂) during sinus rhythm. Note the marked increase in AH interval of S₂ and the very short VA interval during tachycardia.

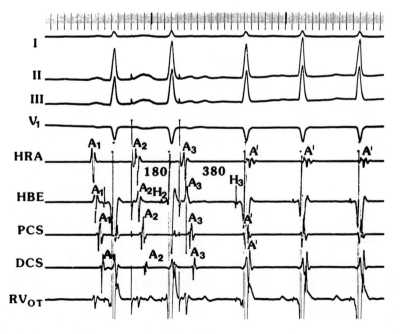

*Figure 17-20*   Initiation of AV node reentry with two atrial extrastimuli (A₂A₃) introduced during sinus rhythm. A₃H₃ shows an increase of 200 ms over A₂H₂.

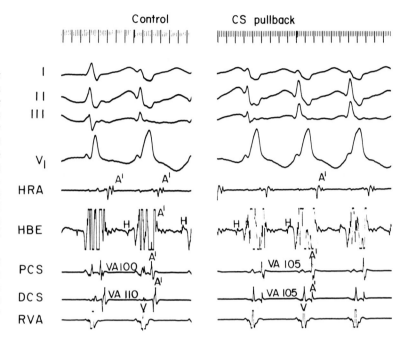

*Figure 17-21* Map of the left AV ring during AV reentry with right bundle branch block. The earliest VA interval (100 ms) is noted on the proximal coronary sinus (PCS) electrogram in the left-hand panel. Note that the VA interval on the distal (DCS) pole is 110 ms. In the right-hand panel, the catheter in the CS is withdrawn to a more proximal location and the VA interval is 105 ms on both the distal and proximal CS electrode pairs. Thus, the earliest retrograde atrial activity during tachycardia was at the previous PCS site; in this patient the pathway was located in the left free wall near the interatrial septum.

tachycardia focus. One method is to identify the earliest electrical activity preceding the QRS complex during VT.[25] Although the electrogram is characteristically abnormal at this site in patients with coronary artery disease, it may be nearly normal in patients with VT without structural heart disease (Fig. 17-22). In patients with previous myocardial infarction, demonstration of middiastolic potentials[26] or a zone of slow conduction[27] during VT has been proposed to localize the origin of tachycardia. Recent data shed doubt on the latter technique.[28] Less useful but ancillary techniques are mapping in sinus rhythm to detect abnormal ventricular electrograms and ventricular pace mapping. During pace mapping, 12-lead electrocardiograms are obtained at multiple pacing sites and compared with the 12-lead electrocardiographic (ECG) morphology of VT.

The mapping scheme noted in Fig. 17-23 can be used to identify various locations in the left ventricle. During tachycardia, the catheter in the left ventricle is positioned at the various sites that are identified using multiple fluoroscopic views, and electrograms are recorded at each site. This technique

does not always allow precise localization of the origin of tachycardia, but reasonable approximations can be made (Fig. 17-22). This is usually adequate if the patient is to undergo surgical ablation of the VT, but more precise mapping is necessary if catheter ablation is to be used.

## Endocardial Catheter Ablation

Many exciting advances have taken place in the technique and clinical application of endocardial catheter ablation as a treatment for cardiac arrhythmias since its original description in 1982.[29,30] This procedure was used initially to ablate tissue in the AV junction in an effort to control refractory supraventricular tachyarrhythmias. However, the indications for catheter ablation quickly expanded to include the treatment of patients with VT and to cure patients with supraventricular tachycardia by ablating, without causing AV block, specific areas of the heart involved in the arrhythmia.[26–28,31–51]

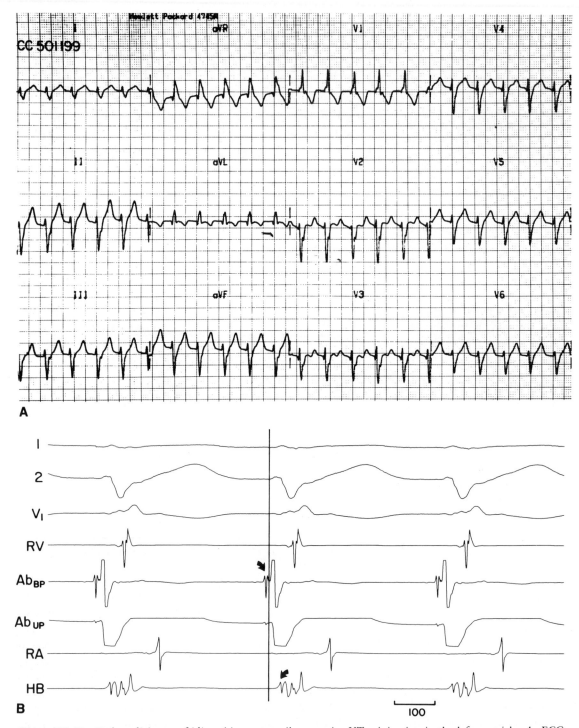

**A**

**B**

*Figure 17-22* Endocardial map of idiopathic, verapamil-responsive VT originating in the left ventricle. *A.* ECG during VT. *B.* At the site of successful endocardial catheter ablation, note the sharp potential (*arrow*) preceding onset of the QRS complex during VT in the bipolar electrogram on the ablation catheter (Ab$_{BP}$). A retrograde His is identified by the lower arrow.

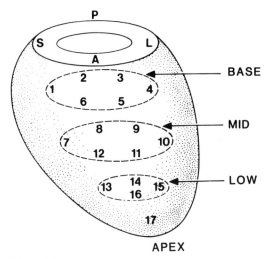

*Figure 17-23*  Schematic for left ventricular mapping. The left ventricle is divided into three rings designated at the base, mid, and low ventricle and at the apex. Electrograms during tachycardia are obtained at each point.

Our intent is to provide an overview of catheter ablation techniques and results; the reader is referred to Refs. 26 to 54 for more details.

The first energy source utilized was high-energy electrical direct current discharges delivered from a standard defibrillator. The shocks are given through the tip of an electrode catheter in the heart, usually serving as the cathode, and directed to an electrode patch positioned on the surface of the chest or back of the patient, usually serving as the anode for the electrical field.[29,30] The tip of the catheter is positioned strategically near the area to be ablated and the shock, which is painful, is delivered during general anesthesia. The major cause of tissue damage is related to the marked electrical field that disrupts cell membranes.

An alternative energy source that has gained in popularity is unmodulated radiofrequency current that causes coagulation necrosis of tissue because of extreme heat and consequent desiccation of tissues in the immediate vicinity.[36,39–43,45–47,49,50,52–54] One major advantage of the delivery of radiofrequency energy is the ability to titrate energy better to produce a smaller and more localized lesion. In addition, general anesthesia is not necessary because

pain during the delivery of the radiofrequency energy is minimal. Both techniques have been successful in various types of arrhythmias, and the use of one energy source versus another may depend on the particular clinical circumstance and operator bias. Further, other energy sources—such as microwave and laser—are being investigated; it is unclear which particular energy delivery system will predominate in the future. Although efficacy has been demonstrated with radiofrequency and direct-current catheter ablation techniques, long-term safety—for example, over more than 10 years—of the lesions introduced at sites around the right and left AV ring remains to be determined, especially long-term sequelae to the coronary artery in the field of energy delivery. Follow-up of patients for several years has yet to demonstrate any significant problems.

## Supraventricular Tachycardia

### Ablation of Atrioventricular Junction

Ablation of the AV junction, often referred to as His bundle ablation, was initially utilized to control a variety of supraventricular tachyarrhythmias.[29,30] Theoretically, any patient with a supraventricular arrhythmia that conducts to the ventricles over the AV node and His-Purkinje system is a potential candidate for AV junctional ablation. At present we reserve this technique for certain atrial tachyarrhythmias, especially atrial fibrillation, in which a primary cure of the arrhythmia with catheter ablation techniques is not currently possible. In these individuals, production of complete heart block will not cure the atrial arrhythmia but will prevent impulses from being conducted to the ventricle. These patients experience a marked improvement in symptoms when their heart rate is controlled by a rate-responsive ventricular pacemaker. For arrhythmias such as AV and AV node reentry, the aim of ablation is to cure the patient by destroying tissue in the reentrant circuit. Preliminary data show that this can also be done for some patients with atrial tachycardia, sinus node reentry, and atrial flutter.[48–51]

An example of radiofrequency ablation of the AV junction is shown in Fig. 17-24. Although this

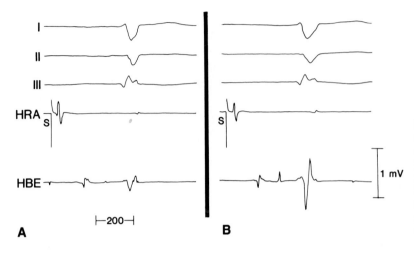

I

II

III

HRA

HBE

├─200─┤

A

B

1 mV

*Figure 17-24*  Successful and unsuccessful sites of atrioventricular junctional ablation. Note the small His potential in the unsuccessful attempt (*A*) but the relatively large His and atrial deflections at the site of successful AV junctional ablation (*B*).

technique was originally designated "His bundle ablation," the main area of block is more likely in the AV node. Thus, catheter recordings at the successful ablation site usually show a substantial-sized atrial as well as His deflection, suggesting energy delivery in the AV node region (Fig. 17-24). When a large His deflection is recorded in conjunction with a very small atrial electrogram, the catheter is more distal in location, as described earlier in this chapter. At this site energy delivery often ablates the right bundle branch but does not cause complete heart block, possibly because the central fibrous body protects the His bundle. Most patients with complete heart block resulting from energy delivered at a more proximal ablation site have a junctional escape rhythm that responds to autonomic interventions, and the QRS complex is very similar to the previously conducted sinus impulses (Fig. 17-25). Although it is rarely necessary, complete heart block can be achieved by ablation on the left ventricular endocardium where the His emerges between the right and noncoronary aortic cusps.

*Ablation of Accessory Pathways*

It is possible to position the tip of an electrode catheter near either the atrial or ventricular insertion site of an accessory pathway and cause destruction of the accessory pathway apparatus with energy delivery

using either high-energy direct current or radiofrequency energy.[37-43] Two approaches are used to ablate left-sided accessory pathways. The retrograde aortic catheterization technique involves introducing the ablation catheter into a femoral artery and advancing it under fluoroscopic guidance across the aortic valve into the left ventricular cavity. We use a catheter with a flexible distal tip for easy maneuverability in the left ventricle. As demonstrated in Fig. 17-26, the site of the accessory pathway is mapped using the coronary sinus catheter and the tip of the ablation catheter is positioned under the mitral valve in the region of the earliest atrial activity noted on the coronary sinus catheter. However, this is only a first approximation, since the area of interest is usually the ventricular insertion site using this method. More precise mapping is performed by subtle movements of the ablation catheter to an area that records an accessory pathway potential, early ventricular activation preceding the surface ECG delta wave in manifest preexcitation, or both (Fig. 17-27). Mapping left-sided manifest accessory pathways can be done with the ablation catheter only, without a coronary sinus catheter. We prefer using multiple catheters to the "single-catheter" technique, which we consider technically more difficult.

It is also possible to ablate the accessory pathway by positioning the catheter ablation electrode above the mitral valve, near the atrial insertion site of the

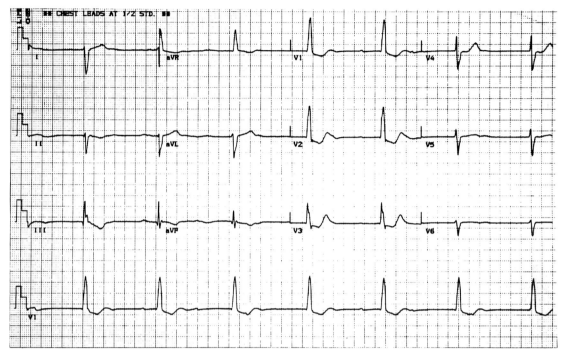

*Figure 17-25*   Junctional escape rhythm after successful ablation of AV junction with complete heart block. Same patient shown in Fig. 17-24.

pathway, using either the retrograde aortic method or the atrial transseptal approach.[43] Right-sided free-wall and septal pathways are typically ablated with a catheter positioned on the atrial side of the tricuspid valve. The ablation catheter is most often inserted into the femoral vein and advanced to the tricuspid annulus, but a superior approach can also be used, with catheter insertion in the subclavian or internal jugular vein. Mapping of concealed accessory pathways with retrograde conduction only is done during

*Figure 17-26*   Radiograph of left ventricular endocardial catheter position resulting in successful ablation of a left lateral accessory pathway. The tip of the ablation catheter (*arrow*) is near the AV ring at the ventricular insertion site of the accessory pathway. Note that the catheter tip is near the middle electrode pole on the coronary sinus catheter, which recorded earliest atrial activity during AV reentry. LAO = left anterior oblique; AP = anteroposterior view..

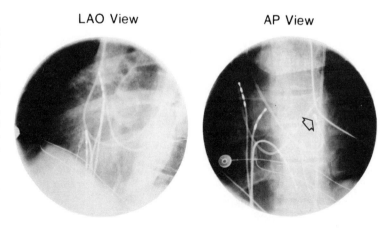

LAO View          AP View

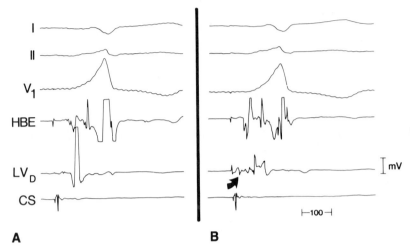

*Figure 17-27*   Successful (*B*) and unsuccessful (*A*) catheter ablation positions (same patient shown in Fig. 17-26). It is important to record atrial activity of reasonable magnitude at the ventricular ablation site, ensuring that the catheter tip is near the base of the ventricle where the pathway inserts. At the unsuccessful site, the catheter tip (LV$_D$) records a ventricular potential that activates with the start of the delta wave on the surface ECG, but only a very small atrial potential is present. At the successful site, there is a substantial-sized atrial deflection (*arrow*), followed by either an accessory pathway deflection and/or very early ventricular activation. mV = 1 millivolt; LV$_D$ = bipolar electrogram on tip of ablation catheter.

AV reentry or ventricular pacing. The ablation catheter is positioned at the AV groove to record adequate atrial and ventricular electrograms. Success occurs at sites that demonstrate the earliest VA intervals for a given patient and continuous electrical activity bridging the ventricular and atrial electrograms, with or without the presence of a discrete accessory pathway potential. Figures 17-28 to 17-30 are examples of accessory pathway ablation.

It is not always clear why a particular lesion causes loss of conduction over the accessory pathway. As demonstrated in Fig. 17-31, which is a schematic representation of the potential mechanism for successful catheter ablation of accessory pathways, the accessory pathway "apparatus" includes the atrial and ventricular insertion sites and the accessory pathway itself. In Fig. 17-31, a catheter is positioned near the AV ring, where an early ventricular activation point has been recorded. Radiofrequency energy presumably destroys atrial and ventricular tissue in this region but might also directly ablate the accessory pathway. Regardless, complete disruption of any part of the accessory pathway apparatus should result

in lack of conduction over the pathway from the atrium to the ventricle. It is theoretically possible that in some patients the accessory pathway remains unharmed by this technique but conducts into a blind alley of dead ventricular or atrial tissue. In fact, in some of our patients accessory pathway potentials have been recorded before and after successful catheter ablation, although ventricular preexcitation is lost.

### Ablation Cure of AV Node Reentry

The anatomic reentrant circuit used in AV node reentry is still unclear. The traditional concept is that anterograde conduction is over a slowly conducting pathway within the AV node and retrograde conduction is over a rapidly conducting pathway presumably in the AV node or utilizing at least part of the AV node and possibly atrial tissue. Energy delivery at discrete sites in the posterior and anterior septum can modify AV node function and prevent inducibility and spontaneous recurrences of AV node reentry.[44–47] These observations suggest that in most

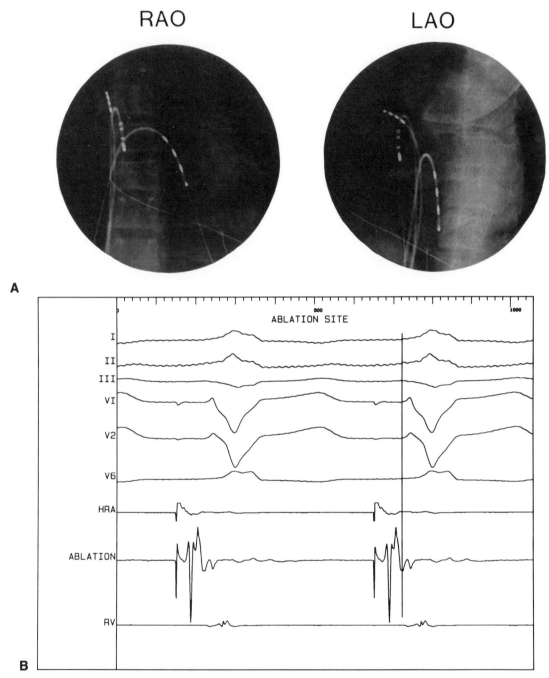

**Figure** *17-28* Ablation of a right free-wall accessory pathway. *A*. Radiograph of the ablation catheter position (*middle catheter*) in the right (RAO) and left (LAO) oblique views. The upper and lower catheters are in the high right atrium and right ventricular apex, respectively. *B*. Right atrial pacing to maximize ventricular preexcitation. The electrogram on the ablation catheter shows an initial large atrial deflection followed by a probable accessory pathway potential and ventricular activity preceding the onset of the delta wave (*vertical line*). *C*. Initiation of radiofrequency current instantaneously abolishes conduction over the accessory pathway, as noted by the normalization of the fifth QRS complex. AMP = amperes.

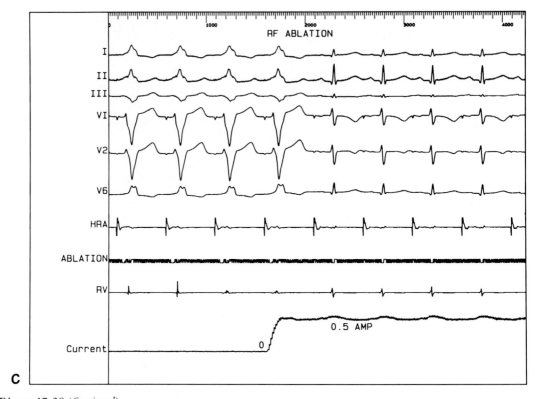

*Figure* 17-28 *(Continued)*

patients at least a portion of the atrium is used in the AV node reentrant circuit (Fig. 17-32). This has led to two approaches to cure AV node reentry (Fig. 17-33).

The anterior approach to modify AV node conduction involves energy delivery through a catheter positioned in the anterior interatrial septum.[44] The ablation tip records a large atrial deflection, a His bundle deflection usually <35 microvolts, and an atrial electrogram at least two times the ventricular amplitude (Fig. 17-34). The ablation site is very close to the AV node, and a successful outcome typically results in a permanent prolongation of the PR interval and either poor or absent retrograde conduction. It has been postulated that this is due to ablation of the fast AV node pathway, with subsequent conduction over the slowly conducting AV node pathway. An example using this approach is shown in Fig. 17-35. This patient required isoproterenol for induction of AV node reentry, which is a requisite at electrophysiologic study in approximately 20 percent of patients with this arrhythmia (Fig. 17-35A). Prior to ablation, the patient demonstrates a normal PR interval (Fig. 17-35B); but after ablation, there is complete VA block and no inducible AV node reentry, while the PR interval is prolonged (Fig. 17-35C).

The aim of the posterior approach is to eliminate conduction over the slow AV node pathway.[45] The tip of the ablation catheter is positioned initially in the right posterior septum near the os of the coronary sinus (Figs. 17-33 and 17-36). A site is chosen that has a large ventricular and small atrial electrogram (Fig. 17-37). Often one can record two distinct atrial

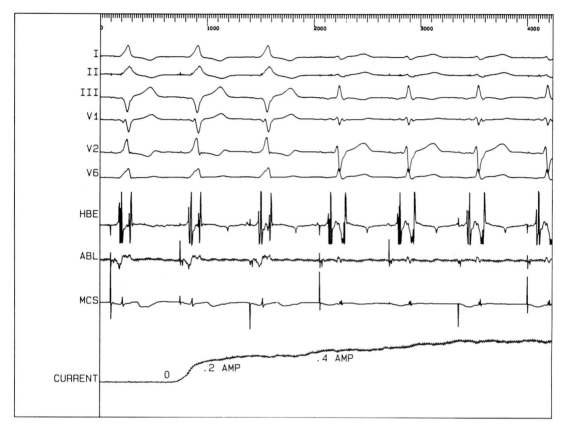

*Figure 17-29*   Ablation of posteroseptal accessory pathway. As the current is being increased to 0.5 A, accessory pathway conduction disappears at about 0.4 A (fourth QRS complex). (*From Prystowsky EN, Noble RJ: Heart Dis Stroke 1:188, 1992. Reproduced by permission.*)

potentials at the site of successful ablation (Fig. 17-37), but success does not depend on ablation at a site with this finding. Jackman et al.[45] suggest that the second atrial electrogram recorded during sinus rhythm may represent the atrial connection with the slow pathway. Thus, ablation of this area could prevent conduction from the atrium to the slow AV node pathway, thereby preventing initiation of AV node reentry. Clearly, destruction of atrial tissue at multiple critical points leading to the posterior AV node input can yield similar success.[46]

There is an alternative explanation for the high rate of success in treating AV node reentry with ablation at the site of two separate atrial electrograms. The target site with two distinct atrial electrograms may represent the posterior turnaround point of the AV node reentrant circuit. This would involve atrial tissue conducting in longitudinal and transverse directions. According to anisotropic conduction, the first low-amplitude atrial depolarization represents transverse atrial conduction, and the second larger atrial deflection with a more rapid upstroke is due to longitudinal conduction. The observations are consistent with the proposed hypothesis. Unlike the anterior approach, successful posterior ablation causes little or no change in the PR interval. However, conduction over the slow AV node pathway is either eliminated or markedly impaired (Fig. 17-38).

### Ablation Cure of Atrial Flutter and Atrial Tachycardia

Preliminary data are encouraging for catheter ablation to cure typical atrial flutter and atrial tachycardia.[48-51] Typical or type 1 atrial flutter in humans appears to have a caudocranial activation sequence that includes the posteroseptal right atrium in the reentrant circuit.[49] Radiofrequency energy applied to atrial tissue inferior or posterior to the coronary sinus ostium successfully terminated atrial flutter in 10 of 12 patients.[49] Successful ablation of atrial tachycardia has been performed in a small group of patients[50,51] (Fig. 17-39). Long-term follow-up is not yet available for most of these patients.

### Ablation of the Focus of Ventricular Tachycardia

A catheter can be positioned in the ventricle near the presumed site of origin of VT and energy delivered to this area.[26-28,32-36,54] Because of the

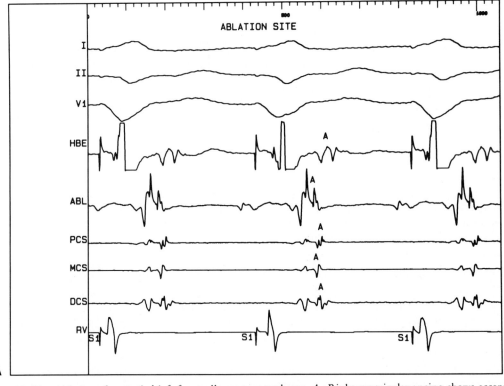

**A**

*Figure 17-30*   Ablation of concealed left free-wall accessory pathway. *A.* Right ventricular pacing shows eccentric retrograde atrial activation sequence with coronary sinus (CS) preceding His bundle (HBE) atrium (A). Earliest A activity is on the ablation catheter (Abl), with a probable accessory pathway potential between the initial ventricular and atrial deflection. *B.* During radiofrequency current delivery, there is a sudden change in the retrograde atrial activation sequence on the third beat. Note the VA increase on the CS leads, e.g., 158 to 220 ms on the mid-CS electrogram. Retrograde conduction is now concentric over the normal conducting system with the earliest A on the HBE lead. The constant VA interval on the HBE electrogram confirms that during ventricular pacing, the atrial septum is activated over the normal ventriculoatrial conducting system and not via the left-sided accessory pathway.

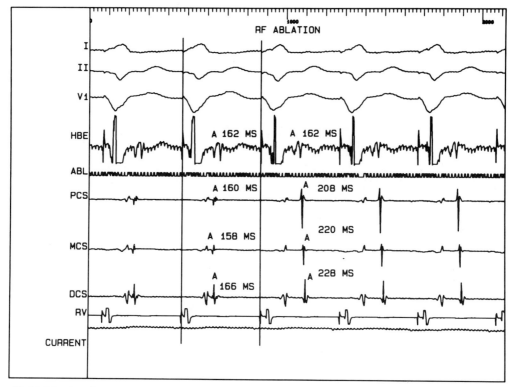

RF ABLATION

I

II

V1

HBE    A 162 MS    A 162 MS

ABL

PCS    A 160 MS    A 208 MS

MCS    A 158 MS    A 220 MS

DCS    A 166 MS    A 228 MS

RV

CURRENT

**B**

***Figure** 17-30 (Continued)*

relatively small size of the ablation lesions, it is often difficult, even with multiple ablation attempts using high-energy direct current, to cure patients with heart disease of their sustained VT. Radiofrequency energy has also been used to treat patients with VT, but minimal data are currently available regarding this approach in patients with heart disease. Catheter ablation techniques are very successful in patients with no obvious structural heart disease who have VT (Chap. 9).[36,54] These patients usually have VT with a left bundle branch block and inferior axis, or right bundle branch block and left axis morphology. The former is located in the right ventricular outflow tract and the latter in the left ventricle in the inferior septal region. A select group of patients with bundle branch reentrant tachycardia in which the right bundle branch is a requisite part of the tachycardia

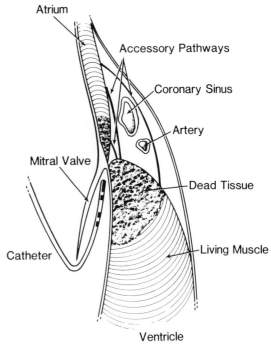

***Figure** 17-31* Schematic of potential mechanism for loss of conduction over accessory pathway with catheter ablation. *(See text for details.)* ⟶

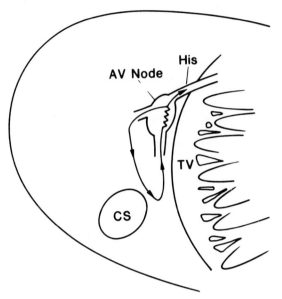

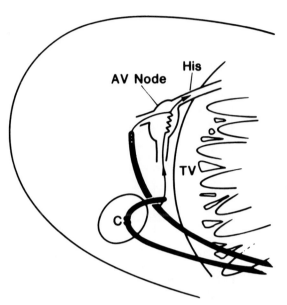

**Figure 17-32**   Proposed AV node reentrant circuit. As diagrammed, at least part of the circuit is outside of the AV node, in particular the connection from the retrograde fast pathway to the anterograde intranodal slow pathway (*zigzag line*). CS = os of coronary sinus; TV = tricuspid valve. Atrial septum shown in a right anterior oblique view.

**Figure 17-33**   Anterior and posterior catheter ablation sites for cure of AV node reentry.

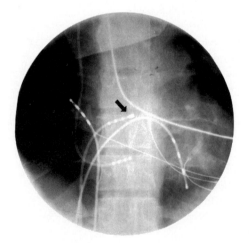

**Figure 17-34**   Radiograph of successful AV node modification site (*arrow*) to cure AV node reentry. (*See text for details.*) Arrow is site of energy delivery.

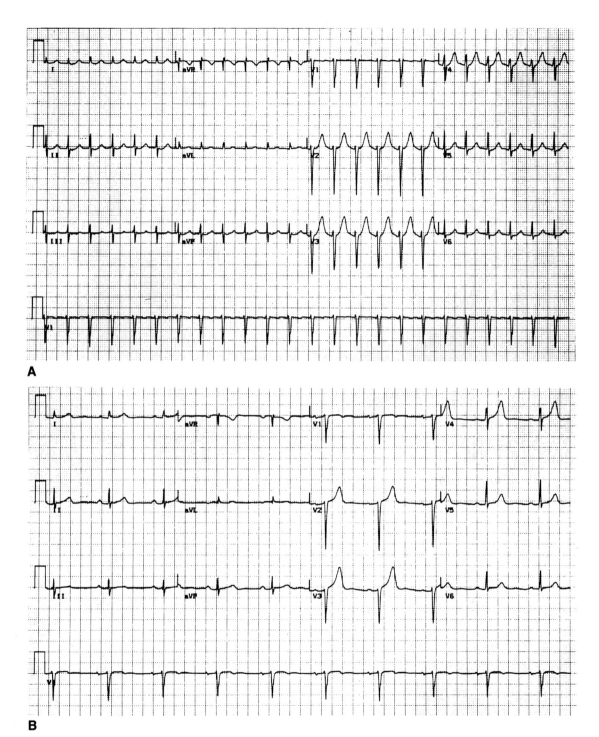

**A**

**B**

*Figure 17-35* Electrocardiogram before and after successful radio-frequency anterior modification of AV node conduction (same patient as in Fig. 17-34). *A*. AV node reentry (isoproterenol, 1 μg/min) *B*. ECG before ablation (control). *C*. ECG after ablation (post AVN modification). Note the increase in PR interval.

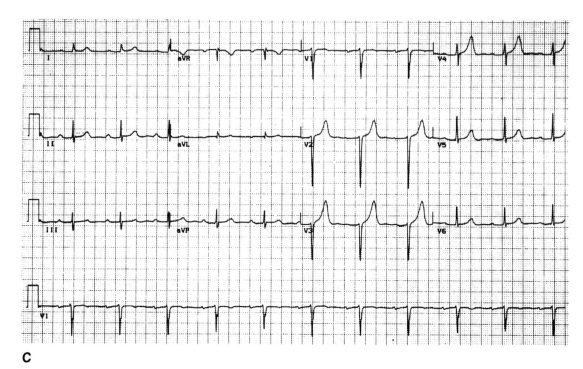

**C**

*Figure* 17-35 (*Continued*)

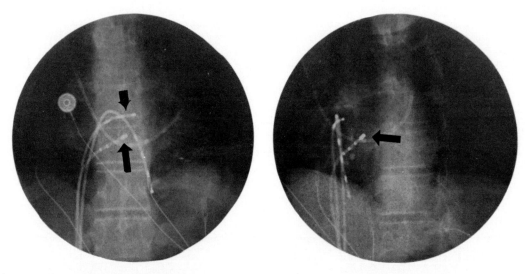

*Figure* 17-36   Radiograph of posterior catheter ablation site to cure AV node reentry. The left panel is a slight right anterior oblique view and the right panel is a left anterior oblique view. The large arrows point to the distal electrode on the ablation catheter positioned near the os of the coronary sinus on the posterior right interatrial septum. Note the substantial distance between the ablation site and the anterior AV node area identified by the distal electrode pair on the His bundle catheter (*small arrow*).

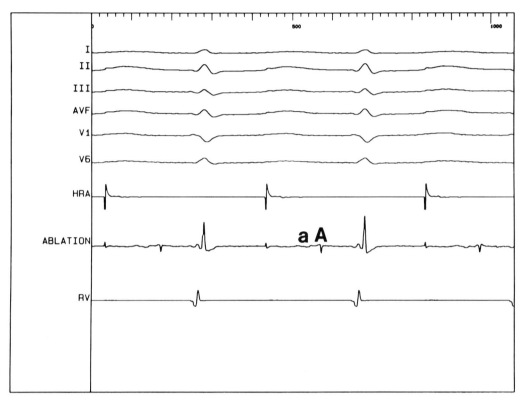

*Figure* 17-37   Electrograms recorded on the distal bipolar electrodes of the ablation catheter at the site of energy delivery. There are two distinct atrial potentials. The first has low amplitude and a slow upstroke (a), and the second has greater amplitude and relatively rapid upstroke (A). (*See text for details.*)

*Figure* 17-38   AV node refractory curves before (Pre) and after (Post) successful ablation using the posterior approach to cure AV node reentry. The interval between the His depolarization of the last beat of the atrial drive train ($H_1$) to the His of the atrial premature beat ($H_2$) is plotted as a function of the atrial premature interval ($A_1A_2$) measured on the His bundle electrogram (HBE). Before ablation, there is a sudden "jump" in the $H_1H_2$ interval at a critical $A_1A_2$ interval. AV node reentry began with this sudden block in conduction over the fast pathway and subsequent conduction over the slow pathway. Successful ablation eliminated conduction over the slow pathway (no jump) and AV node reentry could not be initiated.

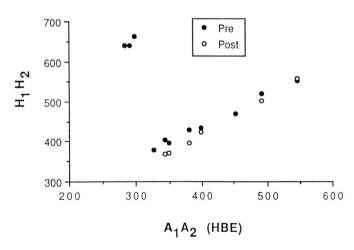

5.  Franz MR: Long-term recording of monophasic action potentials from human endocardium. *Am J Cardiol* 51:1629, 1983.

6.  Gallagher JJ et al: Epicardial mapping in the Wolff-Parkinson-White syndrome. *Circulation* 57:854, 1978.

7.  Prystowsky EN: The sick sinus syndrome—Diagnosis and treatment, in Donoso E (ed): *Advances and Controversies in Cardiology* New York, Thieme-Stratton, 1981, p 95.

8.  Mandel WJ et al: Assessment of sinus node function in patients with sick sinus syndrome. *Circulation* 46:761, 1972.

9.  Strauss HC et al: Premature atrial stimulation as a key to the understanding of sinoatrial conduction in man. *Circulation* 47:86, 1973.

10. Lange G: Action of driving stimuli from intrinsic and extrinsic sources on in situ cardiac pacemaker cells. *Circ Res* 17:449, 1965.

11. Browne KF et al: Factors influencing specificity of sinus node recovery time in man. *Circulation* 68(III):III-382, 1983.

12. Benditt DG et al: Analysis of secondary pauses following termination of rapid atrial pacing in man. *Circulation* 54:436, 1976.

13. Narula OS et al: A new method for mesurement of sinoatrial conduction time. *Circulation* 58:706, 1978.

14. Reiffel JA et al: The human sinus node electrogram: A transvenous catheter technique and a comparison of directly measured and indirectly estimated sinoatrial conduction time in adults. *Circulation* 62:1324, 1980.

15. Gomes JAC et al: New application of direct sinus node recordings in man; assessment of sinus node recovery time. *Circulation* 70:663, 1984.

16. Gomes JAC et al: The sinus node electrogram in patients with and without sick sinus syndrome: Techniques and correlation between directly measured and indirectly estimated sinoatrial conduction time. *Circulation* 66:864, 1982.

17. Kerr CR et al: Characterization of refractoriness in the sinus node of the rabbit. *Circ Res* 47:742, 1980.

18. Kerr CR, Strauss HC: The measurement of sinus node refractoriness in man. *Circulation* 68:1231, 1983.

19. Dhingra RC et al: Significance of block distal to the His bundle induced by atrial pacing in patients with chronic bifascicular block. *Circulation* 60:1455, 1979.

20. Damato AN et al: Functional 2:1 A-V block within the His-Purkinje system: Simulation of type II second degree A-V block. *Circulation* 47:534, 1973.

21. Prystowsky EN et al: Electrophysiologic assessment of the atrioventricular conduction system after surgical correction of ventricular preexcitation. *Circulation* 59:789, 1979.

22. Schuilenburg RM: Patterns of V-A conduction in the human heart in the presence of normal and abnormal A-V conduction, in Wellens HJJ, Lie KI, Janse MJ (eds): *The Conduction System of the Heart.* Philadelphia, Lea & Febiger, 1976, p 485.

23. Prystowsky EN et al: Induction of ventricular tachycardia during programmed electrical stimulation: Analysis of pacing methods. *Circulation* 73:II-32, 1986.

24. Gallagher JJ et al: New catheter techniques for analysis of the sequence of retrograde atrial activation in man. *Eur J Cardiol* 6(1):1, 1977.

25. Josephson ME et al: Recurrent sustained ventricular tachycardia: 2. Endocardial mapping. *Circulation* 57:440, 1978.

26. Fitzgerald DM et al: Electrogram patterns predicting successful catheter ablation of ventricular tachycardia. *Circulation* 77:806, 1988.

27. Morady F et al: Identification and catheter ablation of a zone of slow conduction in the reentrant circuit of ventricular tachycardia in humans. *J Am Coll Cardiol* 11:775, 1988.

28. Morady F et al: Concealed entrainment as a guide for catheter ablation of ventricular tachycardia in patients with prior myocardial infarction. *J Am Coll Cardiol* 17:678, 1991.

29. Gallagher JJ et al: Catheter technique for closed-chest ablation of the atrioventricular conduction system. *N Engl J Med* 306:194, 1982.

30. Scheinman MM et al: Catheter-induced ablation of the atrioventricular junction to control refractory supraventricular arrhythmias. *JAMA* 248:851, 1982.

31. Scheinman MM: Catheter ablation: Present role and projected impact on health care for patients with cardiac arrhythmias. *Circulation* 83:1489, 1991.

32. Hartzler GO: Electrode catheter ablation of refractory focal ventricular tachycardia. *J Am Coll Cardiol* 2:1107, 1983.

33. Fontaine G et al: Treatment des tachycardies ventriculaires rebelles par fulguration endocavitaire associee aux anti-arhthmiques. *Arch Mal Coeur* 79:1152, 1986.

34.  Tchou P et al: Transcatheter electrical ablation of the right bundle branch: A method of treating macroreentrant ventricular tachycardia attributed to bundle branch reentry. *Circulation* 78:246, 1988.

35.  Morady F et al: Long-term results of catheter ablation of idiopathic right ventricular tachycardia. *Circulation* 82:2093, 1990.

36.  Page RL et al: Radiofrequency catheter ablation of idiopathic recurrent ventricular tachycardia with right bundle branch block, left axis morphology. *PACE* 16:327, 1993.

37.  Morady F et al: Long-term results of catheter ablation of a posteroseptal accessory atrioventricular connection in 48 patients. *Circulation* 79:1160, 1989.

38.  Warin JF et al: Catheter ablation of accessory pathways: Technique and results in 248 patients. *PACE* 13:1609, 1990.

39.  Borggrefe M et al: High frequency alternating current ablation of an accessory pathway in humans. *J Am Coll Cardiol* 10:576, 1987.

40.  Jackman WM et al: Catheter ablation of accessory atrioventricular pathways (Wolff-Parkinson-White syndrome) by radiofrequency current. *N Engl J Med* 324:1605, 1991.

41.  Kuck KH et al: Radiofrequency current catheter ablation of accessory atrioventricular pathways. *Lancet* 337:1557, 1991.

42.  Calkins H et al: Diagnosis and cure of the Wolff-Parkinson-White syndrome or paroxysmal supraventricular tachycardias during a single electrophysiologic test. *N Engl J Med* 324:1612, 1991.

43.  Natale A et al: Atrial and ventricular approaches for radiofrequency catheter ablation of left-sided accessory pathways. *Am J Cardiol* 70:114, 1992.

44.  Haissaguerre M et al: Closed-chest ablation of retrograde conduction in patients with atrioventricular nodal reentrant tachycardia. *N Engl J Med* 320:426, 1989.

45.  Jackman WM et al: Treatment of supraventricular tachycardia due to atrioventricular nodal reentry by radiofrequency catheter ablation of slow-pathway conduction. *N Engl J Med.* 327:313, 1992.

46.  Jazayeri MR et al: Selective transcatheter ablation of the fast and slow pathways using radiofrequency energy in patients with atrioventricular nodal reentrant tachycardia. *Circulation* 85:1318, 1992.

47.  Wathen M et al: An anatomically guided approach to atrioventricular node slow pathway ablation: *Am J Cardiol* 70:886, 1992.

48.  Saoudi N et al: Catheter ablation of the atrial myocardium in human type I atrial flutter. *Circulation* 81:762, 1990.

49.  Feld GK et al: Radiofrequency catheter ablation for the treatment of human type 1 atrial flutter. *Circulation* 86:1233, 1992.

50.  Walsh EP et al: Transcatheter ablation of ectopic atrial tachycardia in young patients using radiofrequency current. *Circulation* 86:1138, 1992.

51.  Silka MJ et al: Transvenous catheter ablation of a right atrial automatic ectopic tachycardia. *J Am Coll Cardiol* 5:999, 1985.

52.  Huang SKS et al: Chronic incomplete atrioventricular block induced by radiofrequency catheter ablation. *Circulation* 80:951, 1989.

53.  Langberg JL et al: Catheter ablation of the atrioventricular junction with radiofrequency energy. *Circulation* 80:1527, 1989.

54.  Klein LS et al: Radiofrequency catheter ablation of ventricular tachycardia in patients without structural heart disease. *Circulation* 85:1666, 1992.

# Chapter 18

# *Noninvasive Methods*

Invasive electrophysiologic testing has many advantages, such as the ability to initiate a tachyarrhythmia and at the same time confirm the diagnosis. In addition, electrophysiologic testing is an excellent way to judge the efficacy of nonpharmacologic and pharmacologic therapy. It is less helpful in defining marked abnormalities of the sinus node and AV conduction system that cause episodic syncope.[1,2] Intermittent sinus node dysfunction is commonly not detected, whereas AV conduction abnormalities are often at least partially manifest during study.

Noninvasive methods can be extremely valuable and provide unique and complementary information to electrophysiologic testing. Signal-averaged electrocardiography (SAECG) and heart rate variability (HRV) are tests to assess relative risk to develop sustained ventricular tachycardia (VT) or ventricular fibrillation (VF). Exercise testing and head-up tilt are used to initiate arrhythmias and diagnose neurally mediated syncope, respectively. Long-term electrocardiographic (ECG) monitoring and recording techniques can document the cause of palpitations, presyncope, and syncope, which is often elusive at electrophysiologic study. Esophageal electrograms can be diagnostic, and esophageal pacing can terminate a variety of tachyarrhythmias. These techniques and suggested applications are reviewed in this chapter.

## *Electrocardiographic Recordings*

Technology has advanced significantly since Holter described a portable magnetic tape recorder that could continuously record a patient's ECG for as long as 10 h.[3] Long-term ambulatory ECG (Holter) recorders can now record two ECG leads continuously for 24 to 48 h.[4] In addition, other technologies such as event recorders with or without a memory loop are available and have important diagnostic capabilities. Possibly the most common type of recording used clinically is continuous ECG monitoring in a telemetry unit in hospital. Before describing the various techniques, some example of artifacts common to any lead technology are discussed.

Figure 18-1 is taken from a patient in the electrophysiology laboratory. The intracardiac recordings confirm normal sinus rhythm at a time when a relatively regular rapid ventricular tachyarrhythmia is apparently present on the ECG leads. The artifactual VT was produced by manually jiggling the ECG recording cable. The ECG strip should always be analyzed to determine if regular QRS activity appears to be "marching through" the underlying "arrhythmia" (Fig. 15-4), which is not present in this example. This observation confirms an artifact in recording techniques. In addition, determination of the status of the patient at the time the recording was made may be helpful to diagnose artifact. Motion artifact is relatively common and occurs frequently with activity that involves movement of the upper torso, such as brushing teeth.

Figure 18-2 shows a "toothbrush arrhythmia" that occurred only in one ECG lead. The patient has sinus rhythm with premature ventricular complexes on the top tracing, but there is an apparent atrial arrhythmia on the bottom tracing due to artifact recorded during arm motion while the patient was brushing his teeth. Electrodes can become loose or disconnected, resulting in no or very small recorded signals. Commonly a shift in the baseline occurs and certain diagnostic clues may be found. In Fig. 18-3,

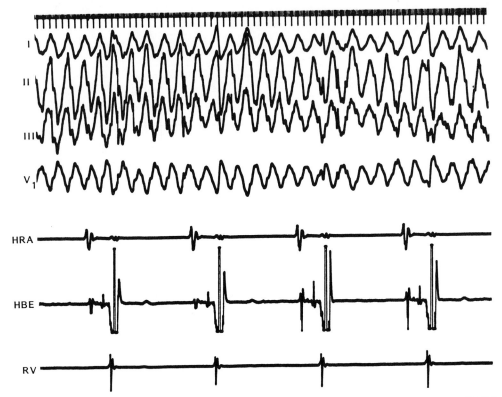

*Figure 18-1*   Artifact due to manipulation of ECG recording cable. Simultaneous tracings are ECG leads I, II, III, V$_1$, and intracardiac leads from the high right atrium (HRA), His bundle area (HBE), and right ventricle (RV). The patient is in sinus rhythm, as noted from the intracardiac tracings.

there is continuous ECG activity in the top tracing but a period of apparent asystole in the bottom tracing. In the latter lead, note that the baseline suddenly moves upward and, importantly, there is evidence of depolarization and repolarization when the baseline returns toward normal. On occasion, only the QRS complex is lost but repolarization remains, clearly a recording artifact. Another type of artifact occurs when extraneous electrical signals are sensed by the recording device, such as a bedside intravenous infusion pump. If it is safe to do so, it is useful to turn off the electrical equipment to identify the source of artifact. In Fig. 18-4, a fluoroscope was documented to be the cause of the artifact that mimicked an atrial tachycardia.

### Telemetry Unit Monitoring

Continuous ECG monitoring in hospital provides for patient safety and may yield diagnostic information. In our experience, it is uncommon to diagnose the cause of a patient's symptoms with this technique unless an arrhythmia occurs quite frequently. However, we recommend constant ECG monitoring for any in-hospital patient who is undergoing evaluation or treatment for a cardiac arrhythmia. This approach is also used in patients considered at risk for development of an arrhythmia—for example, after acute myocardial infarction. Figures 18-5 and 18-6 are from two patients undergoing evaluation for syncope. The patient in Fig. 18-5 became presyncopal, with the sudden onset of complete heart block and ventric-

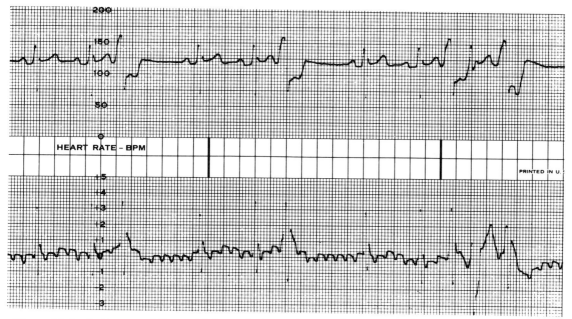

*Figure 18-2*  Artifact resembling atrial flutter during Holter recording. *(See text for details.)*

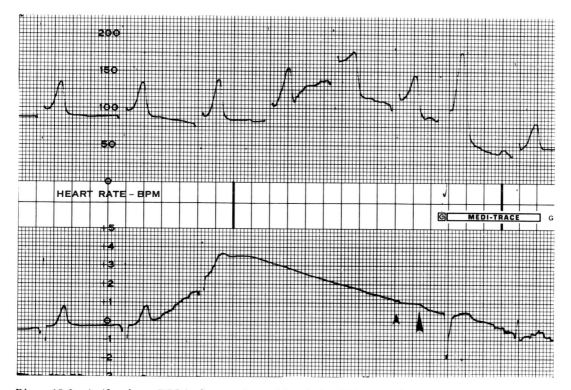

*Figure 18-3*  Artifact due to ECG lead connection problem during Holter recording. The small arrowhead denotes the diminutive QRS complex and the large arrowhead the T wave as noted from the simultaneous tracing above. *(See text for details.)*

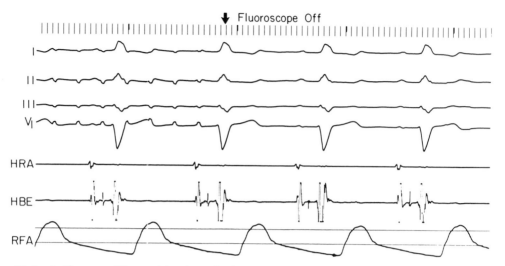

**↓ Fluoroscope Off**

I

II

III

V₁

HRA

HBE

RFA

***Figure 18-4***   Artifact resembling atrial tachycardia due to proximity of recording apparatus to external electrical interference. The patient is in sinus rhythm, as noted by the intracardiac recordings. When the fluoroscope was turned off, the artifact disappeared. RFA = right femoral artery pressure tracing.

ular asystole. The patient in Fig. 18-6 had episodes of both rapid nonsustained VT and finally sustained VT that required cardioversion.

Recent technology has enabled quantification of arrhythmias, and 24-h trend plots can be generated for several variables including heart rate, ectopy, and specific arrhythmias such as VT. These analyses are quite useful in some patients to judge drug efficacy and preclude the need for additional 24-h ECG recordings in many cases.

### Long-Term Continuous Electrocardiographic (Holter) Recordings

Several techniques are available for long-term ECG recordings.[4,5] Most commonly, two ECG leads from the patient are connected to a battery-powered reel-to-reel or cassette tape recorder and data are acquired for 24 h or longer. The recorder has an internal clock and an event marker that can be activated by the patient. The data are analyzed on machines with variable sophistication, but most allow quantitative

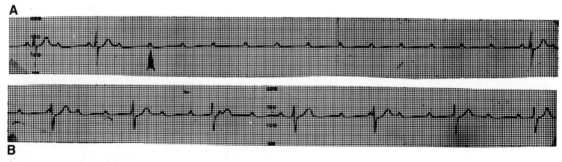

**A**

**B**

***Figure 18-5***   Paroxysmal AV block during continuous ECG recording. In ECG strip *A*, the initial rhythm is sinus with 2:1 AV block. The arrowhead notes the initiation of complete AV block and at the end of this strip an escape junctional focus occurs. Complete heart block is noted in ECG strip *B*.

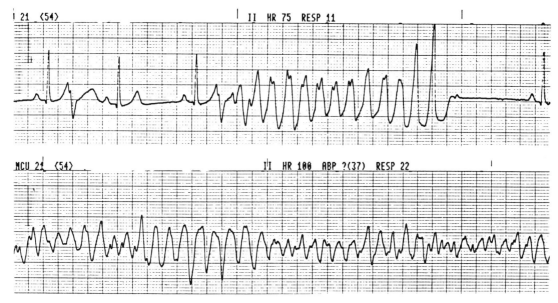

*Figure 18-6*   Continuous ECG monitoring with rapid nonsustained VT in the top strip and VT/VF in the bottom strip.

analysis of heart rate and ventricular ectopy with reasonable accuracy. In our experience, arrhythmias, especially atrial arrhythmias, are often misclassified; therefore these areas of the ECG need to be printed out and analyzed separately. Similarly, determination of complex pacemaker function requires overreading by the physician. Real-time recorders contain a microprocessor that enables the ECG to be analyzed immediately upon acquisition. Presently, these devices have limited storage capacity and only some data are retained, thus limiting their quantitative ability. Further, the diagnostic capabilities of the unit must be relied on to capture all pertinent arrhythmias. These limitations may be overcome by future generations of these devices, but at present we prefer recorders that capture electrical events throughout the entire time period under investigation.

We find this technique particularly helpful when quantitative arrhythmia data are needed. It is also useful to evaluate changes in spontaneous arrhythmia frequency to judge drug efficacy, although we prefer serial electrophysiologic-pharmacologic testing to judge efficacy of drug therapy in patients

with sustained ventricular tachyarrhythmias.[6] It is a very good method to diagnose and quantitate arrhythmias that occur frequently (Fig. 18-7), but it is usually nondiagnostic in the workup of patients with infrequent palpitations, syncope, or presyncope. Long-term ECG recordings are helpful to evaluate pacemaker function, especially with rate-responsive pacemakers, where recordings throughout the day may be necessary to determine whether the pacemaker settings are correct. Events that are present during sleep are also evaluated best with this method. Infrequent symptoms possibly due to an arrhythmia can be correlated with an ECG strip more efficiently with patient-activated event recorders, described in the next section.

### Patient-activated Short-Term Event Recorders

Short-term event recorders offer a useful alternative to Holter recorders to correlate cardiac rhythm with infrequent symptoms. In one study,[7] the type of symptom affected the diagnostic yield. Less than 25 percent of patients with syncope had an event during an average of 6.4 weeks of monitoring. In

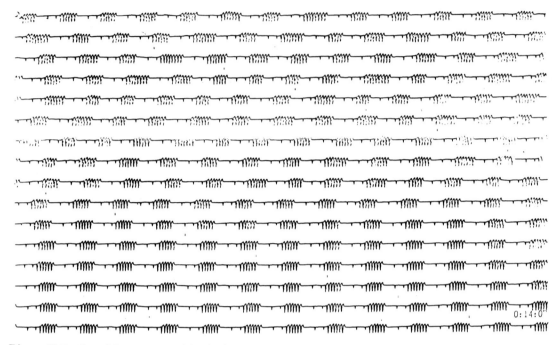

*Figure 18-7*    Repetitive monomorphic VT diagnosed during 24-h ECG ambulatory recording.

contrast, presyncope occurred during monitoring in 25 and 59 percent of patients with and without heart disease, respectively. The cause of palpitations, which typically occur more frequently than presyncope or syncope, was diagnosed in approximately two-thirds of patients.

Two types of patient-activated short-term event recorders are available. One is a hand-held device that patients carry on their person and activate only as needed. Thus, the device will record the patient's rhythm only when the patient applies the device directly to his or her body, usually the chest area. The advantage of this technique is that the patient does not need to wear electrode patches, which are inconvenient and often irritating, continuously. However, the symptom must last long enough for the patient to be able to position and activate the device, which can be useful in palpitations and presyncope (Fig. 18-8) but not in syncope. The stored information can then be transmitted by telephone for analysis. These devices are sometimes referred to as "postsymptom" event recorders, since the ECG is

obtained only after the symptom occurs. Recently, a wristwatch-like recording device has become available that may be used in lieu of the hand-held recorder.

An extremely valuable addition to the armamentarium of event recorders is the memory loop recorder.[7-10] These devices are connected to the patient with electrode patches. They are capable of continuous ECG recordings for short time intervals, up to 5 min with some currently available models. Loop event recorders can be worn by the patient for a month or more and are smaller in size and with longer battery life than a Holter recorder. Although monitoring for months is possible, patient compliance, in our experience, usually does not exceed 4 to 6 weeks.

The loop recorder is the most helpful and practical method of detecting infrequent short-lasting arrhythmias (Fig. 18-9). Devices with 5 min of recording time are used to document the cause of syncope. For example, the recorder can be programmed to save approximately 4 min of retrograde information and 1 min of prospective data when

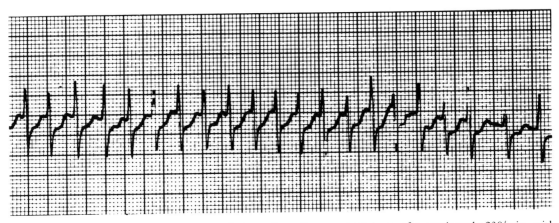

*Figure 18-8*   ECG recording of a supraventricular tachycardia at an initial rate of approximately 230/min, with variable block noted at the end of the tracing. This was obtained with a hand-held event recorder at the time of presyncope.

activated by the patient. Most patients with an arrhythmic cause for syncope regain consciousness in time to activate the device and record the arrhythmia. Since the recording occurs before the symptom, these devices are often called *presymptom* recorders. If a patient has a history of prolonged syncope, the short-term event recorder is useless. A recently described small implantable ECG recorder may prove ideal for these patients.[11]

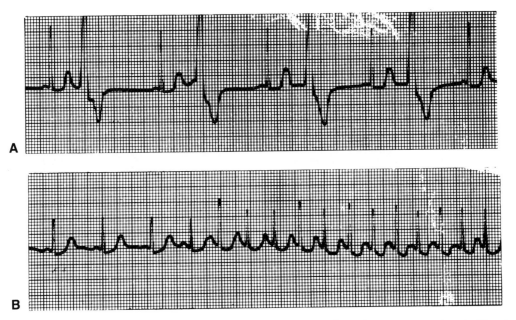

*Figure 18-9*   Two separate arrhythmias documented with symptoms using a loop event recorder. *A*. Ventricular bigeminy associated with heavy palpitations. *B*. Sensation of fluttering or fast heart rate occurred during supraventricular tachycardia.

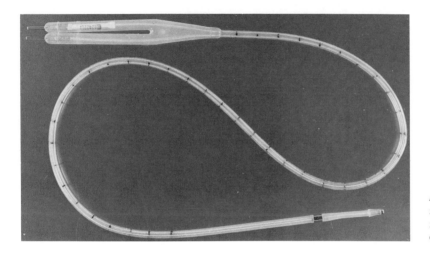

*Figure 18-10*  Bipolar permanent endocardial pacemaker lead used to record esophageal electrogram.

## Esophageal Electrocardiography

The esophagus is in close proximity to the interatrial septum and left atrium through part of its intrathoracic course. An esophageal lead placed with the electrodes approximately 40 cm from the nares will record excellent discreet atrial electrograms.[12-15] The recorded atrial activity may originate from multiple areas in the atria.[15] Continuous esophageal recordings can be obtained using a pill electrode that is connected to a long-term recording device.[16] Alternatively, esophageal electrograms are obtained acutely when needed for diagnostic purposes. We use a bipolar endocardial pacing lead (Fig. 18-10) positioned behind the atria (Fig. 18-11). Bipolar electrogram recordings are stable, and atrial pacing can be used to terminate certain types of tachycardia—for example, atrial flutter.

The esophageal ECG is a simple and valuable diagnostic tool. Figure 18-12 is an example of atrial flutter with 2:1 block. In this patient, the diagnosis can be made from analysis of the ECG taken simultaneously with the esophageal tracing. However, in another patient, the esophageal recording demonstrated characteristics of VT that were not evident on the surface 12-lead ECG (Fig. 18-13). Note that there are two ventricular electrograms for each atrial electrogram. The presumed diagnosis is VT with 2:1

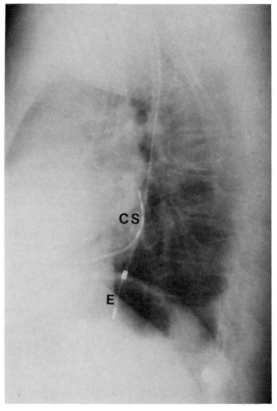

*Figure 18-11*  Lateral chest radiograph demonstrating the esophageal lead (E) behind the heart and the coronary sinus (CS) lead outlining the left AV sulcus.

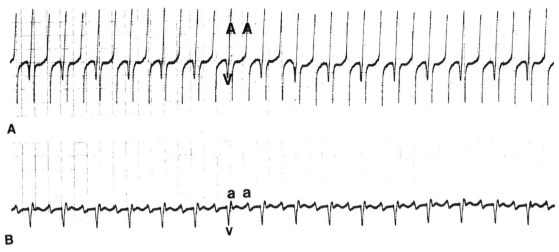

***Figure 18-12***   Simultaneous esophageal (*A*) and ECG (*B*) recordings. The patient has atrial flutter with large-amplitude atrial electrograms (A) and small ventricular electrograms (V) recorded from the esophageal lead. In contrast, atrial (a) depolarizations are much smaller than those from the ventricle (v) in the ECG.

ventriculoatrial (VA) conduction. The rare occurrence of junctional tachycardia with bundle branch block and 2:1 conduction to the atria cannot be absolutely dismissed.

Analysis of the VA interval during supraventricular tachycardia is useful to differentiate AV node reentry from AV (Wolff-Parkinson-White) reentry[17] (Chap. 12). Figure 18-14 is from a patient with a spontaneous episode of narrow QRS complex tachycardia of approximately 150/min. During tachycardia, the atrial and ventricular electrograms are superimposed. The very short VA interval excludes AV reentry. Tachycardia terminates with atrial activation

and no subsequent ventricular activity, strongly suggesting an AV node-dependent arrhythmia. Since AV reentry is excluded, AV node reentry is the logical diagnosis. In another example, an esophageal tracing was recorded from a 16-year-old boy who had a spontaneous episode of tachycardia while being examined in the office (Fig. 18-15). Tachycardia was approximately 195/min and the esophageal VA interval was 100 ms. A Valsalva maneuver terminated tachycardia with atrial activity without conduction to the ventricle (arrow). As noted above, this strongly suggests an AV node-dependent mechanism. The relatively long VA interval is more consistent with

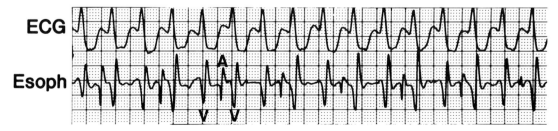

***Figure 18-13***   Simultaneous ECG and esophageal recordings during VT. There are two ventricular (V) electrograms for each atrial (A) electrogram in the esophageal (Esoph) electrogram.

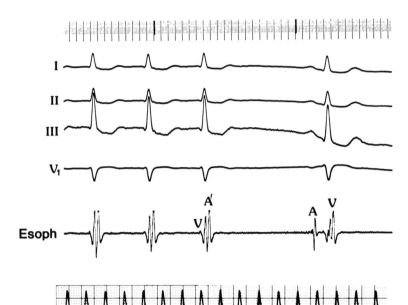

*Figure    18-14*  Simultaneous ECG and esophageal recordings during AV node reentry. A′ = retrograde atrial activity; A = anterograde atrial activity; V = ventricular activity. *(See text for details.)*

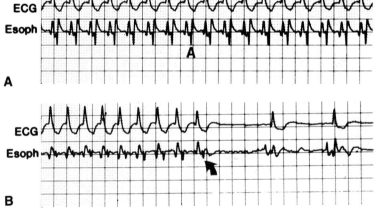

*Figure    18-15*  Simultaneous ECG and esophageal tracings during AV reentry. *A.* Reciprocating tachycardia. The VA interval is 100 ms. *B.* A Valsalva maneuver terminates tachycardia with a recorded atrial deflection (*arrow*) but no subsequent QRS complex.

AV reentry but does not exclude AV node reentry. This patient underwent electrophysiologic evaluation. AV reentry using a concealed left free-wall accessory pathway for VA conduction was diagnosed.

## Signal-averaged Electrocardiography

Reentry is considered the mechanism for most cases of VT, especially in patients who have coronary artery disease with a previous myocardial infarction. Fragmented and prolonged electrograms have been recorded from areas of slow conduction in damaged ventricles in animal experiments and in humans with VT.[18-22] Signal-averaged ECG is a noninvasive method to detect presumed areas of slow conduction in the ventricle through surface ECG recordings.

Signal-averaged ECG is used to reduce noise, most importantly skeletal muscle activity, so that low-amplitude, high-frequency electrical signals from the heart can be detected.[23,24] Three surface bipolar ECG leads (X, Y, Z) are recorded for approximately

200 heartbeats and the voltage of the ECG is fed through a high-gain (× 1000) amplifier. The signal is averaged by a computer, and a high-pass filter is used to minimize the contribution of the large-amplitude but low-frequency content activity occurring during repolarization. The most commonly employed high-pass filters are 25 and 40 Hz. The signals can be processed by frequency or, more commonly, time-domain analysis. In most systems, the X, Y, and Z leads are combined into a vector magnitude referred to as the filtered QRS complex (Fig. 18-16). Acquiring enough beats to average the signal is extremely important and necessary to reduce the noise level. Noise can be mistaken for abnormal activity, as noted in Fig. 18-17. In this patient a SAECG was obtained after two beats (Fig. 18-17*A*) that is abnormal due to noise. When enough beats were averaged (Fig. 18-17*B*) to eliminate noise, which is random, the SAECG is normal. In summary,

signal averaging is performed to eliminate noise and filtering is done to enable analysis of the high-frequency content.

The SAECG in Fig. 18-16 has an abnormal filtered QRS duration, low-amplitude signal duration, and root-mean-square (RMS) voltage-—all three time-domain parameters used to evaluate the SAECG. There are still no universally accepted normal values for these three parameters at the 25- and 40-Hz high-pass filter settings. The definition of a late potential—which is the high-frequency, low-amplitude signal continuous with the end of the QRS complex—also has not been standardized. Representative criteria for an abnormal SAECG at a 40-Hz high-pass filter setting are a filtered QRS duration >114 ms; RMS of the last 40 ms of the vector magnitude complex <20 μV; and terminal low-amplitude signal (LAS) below 40 μV >38 ms. Criteria at 25 Hz are a filtered QRS complex

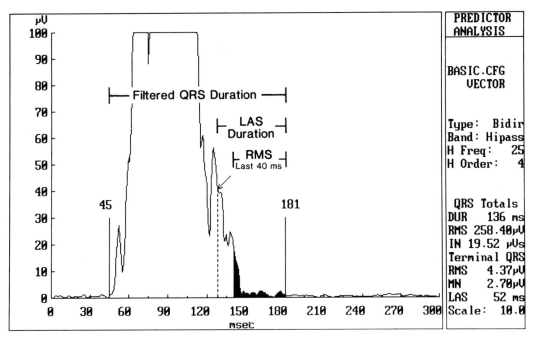

*Figure 18-16*  Signal-averaged ECG in a patient with sustained VT. The three parameters evaluated are the filtered QRS duration; the duration of the low-amplitude signal (LAS), which is that signal under 40 μV to the end of the QRS duration; and the root-mean-square (RMS) voltage of the last 40 ms of the QRS duration. (*See text for details.*)

>114 ms; RMS <25 μV; and LAS >32 ms. Each laboratory should define its own normal values until standardized criteria are established.

Several studies have shown that the SAECG is a useful test to identify patients after myocardial infarction at greatest risk to develop sustained ventricular tachyarrhythmias.[23-28] Gomes and coworkers[26] investigated the relative predictive value of the SAECG and left ventricular ejection fraction in anterior-wall versus inferior-wall myocardial infarction. As noted in other studies, the SAECG had greater sensitivity in patients with an inferior-compared with an anterior-wall myocardial infarction. The predictive value of the SAECG compared with ejection fraction was superior in patients with an anterior infarction but similar in patients with an inferior infarction.[26]

In our experience, an abnormal SAECG occurs commonly in patients with sustained VT who have coronary artery disease but much less frequently in patients who have survived an episode of cardiac arrest. Its predictive ability is not as well studied in patients with non-coronary artery disease who have sustained VT or are survivors of cardiac arrest. The problem is compounded in patients with cardiomyopathy who often have conduction defects, including left bundle branch block. Patients with QRS durations ≥ 120 ms on the 12-lead ECG have abnormally prolonged filtered QRS durations with or without an abnormal RMS. In particular, it is very difficult to evaluate an SAECG in the presence of left bundle branch block (Fig. 18-18). Techniques such as spectrotemporal mapping[29] or frequency analysis[30] may be more helpful in these patients.

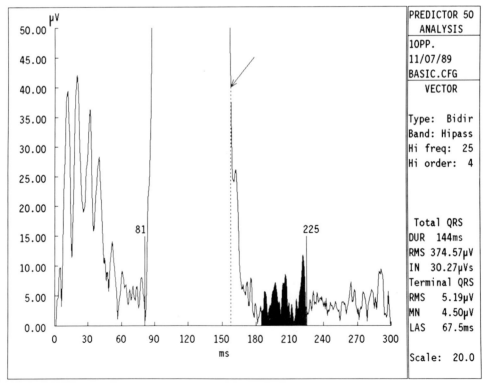

**A**

*Figure 18-17*    Effect of number of beats averaged on noise reduction. *A*. Only two QRS complexes are averaged and a false-positive result is noted. *B*. 205 QRS complexes are averaged and the tracing is normal.

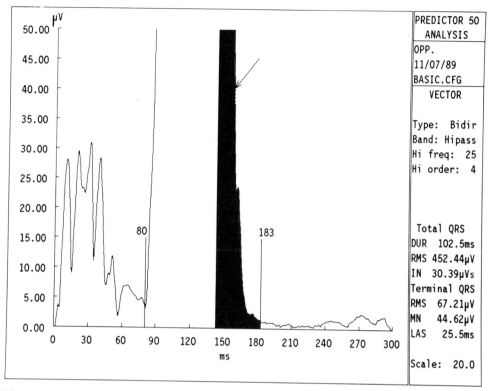

*Figure 18-17 (Continued)*

Signal-averaged electrocardiography is a useful test in patients with a history of syncope.[31-33] It is frequently positive in patients in whom sustained VT is induced at electrophysiologic study or occurs spontaneously. However, one major problem is the rather high prevalence of false-positive results in patients with syncope. In other words, many patients with syncope unrelated to sustained VT will have a positive SAECG. As a general rule, a positive SAECG in a patient with normal ventricular function should be considered a false-positive result—these individuals rarely have sustained VT. Of note, sensitivity of SAECG is excellent and false-negative tests are extremely uncommon.

Antiarrhythmic drugs can alter the SAECG even when there is no measurable change on the surface ECG. Figure 18-19A demonstrates a normal SAECG in a patient with a previous myocardial

infarction and no spontaneous or inducible sustained VT at electrophysiologic study. The patient required antiarrhythmic drug therapy to suppress frequent ventricular ectopy that caused intolerable palpitations. In the presence of quinidine therapy, the SAECG became positive (Fig. 18-19B). Thus, the SAECG should be obtained with the patient in the drug-free state. In our experience, appearance or disappearance of a late potential during drug therapy has no relevance to drug efficacy.

## Exercise Testing

During exercise, there is a marked change in autonomic tone with increased sympathetic and decreased parasympathetic activity. Under usual circumstances, the cardiac output increases, primarily due to an increase in heart rate, and myocardial oxygen consumption also increases. Myocardial ischemia may occur and depends on the degree of coronary artery obstruction or other factors such as myocardial hypertrophy. Exercise testing may be useful (1) to initiate certain arrhythmias, usually those that occur spontaneously during strenuous activity; (2) to judge drug efficacy or proarrhythmic effects, especially with agents such as flecainide[34]; (3) to determine the effect of drug therapy given to prevent excessive ventricular

rates during atrial fibrillation in some patients; and (4) to evaluate rate-responsive pacemaker settings.

Both ventricular and supraventricular tachyarrhythmias can be initiated during exercise testing. In our experience, sustained supraventricular or ventricular tachycardia that occurs *only* during exercise is very uncommon. Typically, these arrhythmias are very difficult to induce during electrophysiologic testing in the baseline state, but they commonly emerge during graded infusions of isoproterenol with or without programmed electrical stimulation. Exercise-induced VT commonly occurs in patients

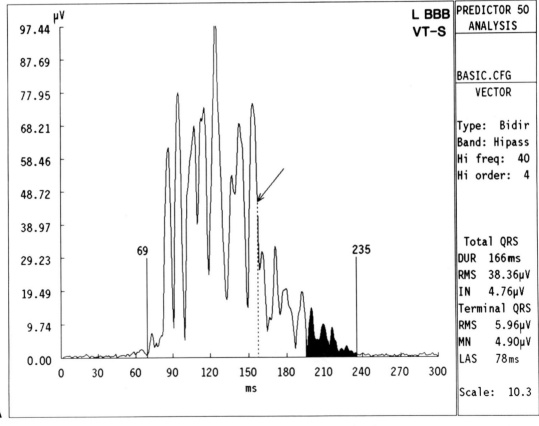

*Figure 18-18*  Signal-averaged ECG in the presence of left bundle branch block. *A.* In the patient with a history of sustained VT (VT-S) and left bundle branch block (LBBB), all three SAECG parameters are abnormal. The filtered QRS duration is 166 ms, the RMS is 5.96 μV, and the LAS is 78 ms. *B.* All three parameters are also abnormal in a patient with LBBB and no spontaneous or inducible VT.

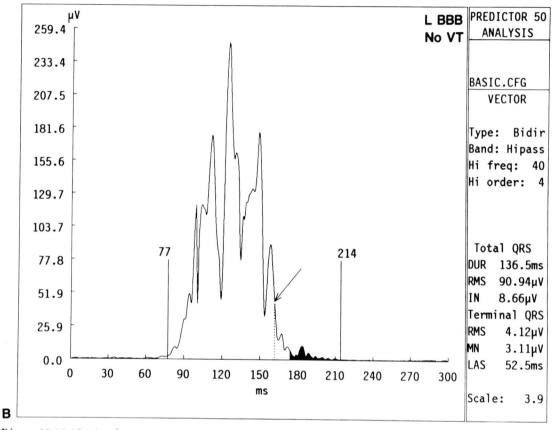

**B**

*Figure 18-18 (Continued)*

with right ventricular outflow tract VT and normal ventricular function. In some patients, exercise as well as programmed electrical stimulation initiate VT, and spontaneous VT occurs at rest or with activity.

Although some investigators[35] have advocated routine use of exercise testing to judge drug efficacy, we have not found this to be particularly helpful in most patients. In a prospective study of 119 patients with VT, programmed ventricular stimulation initiated VT in 71 percent, compared with 27 percent of patients induced with exercise.[36] More importantly, in this patient population, sustained VT or VF rarely occurred during treadmill testing, even in patients with a history of these arrhythmias. In fact,

only one episode of VF occurred during treadmill testing in patients presenting with cardiac arrest without acute myocardial infarction (Fig. 18-20). Since induction of the clinical arrhythmia in the absence of drug therapy occurs so uncommonly, we do not routinely use exercise testing to judge drug efficacy. Increased sympathetic tone can antagonize the effects of antiarrhythmic drugs, but this is often more easily demonstrated during isoproterenol infusion at electrophysiologic study than with exercise testing.

An exercise study should be part of the evaluation of a patient in whom symptoms occur during exertion. An example is demonstrated in Fig. 18-21. This patient had exercise-induced presyncope and

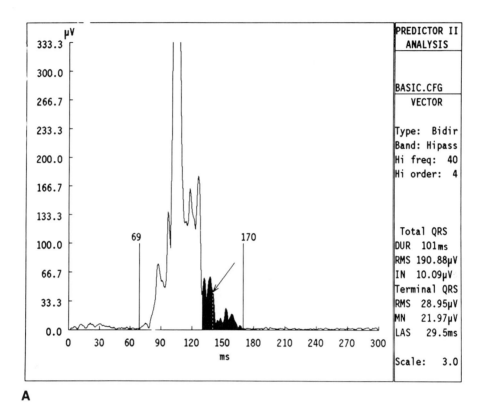

**A**

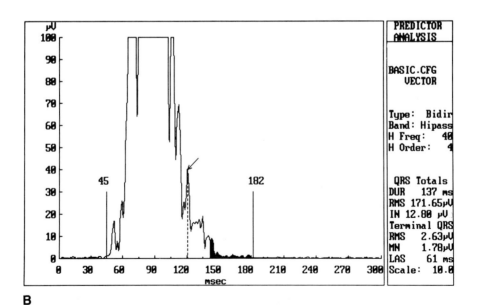

**B**

*Figure 18-19* Effect of quinidine on the SAECG. *A.* No drug. *B.* Quinidine. *(See text for details.)*

SUSTAINED ➡

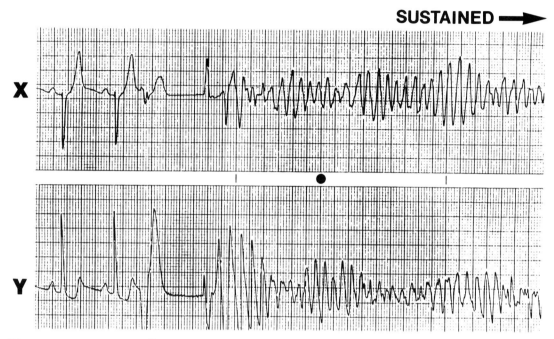

*Figure 18-20*   Ventricular fibrillation occurring shortly after the end of exercise testing. *(See text for details.)* Recorded are ECG leads X and Y.

her resting ECG was only mildly abnormal, with intermittent first-degree AV block (Fig. 18-21A). The patient underwent exercise testing as shown in Fig. 18-21B. Standing prior to exercise worsened conduction, and Mobitz type I second-degree AV block occurred. Throughout exercise, the extent of block increased and the patient became dizzy with more strenuous activity. During recovery 2:1 block resumed and finally 1:1 conduction reappeared. The QRS complex was normal, and at electrophysiologic study intra-His block was demonstrated during graded doses of isoproterenol infusion. It is rare for AV nodal block to occur with exertion (see Chap. 1). One should always suspect intra-His disease when exercise-induced AV block occurs in a patient with a narrow QRS complex.

## Head-up Tilt Testing

Head-up tilt-table testing is an excellent method to diagnose neurally mediated syncope.[37–40,42,43] This

form of syncope is often associated with normal ventricular function. Assumption of an upright posture causes redistribution of part of the blood volume to the dependent areas of the body.[37] As a consequence, there is a decrease in ventricular filling and stroke volume with a compensatory baroreceptor-mediated constriction of vascular smooth muscle and an increase in inotropy and heart rate. In patients with neurally mediated syncope, these compensatory mechanisms fail, resulting in hypotension, bradycardia, or both. Typically, echocardiographic measurements taken during head-up tilt demonstrate a significant decrease in left ventricular end-systolic dimensions and an increase in fractional shortening compared with patients without syncope.[41] Thus, hypotension and bradycardia appear to be related to overactivity of cardiac mechanoreceptors, resulting in a decrease in sympathetic and an increase in parasympathetic excitation.

Methods of tilt-table testing are not yet standardized. In fact, few publications contain the same protocol, which may explain some of the reported

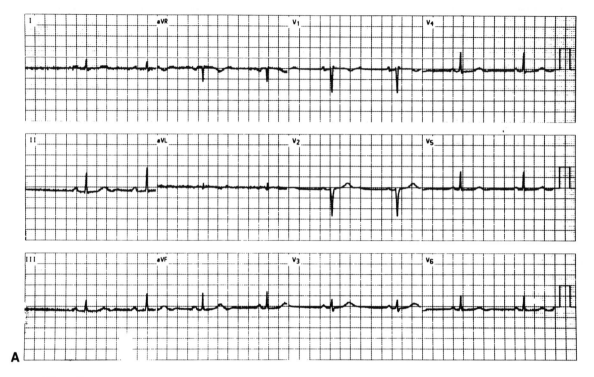

**A**

**Standing**

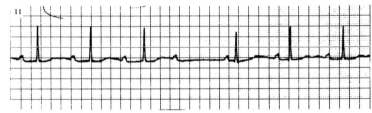

**Stage 3 TM**

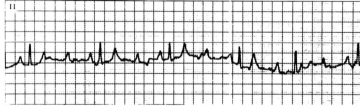

**Recovery**

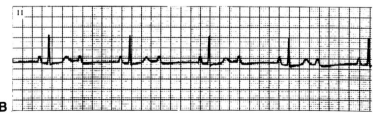

**B**

*Figure 18-21* Exercise-induced AV block. *A*. Minimal abnormalities are noted on the resting ECG. *B*. Mobitz type I second-degree AV block occurs with standing, and the degree of block increases with exercise on the treadmill (TM). During recovery, 2:1 block occurred initially, and finally 1:1 conduction resumed. A DDD pacemaker eliminated symptoms in this patient. *(See text for details.)*

variability in sensitivity and specificity of this test. Since an increase in false-positive results can occur using a saddle tilt table,[40] we and others[40,42] recommend a tilt table with a footboard support (Fig. 18-22). The angle of tilt should be 60° or greater.[42] Duration of tilt is highly variable. Fitzpatrick et al.[40] used 60 min at 60° tilt and demonstrated a positive result in 75 percent of patients with unexplained syncope; only 7 percent of control subjects had an abnormal test. Benditt et al.[42] suggest a tilt duration of at least 45 min in the absence of isoproterenol provocation. In one study, a positive response occurred at a mean of 24.5 ± 10 min.[40] Figure 18-23 is an example of neurally mediated syncope during tilt in the absence of isoproterenol.

Isoproterenol provocation during head-up tilt testing is controversial. Advocates claim it increases sensitivity without a substantial decrease in specificity.[38,39,42,44] In contrast, Kapoor and Brant[45] discourage the use of isoproterenol, which they state markedly lowers specificity of the tilt test. In other words, the use of isoproterenol would increase false-positives to an unacceptable degree. Fitzpatrick et al.[40] reported a reasonable sensitivity of 75 percent with head-up tilt without isoproterenol. Because of the

substantial variability in testing procedures, including the degree and duration of tilt and isoproterenol dose, it is difficult to compare data from the various studies. However, our current approach is to perform head-up tilt at 80° in the absence of isoproterenol for 45 min. If the test is negative, we administer isoproterenol at 1 μg/min and tilt the patient for another 10 min. This can be repeated at 3 μg/min for another 10-min tilt duration. It is very important to analyze symptoms preceding syncope or presyncope. By comparing the patient's clinical symptoms with those at head-up tilt, false-positive results can be minimized. In other words, it is not unreasonable to use isoproterenol provocation, but every effort should be made to ascertain whether the symptoms associated with a positive tilt test are similar to symptoms with spontaneous syncope or presyncope. In any case, it is possible for a patient to have syncope caused by more than one mechanism.

## Heart-Rate Variability

High levels of vagal tone have a beneficial effect on the electrophysiologic properties of the ventricle to prevent emergence of sustained VT or VF in some instances.[46] Canine studies have demonstrated that enhanced vagal tone can increase the VF threshold.[47] In humans, increased parasympathetic tone antagonizes the effect of enhanced sympathetic tone to shorten ventricular refractoriness.[48] LaRovere and colleagues[49] injected phenylephrine into humans after myocardial infarction and noted that a low baroreceptor sensitivity index identified a group of patients at increased risk for dying. One model of parasympathetic denervation is long-standing diabetes mellitus. In these patients, there is a substantial reduction in sinus arrhythmia and other measures of vagal tone and there is also an increased risk of sudden death. Therefore, several lines of evidence suggest that enhanced vagal tone may provide an antiarrhythmic state for the ventricle regarding occurrence of VF.

Analysis of heart rate variability (HRV) has

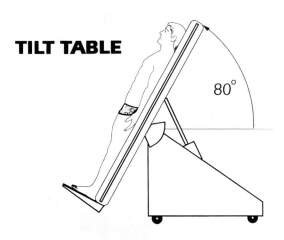

**TILT TABLE**

80°

*Figure 18-22*  Tilt table with footboard support used for head-up tilt testing. The patient is shown in an upright tilt at 80°. *(See text for details.)*

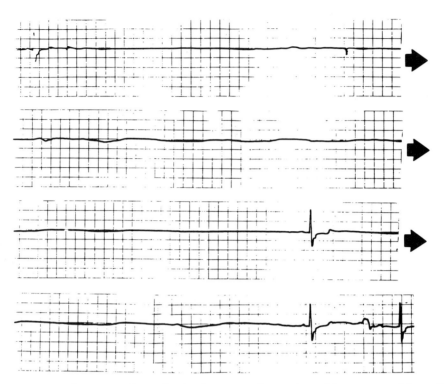

*Figure 18-23*   Syncope during tilt-table evaluation for syncope in a patient with no structural heart disease. Prior to asystole, there was a sudden marked fall in systolic blood pressure associated with symptoms of nausea and diaphoresis. An extremely long period of asystole resulted. This patient had a history of syncope preceded by nausea and diaphoresis, and these symptoms were reproduced with tilt evaluation. No further syncope has occurred during beta-blocker therapy.

been performed for several clinical situations. In essence, HRV evaluates sympathovagal balance.[50,51] Some of the initial methods to evaluate HRV are simple. One test involves breathing at a fixed rate of 5 to 6/min with determination of changes in heart rate. Another method is the Valsalva index, which measures the ratio of the shortest RR interval recorded during phase 2 divided by the maximal RR interval during phase 4. Recent investigations have analyzed long periods of ECG recording—for example, 24-h Holter ECGs—to measure HRV. Analysis has involved both frequency and time domain characteristics.

Most research in HRV has been directed at identification of patients at risk for sudden death after acute myocardial infarction. Some reports suggest that abnormalities of HRV are useful in this regard.[52,53] However, Vybiral et al.[54] were unable to detect any unusual trends in HRV prior to VF in a group of patients who had VF recorded during 24-h Holter monitoring. Thus, although the predictive aspects of HRV determined soon after myocardial infarction may be useful for risk stratification, its use in patients with chronic coronary artery disease is unclear. Importantly, the lack of substantial differences in HRV prior to the onset of VF compared with other times during the day do not support a cause-and-effect relationship between HRV and VF.[54]

Heart rate variability is a promising tool to identify patients at risk for sudden death, but many questions remain to be answered. At present, there are many methods to calculate HRV and no agreement on which one is best. Normal values are not known for most patient groups. The sensitivity, specificity, and positive and negative predictive accuracy of HRV will require more investigation before HRV can be used as a routine clinical test.

## Commentary

Several noninvasive tests are available, and more than one test may be useful in some patients. Tests should be performed in a hierarchical sequence, beginning with the one most likely to yield key diagnostic data. An example is the workup of a patient with short episodes of dizziness associated with palpitations

that occur every few days. A loop event recorder should be tried first. A Holter recorder could be useful, but the event would have to occur on the day the patient was being monitored. An SAECG would provide ancillary data only. Regardless of what test is ordered, it is critical to know its sensitivity and specificity. Otherwise, incorrect interpretation of the result may lead to unwarranted additional tests or therapy or produce a false sense of security. For example, a patient with heart disease and syncope may have a positive head-up tilt test during isoproterenol infusion. This patient may also have sustained VT as the actual cause of syncope. No further workup could lead to the wrong therapy and potentially dire consequences for the patient.

## References

1.  Prystowsky EN: Electrophysiologic testing, in Kelley WM (ed): *Textbook of Internal Medicine*, vol 1. Philadelphia, Lippincott, 1989, p 344.

2.  Fujimura O et al: The sensitivity of electrophysiologic testing in patients with syncope caused by transient bradycardia. *N Engl J Med* 21:1703, 1989.

3.  Holter NJ: New method for heart studies. *Science* 134:1214, 1961.

4.  DiMarco JP, Philbrick JT: Use of ambulatory electrocardiographic (Holter) monitoring. *Ann Intern Med* 113:53, 1990.

5.  Leclercq JF, Coumel P: Ambulatory electrocardiogram monitoring, in MacFarlane PW, Lawrie TDV (eds): *Comprehensive Electrocardiography: Theory and Practice in Health and Disease.* New York, Pergamon Press, 1989, p 1063.

6.  Mason JW et al: A comparison of electrophysiologic testing with Holter monitoring to predict antiarrhythmic drug efficacy for ventricular tachyarrhythmias. *N Engl J Med* 329:445, 1993.

7.  Fogel RI et al: Are event recorders useful and cost effective in the diagnosis of palpitations, presyncope, and syncope? *J Am Coll Cardiol* 21:358A, 1993.

8.  Brown AP, et al: Detection of arrhythmias: Use of a patient-activated ambulatory electrocardiogram device with a solid-state memory loop. *Br Heart J* 58:251, 1987.

9.  Schmidt SB, Jain AC: Diagnostic utility of memory equipped transtelephonic monitors. *Am J Med Sci* 296:299, 1988.

10. Linzer M et al: Incremental diagnostic yield of loop electrocardiographic recorders in unexplained syncope. *Am J Cardiol* 66:214, 1990.

11. Lee BB et al: First results using an implantable arrhythmia monitor. *PACE* 16(II):893, 1993.

12. Cremer M: Ueber die direkte Ableitung der Aktionsstrome des menslichen Herzens vom Oesophagus und über das Elektrokardiogram des Fotus. *Münch Med Wochenschr* 53:811, 1906.

13. Enselberg CD: The esophageal electrocardiogram in the study of atrial activity and cardiac arrhythmias. *Am Heart J* 41:382, 1951.

14. Barold SS: Filtered bipolar esophageal electrocardiography. *Am Heart J* 83:431, 1972.

15. Prystowsky EN et al: Origin of the atrial electrogram recorded from the esophagus. *Circulation* 61:1017, 1980.

16. Jenkins JM et al: Computer diagnosis of supraventricular and ventricular arrhythmias: A new esophageal technique. *Circulation* 60:977, 1979.

17. Gallagher JJ et al: Use of the esophageal lead in the diagnosis of mechanisms of reciprocating supraventricular tachycardia. *PACE* 3:440, 1980.

18. Boineau JP, Cox JL: Slow ventricular activation in

acute myocardial infarction: A source of reentrant premature ventricular contraction. *Circulation* 48:702, 1973.

19. Waldo AL, Kaiser GA: A study of ventricular arrhythmias associated with acute myocardial infarction in the canine heart. *Circulation* 47:1222, 1973.

20. El-Sherif N et al: Reentrant ventricular arrhythmias in the late myocardial infarction period: I. Conduction characteristics in the infarction zone. *Circulation* 55:686, 1977.

21. Simson MB et al: Relation between late potentials on the body surface and directly recorded fragmented electrograms in patients with ventricular tachycardia. *Am J Cardiol* 51:105, 1983.

22. Berbari EJ et al: Recording from the body surface of arrhythmogenic ventricular activity during the ST segment. *Am J Cardiol* 41:697, 1978.

23. Simson MB, MacFarlane PW: The signal-averaged electrocardiogram, in MacFarlane PW, Lawrie TDV (eds): *Comprehensive Electrocardiography: Theory and Practice in Health and Disease.* New York, Pergamon Press, 1989, p 1199.

24. Prystowsky EN: Approach to patients with asymptomatic ventricular arrhythmias after myocardial infarction, in Francis G, Alpert J (eds): *Modern Coronary Care.* Boston, Little, Brown, 1990, p 167.

25. Kanovsky MS et al: Identification of patients with ventricular tachycardia after myocardial infarction: Signal-averaged electrocardiogram, Holter monitoring, and cardiac catheterization. *Circulation* 70:264, 1984.

26. Gomes JA et al: The prognostic significance of quantitative signal-averaged variables relative to clinical variables, site of myocardial infarction, ejection fraction and ventricular premature beats: A prospective study. *J Am Coll Cardiol* 13:377, 1989.

27. Kuchar DL et al: Prediction of serious arrhythmic events after myocardial infarction: Signal-averaged electrocardiogram, Holter monitoring and radionuclide ventriculography. *J Am Coll Cardiol* 9:531, 1987.

28. Denniss RA et al: Prognostic significance of ventricular tachycardia and fibrillation induced at programmed stimulation and delayed potentials detected on the signal-averaged electrocardiograms of survivors of acute myocardial infarction. *Circulation* 74:731, 1986.

29. Haberl R et al: Top-resolution frequency analysis of electrocardiogram with adaptive frequency determination: Identification of late potentials in patients with coronary artery disease. *Circulation* 82:1183, 1990.

30. Lindsay BD et al: Identification of patients with sustained ventricular tachycardia by frequency analysis of signal-averaged electrocardiograms despite the presence of bundle branch block. *Circulation* 77:122, 1988.

31. Kuchar DL et al: Signal-averaged electrocardiogram for evaluation of recurrent syncope. *Am J Cardiol* 58:949, 1986.

32. Gang ES et al: Detection of late potentials on the surface electrocardiogram in unexplained syncope. *Am J Cardiol* 58:1014, 1986.

33. Winters SL et al: Signal-averaging of the surface QRS complex predicts inducibility of ventricular tachycardia in patients with syncope of unknown origin: A prospective study. *J Am Coll Cardiol* 10:775, 1987.

34. Falk RN: Flecainide-induced ventricular tachycardia and fibrillation in patients treated for atrial fibrillation. *Ann Intern Med* 111:107, 1989.

35. Graboys TB et al: Long-term survival of patients with malignant ventricular arrhythmia treated with antiarrhythmic drugs. *Am J Cardiol* 50:437, 1982.

36. Evans JJ et al: Comparison of ventricular tachycardia induction between exercise and electrophysiologic testing in patients with ventricular tachycardia. *Circulation* 70(II):II-243, 1984.

37. Prystowsky EN et al: Diagnostic evaluation and treatment strategies for patients at risk for serious cardiac arrhythmias: Part 1. Syncope of unknown origin. *Mod Concepts Cardiovasc Dis* 60(9):49, 1991.

38. Almquist A et al: Provocation of bradycardia and hypotension by isoproterenol and upright posture in patients with unexplained syncope. *N Engl J Med* 320:346, 1989.

39. Waxman MB et al: Isoproterenol induction of vasodepressor-type reaction in vasodepressor-prone persons. *Am J Cardiol* 63:58, 1989.

40. Fitzpatrick AP et al: Methodology of head-up tilt testing in patients with unexplained syncope. *J Am Coll Cardiol* 17:125, 1991.

41. Shalev Y et al: Echocardiographic demonstration of

decreased left ventricular dimensions and vigorous myocardial contraction during syncope induced by head-up tilt. *J Am Coll Cardiol* 18:746, 1991.

42.  Benditt DG et al: Tilt table testing for evaluation of neurally mediated (cardioneurogenic) syncope: Rationale and proposed protocols. *PACE* 14:1528, 1991.

43.  Grubb BP et al: Tilt table testing in the evaluation and management of athletes with recurrent exercise-induced syncope. *Med Sci Sports Exerc* 25:24, 1993.

44.  Sheldon R et al: Reproducibility of isoproterenol tilt-table tests in patients with syncope. *Am J Cardiol* 69:1300, 1992.

45.  Kapoor WN, Brant N: Evaluation of syncope by upright tilt testing with isoproterenol. *Ann Intern Med* 116:358, 1992.

46.  Hull SS Jr et al: Heart rate variability before and after myocardial infarction in conscious dogs at high and low risk of sudden death. *J Am Coll Cardiol* 16:978, 1990.

47.  Schwartz PJ et al: Autonomic nervous system and sudden cardiac death: Experimental basis and clinical observations for post-myocardial infarction risk stratification. *Circulation* 85(I):I-77, 1992.

48.  Prystowsky EN et al: Effect of autonomic blockade on ventricular refractoriness and atrioventricular nodal conduction in humans: Evidence supporting a direct cholinergic action on ventricular muscle refractoriness. *Circ Res* 49:511, 1981.

49.  LaRovere MT et al: Baroreflex sensitivity, clinical correlates, and cardiovascular mortality among patients with a first myocardial infarction: A prospective study. *Circulation* 78:816, 1988.

50.  Lombardi F et al: Heart rate variability as an index of sympathovagal interaction after acute myocardial infarction. *Am J Cardiol* 60:1239, 1987.

51.  Saul JP et al: Assessment of autonomic regulation in chronic congestive heart failure by heart rate spectral analysis. *Am J Cardiol* 61:1292, 1988.

52.  Kleiger RE et al: Decreased heart rate variability and its association with increased mortality after acute myocardial infarction. *Am J Cardiol* 59:256, 1987.

53.  Farrell TG et al: Risk stratification for arrhythmic events in postinfarction patients based on heart rate variability, ambulatory electrocardiographic variables and the signal-averaged electrocardiogram. *J Am Coll Cardiol* 18:687, 1991.

54.  Vybiral T et al: Conventional heart rate variability analysis of ambulatory electrocardiographic recordings fails to predict imminent ventricular fibrillation. *J Am Coll Cardiol* 22:557, 1993.

Table 19-1  *Pharmacologic Properties of Antiarrhythmic Drugs*

| Drug | Usual Daily Dosage, mg | Target Plasma Concentration, μg/mL | Elimination Half-Life, h | Major Route of Elimination | Protein Binding, % | Oral Bioavailability, % | Active Metabolites | Supplement after Hemodialysis |
|---|---|---|---|---|---|---|---|---|
| Quinidine | 600–1600 | 2–5 | 4–17 | Hepatic | 80 | 60–80 | Yes | No |
| Procainamide | 2000–4000 | 4–10 | 3–5 | Hepatic/Renal | 20 | 70–85 | Yes | Yes (±) |
| Disopyramide | 400–800 | 2–5 | 6–9 | Renal/Hepatic | 50–65 | 80–90 | Yes | Yes |
| Lidocaine[a] | — | 1.5–5.0 | 1.5–2.0 | Hepatic | 60–80 | — | Yes | No |
| Mexiletine | 450–750 | 0.5–2.0 | 8–17 | Hepatic | 70 | 90 | No | Yes |
| Tocainide | 600–1800 | 3–11 | 8–20 | Renal/Hepatic | 50 | 100 | No | — |
| Phenytoin | 200–400 | 10–20 | 16–24 | Hepatic | 90 | 50–70 | No | No |
| Flecainide | 200–400 | 0.2–1.0 | 20 | Renal | 40 | 95 | No | No |
| Propafenone | 450–900 | — | 3–8 | Hepatic | 90 | 25–75 | Yes | — |
| Moricizine | 600–900 | — | 6–13 | Hepatic | 95 | 35–45 | Probable | — |
| Amiodarone | 200–400 | 1–2.5 | ~53 Days | Hepatic | 96 | 35–50 | Yes | No |
| Bretylium[a] | — | — | 4–16 | Renal | <10 | — | No | Yes |
| Sotalol | 160–480 | 0.5–3.0 | 10–20 | Renal | 0 | 90–100 | No | Yes |
| Digoxin | 0.25 | 0.5–2.0 | 36–48 | Renal | 20–30 | 55–75 | No | No |
| Verapamil | 240–480 | — | 3–7 | Hepatic | 90 | 20–35 | Yes | No |
| Diltiazem[a] | — | — | 4 | Hepatic | 70–80 | — | Probable | — |

[a] Intravenous form approved for antiarrhythmic use.

CHF and some should not be used (Table 19-2). There is reduced liver blood flow that may affect metabolism with certain agents. Relatively minor negative inotropic effects of some dugs may be more marked in the presence of substantial left ventricular dysfunction and CHF. Hypokalemia may occur and is often associated with a greater chance for the development of proarrhythmia.

Many antiarrhythmic drugs undergo biotransformation by hepatic oxidative metabolism through the cytochrome P450 system. This has been a fertile research area, providing many insights into drug metabolism and drug-drug interactions. Cimetidine can inhibit the P450 enzymes, which may lead to an increase in plasma concentration of certain antiarrhythmic drugs, necessitating a decrease in dosage (Table 19-2).[9] In contrast, drugs such as phenytoin and phenobarbital can induce the P450 enzyme system, resulting in increased metabolism of some antiarrhythmic drugs, which may require a larger dose to obtain the desired effect (Table 19-2).[10]

Two important P450 isoenzymes are P4502D6 and P4503A4.[11] The isoenzyme P4502D6 is the major enzyme for biotransformation of propafenone, flecainide, metoprolol, propranolol, and timolol. Some individuals are poor metabolizers, which is genetically determined, and have reduced amounts of P4502D6. In other instances, extensive metabolizers can be converted to poor metabolizers when given a drug that inhibits the activity of P4502D6. The overall effect of drug administration to a poor metabolizer is variable and depends on several factors. These include the degree to which other metabolic pathways can be used for drug elimination, the importance of pharmacologic effects of the parent compound and metabolite(s), and potential toxicity of increased amounts of the parent drug. Very low doses of quinidine can inhibit P4502D6, which could potentially alter pharmacodynamic effects of drugs metabolized by this route.[11–14] For example, enhanced beta blockade during propafenone therapy occurs due to accumulation of the parent compound.[11]

The enzyme P4503A4 is responsible for metabolism of lidocaine and quinidine.[11] It is inhibited by erythromycin and ketoconazole. Of note, terfenadine is also a substrate for P4503A4. Inhibition of P4503A4 with erythromycin, for example, may lead to an increase in plasma terfenadine concentration, prolongation of the QT interval, and the development of torsade de pointes.[15]

The extent of drug metabolism in some individuals may depend on genetically determined polymorphisms of enzymatic reactions.[13] A well-studied example of this is procainamide.[16–17] Hepatic N-acetyl transferase is an enzyme under genetic control, and approximately one-half of Caucasians are rapid acetylators. Patients who are rapid acetylators will have increased plasma concentrations of N-acetyl procainamide (NAPA) compared with slow acetylators. These patients will also have a lower incidence of lupus syndrome, which is probably caused by either procainamide or some metabolite(s) other than NAPA.[17] In general, whether one is a slow or fast acetylator, there will be some mixture of procainamide and NAPA when procainamide is given. This is a good example of the difficulty in trying to identify the reason for antiarrhythmic efficacy when the parent drug and its metabolite have different antiarrhythmic drug actions. Procainamide primarily blocks sodium channels, whereas NAPA primarily blocks potassium channels. In general, one must always be vigilant for drug-drug interactions. These can occur with an antiarrhythmic drug that interacts with nonantiarrhythmic agents as well as with other antiarrhythmic drugs. Further, a parent drug and its metabolite(s) may have additive or inhibitory antiarrhythmic actions with each other.

Further examples of dosage modifications of antiarrhythmic drugs due to common pathophysiologic states or concomitant drugs are listed in Table 19-2. Other drug interactions may occur. For example, amiodarone also inhibits P450 enzymes and can increase plasma concentration of procainamide and probably many other antiarrhythmic drugs.[18] Quinidine increases digoxin concentration.[19] In some instances metabolites of a drug can either augment or negate some of the electrophysiologic effects of the parent compound. For example, glycinexylidide (glycylxylide), a metabolite of lidocaine, decreases the effect of lidocaine.[20]

Table 19-2  *Dosage Modification and Drug Interactions*

| Drug | Heart Failure[a] | Renal Disease | Hepatic Disease | Digoxin | Warfarin | Cimetidine | Phenytoin; Phenobarbital |
|---|---|---|---|---|---|---|---|
| Quinidine | — | — | ↓ Dosage | ↑ Serum digoxin level | ± ↓ Warfarin dosage | ↓ Dosage | ↑ Dosage |
| Procainamide | ± ↓ Dosage | ↓ Dosage | — | — | — | ↓ Dosage | — |
| Disopyramide | Avoid | ↓ Dosage | ± ↓ Dosage | — | — | — | ↑ Dosage |
| Lidocaine | ↓ Dosage | — | ↓ Dosage | — | — | ↓ Dosage | — |
| Mexiletine | — | ↓ Dosage | ↓ Dosage | — | — | ↓ Dosage | ↑ Dosage |
| Tocainide | — | — | — | — | — | — | — |
| Phenytoin | — | ↓ Dosage | ↓ Dosage | — | — | ↓ Dosage | — |
| Flecainide | Avoid | ↓ Dosage | — | ↑ Serum digoxin level | — | ± ↓ Dosage | — |
| Propafenone | Cautious use | — | ↓ Dosage | ↑ Serum digoxin level | ↑ Protime | ± ↓ Dosage | — |
| Moricizine | — | — | ↓ Dosage | — | — | ↓ Dosage | — |
| Amiodarone | — | — | ↓ Dosage | ↑ Serum digoxin level | ↑ Protime | — | — |
| Bretylium | — | ↓ Dosage | — | — | — | — | — |
| Sotalol | Cautious use | ↓ Dosage | — | — | — | — | — |
| Digoxin | — | ↓ Dosage | — | — | — | — | — |
| Verapamil | Cautious use | — | ↓ Dosage | ↑ Serum digoxin level | — | ↓ Dosage | ± ↑ Dosage (phenobarbital) |
| Diltiazem | ↓ Dosage | — | ↓ Dosage | ± ↑ Serum digoxin level | — | ↓ Dosage | — |

[a]Use all drugs cautiously in heart failure.

Drugs are frequently eliminated from the body through the kidney. Consequently, a decrease in renal function may result in an increased plasma drug concentration unless the dosage is decreased (Table 19-2). In addition to hepatic metabolism of drugs, significant excretion of some drugs occurs through the biliary system into the intestines.

## Clinical Pharmacokinetics

### Half-Life; Steady State; Dosing Intervals

The elimination half-life of a drug is the time required for 50 percent of the drug to be eliminated from the body. Thus, 75 and 87.5 percent of the drug is eliminated in two and three half-lives, respectively. Complete elimination of the drug is considered at four to five half-lives. Viewing this process in reverse, the time it takes to attain steady-state drug concentration is approximately five half-lives. The steady-state concentration achieved depends only on clearance and dose of the drug.[21] Importantly, since the time to reach steady state depends on the elimination half-life of the drug, factors that affect clearance—such as hepatic and renal disease—will alter the time it takes to reach

steady state. One such example is a prolonged time to steady state with procainamide in a patient with renal impairment.

In contrast, a loading dose does not shorten the time to steady state. Loading doses are used when it is important to reach a target drug concentration in a short time to control an arrhythmia. Intravenous administration of lidocaine or procainamide to terminate ventricular tachycardia or verapamil to treat supraventricular tachycardia are instances where loading doses are appropriate. Steady-state conditions with intravenous administration of a maintenance dosage will still require five elimination half-lives. Alternatively, oral drug can be given after the intravenous load to achieve steady state.

Drugs are often administered at time intervals based on their half-lives of elimination. Thus, a drug that has a 12-h half-life is usually given twice daily. This is a rather simplistic approach that requires more individualization. For example, if a patient has a wide therapeutic range of drug concentrations, alternative dosing schedules can be used. Figure 19-1 demonstrates this concept. A theoretical drug is shown with a half-life of 2 h. The left-hand portion of the figure shows a wide concentration range with therapeutic efficacy; therefore large doses of the drug are given every 8 h. Even with relatively low drug concentrations, the therapeutic end point is met in

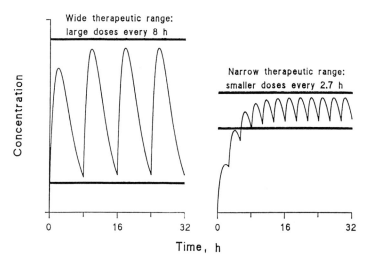

*Figure 19-1* Dosing schemes required to maintain "therapeutic" plasma concentrations (elimination $t_{1/2}$:2 h). See text for details. *(From Ref. 13, with permission.)*

this situation. On the right-hand side, a narrow therapeutic range for this drug is demonstrated. Here smaller doses of the drug must be given frequently to maintain the desired therapeutic plasma concentration. The presence of active metabolites, especially ones that have longer half-lives than the parent compound, may also affect the dosing schedule.

There are practical applications of the above principles. Since three drug half-lives nearly equal steady-state drug concentration, it is reasonable to evaluate drug efficacy or obtain a plasma drug concentration at this time rather than waiting for four to five half-lives. If the drug level is relatively low or efficacy is not achieved, a higher drug dosage should be given as long as toxicity is absent. If the patient is hospitalized during drug administration, this will often shorten the hospital stay. Conditions that alter elimination of drugs should be considered. Patients with heart failure or hepatic and renal dysfunction may need a reduction in dosage of many antiarrhythmic drugs (Table 19-2).

### Therapeutic Range

The upper and lower plasma drug concentrations at which efficacy occurs can be defined as the therapeutic range for that drug. The lowest effective plasma drug concentration is usually defined by some measurable parameter to determine efficacy. The upper level is often more open-ended and frequently defined by drug toxicity or side effects. There are many problems with the concept of therapeutic range as applied to antiarrhythmic drug therapy. Frequently, the proposed therapeutic range was developed for some easily measured parameter of efficacy—for example, suppression of premature ventricular complexes. However, the plasma drug concentrations necessary to suppress 80 percent of premature ventricular complexes might be insufficient to prevent ventricular fibrillation or sustained ventricular tachycardia. Alternatively, "subtherapeutic" plasma drug concentrations might prevent recurrences of supraventricular tachycardia in another patient. In essence, "therapeutic" is a retrospective observation that is deter-

mined with time. The plasma drug concentration that prevents recurrence of an arrhythmia is *therapeutic*. It follows that "therapeutic" plasma drug levels in a patient in whom an arrhythmia recurs are clearly *not* therapeutic.

For these reasons, we suggest "target" rather than "therapeutic" plasma concentrations (Table 19-1). Plasma drug concentrations can be helpful during drug dose titration. As a rule, we do not routinely use the target concentration as the primary determinant to adjust drug dosage. Whenever possible, we increase drug dosage until either side effects are reached or some measure of drug efficacy is obtained. For example, in patients with sustained ventricular tachycardia undergoing serial electrophysiologic-pharmacologic testing, prior to repeat study, the drug dosage is increased using end points such as side effects or abolition of nonsustained ventricular tachycardia. In a patient with frequent paroxysms of atrial fibrillation, the end point is the drug dose that suppresses or markedly reduces the number of episodes of atrial fibrillation.

Plasma drug concentrations are particularly useful in three situations. Some individuals receiving an apparently adequate drug dose demonstrate no signs of efficacy or side effects. A low plasma drug level indicates the need for more drug, whereas a normal to relatively high drug level suggests drug inefficacy. In some patients receiving drugs who have minimal spontaneous arrhythmia, the drug dosage can be adjusted to a desired target plasma concentration. Finally, plasma drug concentrations are useful during follow-up to identify possible reasons for arrhythmia recurrence. A low drug level suggests either patient noncompliance or a change in drug bioavailability or clearance. An example is a patient receiving chronic quinidine therapy with arrhythmia suppression who takes phenytoin and then has a recurrence of arrhythmia (Table 19-2). The plasma quinidine level is low compared with the level obtained before phenytoin was started. In this situation, options are discontinuation of phenytoin, increase in quinidine dosage, or use of an alternative antiarrhythmic drug.

# Antiarrhythmic Drug Classification

## Vaughan Williams Classification of Antiarrhythmic Drug Actions

Classification of antiarrhythmic drug actions was proposed by Vaughan Williams[22] and modified by Harrison[23] (Table 19-3). This scheme divides drug actions into four major classes. Class I includes drugs that block the fast sodium channel. Quinidine, procainamide, and disopyramide are class IA agents. These drugs moderately depress phase zero upstroke of the action potential, moderately slow conduction, and prolong repolarization. Electrocardiographic changes are an increased QRS and QT interval, with minimal increase in the PR interval that is usually caused by a prolonged HV conduction time. Class IB

is represented by lidocaine, mexiletine, tocainide, and phenytoin. Action potential changes are minimal. The electrocardiogram is essentially unchanged. Class IC contains flecainide, propafenone, and probably moricizine. The action potential shows marked depression of phase zero upstroke with substantial slowing of conduction but minimal change in repolarization. Typically, the PR interval is increased and the QRS duration substantially widened. The QT interval may be increased by the prolonged QRS duration, but the JT interval remains unchanged. Of note, the kinetics of interactions with sodium channels support this subdivision of class I. The kinetics are very slow, very fast, and intermediate for IC, IB, and IA, respectively.[24]

Class II agents are beta-adrenergic receptor blockers that prolong the PR interval due to slowing of AV nodal conduction without significant change in the QRS or QT duration. Class III drugs primarily

*Table 19-3   Vaughan Williams Classification of Antiarrhythmic Drug Actions*

| Class | Action | ECG Changes | | | Drugs |
|---|---|---|---|---|---|
| | | PR | QRS | QT | |
| I. | Fast sodium channel blockers | | | | |
| | A.  Phase O depression—moderate  Slow conduction—moderate  Prolong repolarization | ± | ↑ | ↑ | Quinidine Procainamide Disopyramide |
| | B.  Phase O depression—minimal  Slow conduction—minimal  Shorten repolarization | ± | ± | ± ↓ | Lidocaine Mexiletine Tocainide Phenytoin |
| | C.  Phase O depression—marked  Slow conduction—marked  Minimal repolarization changes | ↑ | ↑ ↑ | ± | Flecainide Propafenone Moricizine |
| II. | Beta-adrenergic receptor blockers | ↑ | ± | ± | Propranolol (and others) |
| III. | Prolongation of refractoriness | ± | ± | ↑ ↑ | Amiodarone Bretylium Sotalol |
| IV. | Calcium channel blockers | ↑ | ± | ± | Verapamil Diltiazem |

prolong refractoriness by blocking repolarizing potassium channels; they include amiodarone, bretylium, and sotalol. There is a significant increase in the QT interval with minimal prolongation of QRS duration. The PR interval may be increased, primarily because of other drug actions. This is discussed in more detail below. Class IV includes calcium channel blockers that prolong the PR interval without a change in the QRS or QT interval. Verapamil and diltiazem are currently the only recommended agents in this class with antiarrhythmic efficacy in humans.

*Critique*

The Vaughan Williams classification has many problems and is useful only in the broad context of a general categorization of antiarrhythmic drugs. Arrhythmias most frequently occur in damaged myocardial tissue or in a pathophysiologic milieu. However, the Vaughan Williams classification is based on actions in normal cardiac tissue, especially Purkinje fibers. There are many other problems with this system. Antiarrhythmic drug actions may differ among species. Effects on the autonomic nervous system other than beta blockade are not considered. Alterations in electrolytes and pH can affect antiarrhythmic actions and are not part of this scheme. Antiarrhythmic agents often have more than one drug action; for example, quindinine blocks both sodium and potassium channels and amiodarone has effects that span all four classes. Antiarrhythmic actions of metabolites may differ from the parent compound; for example, NAPA primarily blocks potassium channels, whereas procainamide primarily blocks sodium channels.[24] These factors taken together seriously impair the clinical usefulness of the Vaughan Williams classification of antiarrhythmic drug actions. Regardless, until a more useful classification scheme emerges, it will probably continue to be used.

The effect of heart rate on antiarrhythmic drug action is also not considered in the Vaughan Williams scheme. It has been known for many years that the effect of quinidine on upstroke velocity of the action potential is altered by the stimulation frequency.[25]

A modulated receptor hypothesis regarding antiarrhythmic drug effects with the sodium channel was proposed by Hille[26] and Hondeghem and Katzung.[27] In brief, sodium channels can exist in a resting state (diastole), open or activated state (during action potential upstroke), or inactivated state (plateau of action potential). Clinically useful antiarrhythmic drugs appear to bind to their receptor preferentially during the open state, inactivated state, or both. Lidocaine is thought to block primarily the inactivated state of the sodium channel whereas quinidine appears to block open sodium channels.[24] In addition, sodium channel blocking drugs also have different rates of dissociation from the sodium channel between impulses.[28] In general, for the class I agents, the rates of dissociation seem to correlate with the subclassification of Harrison into A, B, and C. Lidocaine has a rapid recovery from block, quinidine is intermediate, and flecainide is slow.[24] Use-dependent block occurs as channels are used more frequently with increased heart rates. The net block caused by a drug results from the amount of block that occurs with each depolarization and the rate of recovery during diastole.[29] It is not surprising that drugs such as lidocaine, which have a rapid recovery from block, cause minimal change in the QRS duration during normal sinus rhythm; agents such as flecainide, with slow recovery, produce QRS prolongation even at slow rates. During ventricular tachycardia with a rapid rate, one would expect the actions of lidocaine to be much more pronounced. Recent observations in humans have confirmed the kinetics of use-dependent ventricular conduction slowing by antiarrhythmic drugs.[30]

Reverse use dependence can also occur.[31] In this situation the antiarrhythmic effect is most pronounced during slow rates. Of interest, the class III or potassium blocking actions of quinidine to prolong refractoriness are most marked at slow heart rates, whereas the prolongation of conduction, most likely secondary to sodium channel blockade, is pronounced at faster heart rates. Therefore, quinidine demonstrates use dependency for sodium channel blockade and reverse use dependence for potassium channel blockade. Sotalol and NAPA but not amiodarone exhibit reverse use dependence.[31] Reverse use dependency for potassium channel blockade may contribute to the development of torsade de pointes during slow heart rates with a marked increase in QT interval.

### The Sicilian Gambit

A gambit in chess is an opening in which a player sacrifices a piece to obtain an advantage. The "Sicilian Gambit" proposes a new approach to the classification of antiarrhythmic drugs based on their actions on arrhythmogenic mechanisms.[32] The authors of this paper met in Taormina, Sicily, where they developed their gambit on the classification of antiarrhythmic drugs. They present an excellent review of ion-channel activity in cardiac tissue and summarize multiple actions of antiarrhythmic agents on channels, receptors, and pumps in the heart (Figure 19-2). Arrhythmogenic mechanisms in the heart are also reviewed. Suggestions are then made concerning selection of antiarrhythmic drugs based on a vulnerable parameter for a particular arrhythmia in humans.

### Critique

The Sicilian Gambit should be read by anyone interested in antiarrhythmic drug therapy. It is a superb review of basic cardiac electrophysiology and

| DRUG | CHANNELS Na (Fast) | Na (Med) | Na (Slow) | Ca | K | I_f | α | β | M₂ | P | PUMPS Na/K ATPase |
|---|---|---|---|---|---|---|---|---|---|---|---|
| Lidocaine | Low | | | | | | | | | | |
| Mexiletine | Low | | | | | | | | | | |
| Tocainide | Low | | | | | | | | | | |
| Moricizine | High | | | | | | | | | | |
| Procainamide | | A | | | Mod | | | | | | |
| Disopyramide | | A | | | Mod | | | | Mod | | |
| Quinidine | | A | | | Mod | | Low | | | Mod | |
| Propafenone | | A | | | | | | Mod | | | |
| Flecainide | | | A | | Mod | | | | | | |
| Encainide | | | A | | | | | | | | |
| Bepridil | Low | | | High | Mod | | | | | | |
| Verapamil | Low | | | High | | | Low | | | | |
| Diltiazem | | | | Mod | | | | | | | |
| Bretylium | | | | | High | | Agonist/Antag. | Agonist/Antag. | | | |
| Sotalol | | | | | High | | | High | | | |
| Amiodarone | Low | | | Low | High | | Low | Low | | | |
| Alinidine | | | | | Mod | High | | | | | |
| Nadolol | | | | | | | | High | | | |
| Propranolol | Low | | | | | | | High | | | |
| Atropine | | | | | | | | | High | | |
| Adenosine | | | | | | | | | | Agonist | |
| Digoxin | | | | | | | | | Agonist | | High |

*Relative blocking potency*: ◎ Low  ◉ Moderate  ● High  
○ = Agonist  ◑ = Agonist/Antag.  A = Activated state blocker  I = Inactivated state blocker

**Figure 19-2** Summary of the potentially most important actions of drugs in the heart. Sodium channel blockade is subdivided into fast (<300 ms) medium (Med) (200–1500 ms), and slow (>1500 ms) time constants for recovery from block. Receptors are alpha ($\alpha$), beta ($\beta$), muscarinic subtype 2 ($M_2$), and $A_1$ purinergic (P). *(From Ref. 32, with permission.)*

potential actions of drugs on arrhythmogenic mechanisms. In its current form, it has minimal practical use. It is very complex and not organized for clinical application. One primary problem is the incorrect assumption that we understand not only the mechanism but also the underlying ionic, anatomic, and electrophysiologic milieu for most arrhythmias. In the Wolff-Parkinson-White syndrome, the tissue components of the AV reentry tachycardia circuit are well delineated. This is quite different from most arrhythmias. Even in AV reentry, drugs can be selected to target different parts of the circuit. Calcium channel blockers alter AV nodal function, and sodium channel blockers affect the accessory pathway. Thus, even in the most completely understood human arrhythmia, antiarrhythmic efficacy can be achieved using drugs with different ionic targets. Until more data are available on arrhythmogenic mechanisms and antiarrhythmic drug effects in atrial and ventricular tachycardias, the principles of the Sicilian Gambit will be difficult for the clinician to apply in treating cardiac arrhythmias.

### Clinical Antiarrhythmic Drug Classification

Arrhythmias are caused by a disturbance of impulse initiation, conduction, or both. Further, initiation and maintenance of a tachyarrhythmia may have different mechanisms. For example, a premature atrial complex due to enhanced automaticity may initiate AV reentry. Alterations of the autonomic nervous system may be antiarrhythmic or proarrhythmic. In many instances the anatomic basis for the tachyarrhythmia is poorly understood. Therefore, it is not surprising that in most arrhythmias we do not know why an antiarrhythmic drug is effective in one patient yet ineffective or even proarrhythmic in another. Further research, possibly using novel approaches,[33] will hopefully unravel some of these mysteries.

Table 19-4 shows our clinical approach to the drug treatment of cardiac arrhythmias. It is based on a target tissue critical to the maintenance of an arrhythmia and effective drugs demonstrated in

humans. This approach also has weaknesses, because it assumes that antiarrhythmic efficacy results from drug alteration of the electrophysiologic properties of the target tissue. Contrary to this, a drug could be antiarrhythmic by preventing the initiating event without affecting the target tissue. In AV node and AV reentry, propafenone, flecainide, sotalol, and amiodarone may be effective because of alterations in AV nodal properties. They are listed under AV node/atrium (AV node reentry) and accessory pathway (AV reentry) because they would not be prescribed solely to affect AV nodal function. Drugs only given intravenously—for example, lidocaine, bretylium, and adenosine—are discussed later. Uses of digoxin, verapamil, and diltiazem to control ventricular response in atrial fibrillation and flutter are discussed in the text but not listed in Table 19-4. Paramount to use of this classification scheme is a correct arrhythmia diagnosis. Methods to diagnose cardiac arrhythmias are presented in detail in other chapters. Under effective drugs, we have listed agents that we use for these arrhythmias, but alternative drugs might be useful in certain situations. We no longer prescribe tocainide because of its potentially dangerous side-effects profile and minimal clinical usefulness; therefore we have not included it in Table 19-4. The electrophysiologic properties of moricizine suggest it should be useful for supraventricular arrhythmias, but few data are available to substantiate this.

*Atrial tachyarrhythmia* is a general term that includes atrial tachycardia, atrial flutter, and atrial fibrillation. In AV node and AV reentry, there are two separate target-tissue sites. For AV reentry, if drug therapy is chosen in lieu of endocardial catheter ablation, agents that affect the accessory pathway are preferred unless poor anterograde conduction over the accessory pathway is present. For ventricular tachycardia and ventricular fibrillation, mexiletine monotherapy is relegated to a secondary role. In our experience, this drug is more useful in combination with other antiarrhythmic agents. The reader is referred to other chapters in this book for a more detailed discussion of each arrhythmia.

*Table 19-4   Clinical Antiarrhythmic Drug Classification*

| Arrhythmia | Target Tissue | Effective Drugs |
|---|---|---|
| Sinus node reentry | Sinus node | 1. Verapamil, diltiazem<br>2. Beta blockers |
| Inappropriate sinus tachycardia | Sinus node | 1. Beta blockers<br>2. Verapamil, diltiazem<br>3. F, Prop |
| Atrial tachyarrhythmias | Atrium | 1. Q, D, Pr, F, Prop, S, A<br>2. Beta blockers |
| AV node reentry | AV node (anterograde) | 1. Beta blockers<br>2. Verapamil, diltiazem<br>3. Digoxin |
|  | AV node/atrium (retrograde) | 1. Q, D, Pr, F, Prop, S, A |
| AV reentry | AV node | 1. Verapamil, diltiazem<br>2. Beta blockers<br>3. Digoxin[a] |
|  | Accessory pathway | 1. Q, D, Pr, F, Prop, S, A |
| Ventricular tachycardia | Ventricle; His-Purkinje system | 1. Q, D, Pr, F, Prop, Mo, S, A<br>2. Mex<br>3. Verapamil[b]<br>4. Beta blockers[c] |
| Ventricular fibrillation | Ventricle; Purkinje system | 1. Q, D, Pr, F, Prop, Mo, S, A<br>2. Mex |

Abbreviations: A = amiodarone; D = disopyramide; F = flecainide; Mex = mexiletine; Mo = moricizine; Pr = procainamide; Prop = propafenone; Q = quinidine; S = sotalol.

[a]Can be used in patients with concealed accessory pathway, or poor anterograde conduction over manifest accessory pathway.

[b]Very effective in VT with right bundle branch block/left axis and normal ventricle; may be effective in right ventricular outflow tract VT with normal ventricle.

[c]Effective in some patients with exercise-induced VT.

## Individual Antiarrhythmic Drugs

A brief discussion of individual antiarrhythmic agents is included in this section. It is not intended as an exhaustive review of each antiarrhythmic drug. Rather, a summary of antiarrhythmic efficacy, dosing regimen, adverse effects, and our perspective is presented. The reader should refer to specific references, standard texts, 1–3 and Tables 19-1, 19-2, and 19-4 for more detail.

### Quinidine

#### Antiarrhythmic Efficacy

Atrial tachycardia, atrial flutter, atrial fibrillation, AV node reentry, AV reentry, ventricular tachycardia, and ventricular fibrillation.[34-38]

#### Dosing Regimen

The usual daily oral dose is 600 to 1600 mg. One can administer 200 mg of quinidine sulfate every 6 h to initiate therapy. Alternatively, sustained-release formulations can be used and are given every 8 to 12 h. Quinidine gluconate (Quinaglute) has an equivalent of 202 mg of quinidine base in each 324-mg tablet. Quinidine sulfate (Quinidex) has 249 mg of the anhydrous quinidine alkaloid in each 300-mg tablet. It is sometimes useful to switch from one extended preparation to another to obtain the desired antiarrhythmic effect without toxicity. For example, three Quinidex daily equals approximately 750 mg of quinidine. If a higher dose is required but 1500 mg daily is too large, then 2 Quiniglute tablets given three times per day provides an in-between dose of 1200 mg. Some patients may have less gastrointestinal side effects with one preparation versus the other.

Quinidine can also be given intravenously, although extreme caution must be used because of the potential for hypotension.[39] The intravenous loading dose is approximately 6 to 10 mg/kg, given slowly beginning with about 10 mg/min. If hypotension does not occur, the rate of drug administration can be increased to approximately 20 to 30 mg/min with careful monitoring of blood pressure. We rarely use intravenous loading of quinidine and prefer procainamide or lidocaine if a loading dose of a drug is needed to treat an arrhythmia.

### Adverse Effects

Nausea and diarrhea are common side effects and often result in discontinuation of therapy. More serious side effects include thrombocytopenia and proarrhythmia, which is discussed for all drugs later in this chapter.

### Commentary

Quinidine is effective in many arrhythmias. Its limitations are a high rate of intolerance because of gastrointestinal side effects and its proarrhythmic potential. These two factors make it less desirable for patients with supraventricular arrhythmias. When we use quinidine, it is primarily for ventricular tachyarrhythmias.

## Procainamide

### Antiarrhythmic Efficacy

Atrial tachycardia, atrial flutter, atrial fibrillation, AV node reentry, AV reentry, ventricular tachycardia, and ventricular fibrillation.[36,37,40–42]

### Dosing Regimen

The usual daily oral dose is 2000 to 4000 mg. Of note, the 6-h dosing regimen applies only to the sustained-release forms (Pronestyl SR, Procan SR). Intravenous administration is relatively common and useful in both ventricular and supraventricular arrhythmias. A loading dose of 10 to 14 mg/kg is given, with a total dose usually $\leq 1000$ mg. Hypotension is common, and the rate of drug delivery should not exceed 50 mg/min. Blood pressure should be taken every 1 to 2 min during drug administration. Administration of procainamide should be discontinued temporarily if significant hypotension occurs. Intravenous fluids will usually correct the hypotension and allow a slower infusion rate to continue. Maintenance dosage is usually 1 to 4 mg/min.

### Adverse Effects

The development of a lupus syndrome during long-term administration of oral procainamide is relatively common and limits its use. Positive antinuclear antibodies occur frequently and earlier in patients who are slow acetylators.[17] The development of antinuclear antibodies without the lupus syndrome does not require discontinuation of treatment. Nausea is another common side effect.

More serious adverse effects are the rare occurrence of agranulocytosis, possibly more frequent with sustained-released preparations, and proarrhythmia.

### Commentary

Intravenous procainamide is useful in the acute treatment of patients with ventricular tachycardia and to convert some patients with atrial fibrillation.

We infrequently prescribe oral procainamide because of the relatively common occurrence of drug intolerance and the need for frequent dosing.

## Disopyramide

### Antiarrhythmic Efficacy

Atrial tachycardia, atrial flutter, atrial fibrillation, AV node reentry, AV reentry, ventricular tachycardia, and ventricular fibrillation.[43–46]

### Dosing Regimen

The usual daily oral dose is 400 to 800 mg. Disopyramide can be administered every 6 h or twice daily as a slow-release preparation (Norpace CR).

### Adverse Effects

The most common side effects are anticholinergic and include constipation, dry mouth, urinary retention, and blurred vision, Of note, the controlled-release preparation of disopyramide appears to have less anticholinergic side effects.[44] Sustained-release pyridostigmine, 90 to 180 mg twice daily, can reverse the anticholinergic side effects in most patients without affecting antiarrhythmic efficacy.[47] It is important to use the sustained-release form of pyridostigmine. Serious side effects include aggravation or new onset of CHF and proarrhythmia. Onset of CHF during disopyramide therapy occurs in patients with a history of CHF and is very infrequent in those without a history of CHF.[48]

### Commentary

Anticholinergic side effects and worsening of CHF are the major limitations of using disopyramide. However, it is an effective antiarrhythmic agent and can be given twice daily. Our primary use of this drug is in patients without a history of CHF and in men without prostatism. It is used most commonly for atrial tachyarrhythmias.

## Lidocaine

### Antiarrhythmic Efficacy

Ventricular tachycardia and ventricular fibrillation.

### Dosing Regimen

Lidocaine is given intravenously because of its extensive first-pass metabolism when given by mouth. Various dosing regimens have been suggested. The loading dose should be approximately 2 to 4 mg/kg during the first 30 min. One method is to administer 75 mg over 2 min, followed by two to three additional 50 mg boluses given every 5 to 7 min. The maintenance infusion is usually 1 to 4 mg/min.

### Adverse Effects

Central nervous system toxicity is the most common side effect of lidocaine. This is concentration-related and includes paresthesias, tremor, slurred speech, and confusion. Seizures can also occur, but these are usually due to a very high plasma concentration with too rapid an infusion of the loading dose. In CHF, lower loading and maintenance doses should be used. In hepatic insufficiency, a normal loading dose can be given but the maintenance infusion should be decreased.

### Commentary

Intravenous lidocaine is useful to prevent the emergence of ventricular tachycardia or ventricular fibrillation. In our experience, intravenous procainamide is more effective than lidocaine to terminate sustained ventricular tachycardia. We do not recommend routine use of lidocaine to suppress asymptomatic ventricular arrhythmias during the first few days after acute myocardial infarction.

## Mexiletine

### Antiarrhythmic Efficacy

Ventricular tachycardia and ventricular fibrillation.[49–53]

*Dosing Regimen*

The usual daily oral dose is 450 to 750 mg. The drug is administered every 8 h or three times per day.

*Adverse Effects*

The most frequent side effects are neurologic and include nausea, vomiting, tremor, dizziness, and diplopia. The incidence of side effects is decreased when mexiletine is taken with food. Daily doses greater than 750 mg are commonly associated with intolerable side effects, especially in older individuals.

*Commentary*

We and others[54] have had minimal success using mexiletine to treat patients with sustained ventricular tachycardia or ventricular fibrillation. It is more effective in these patients when combined with other antiarrhythmic agents.[49-52] Mexiletine alone may be successful to suppress spontaneous symptomatic ventricular arrhythmias.

## Tocainide

Tocainide has minimal efficacy in patients with sustained ventricular tachycardia or ventricular fibrillation. Its electrophysiologic properties are similar to those of mexiletine, and it offers few if any advantages over this drug. However, some very serious long-term side effects—such as agranulocytosis and interstitial pneumonitis[55,56]—preclude our use of tocainide.

## Phenytoin

There are few data on the clinical effectiveness of phenytoin in large numbers of patients with cardiac arrhythmias. Suggested efficacy has been in the therapy of atrial and ventricular arrhythmias caused by digitalis toxicity, and it may be useful in some patients with the long QT syndrome.[57,58] We infrequently use this agent. Patients with serious digitalis-

induced arrhythmias are candidates for digitalis-specific antibody therapy. Beta-adrenergic blockers and nonpharmacologic therapy are the treatments of choice for patients with the long QT syndrome.

## Flecainide

*Antiarrhythmic Efficacy*

Inappropriate sinus tachycardia (resistant cases), atrial tachycardia, atrial flutter, atrial fibrillation, AV node reentry, AV reentry, ventricular tachycardia, and ventricular fibrillation.[59-63]

*Dosing Regimen*

The usual daily oral dose is 200 to 400 mg, given twice daily.

*Adverse Effects*

The most serious effects are CHF and proarrhythmia. At higher doses, dizziness, headache, and visual disturbances can occur.

*Commentary*

Publication of the Cardiac Arrhythmia Suppression Trial (CAST)[64] markedly altered the use of flecainide and prompted the manufacturers of encainide to withdraw it from the market. Mortality was greater in patients treated with encainide or flecainide compared with placebo after acute myocardial infarction.[64]

A subsequent study demonstrated the inefficacy and substantial proarrhythmic effect of flecainide in patients treated for sustained ventricular tachycardia or ventricular fibrillation.[65] Because of these data, we rarely use flecainide in patients with ventricular arrhythmias who have ventricular dysfunction. However, the Food and Drug Administration has recently approved flecainide for the treatment of patients with supraventricular tachycardia in the presence of normal cardiac function. In these individuals, the drug is often effective and has minimal long-term toxicity.

## Propafenone

### Antiarrhythmic Efficacy

Inappropriate sinus tachycardia (resistant cases), atrial tachycardia, atrial flutter, atrial fibrillation, AV node reentry, AV reentry, ventricular tachycardia, and ventricular fibrillation.[66-71]

### Dosing Regimen

The usual daily oral dose is 450 to 900 mg. Most patients require three-times-a-day dosing, although propafenone can be given twice daily in some patients.

### Adverse Effects

The most serious side effects are heart failure and proarrhythmia. Noncardiac side effects are usually dose-related and most commonly include a metallic taste in the mouth, constipation, visual blurring, dizziness, and nausea. The drug is usually well tolerated at ≤600 mg/day.

### Commentary

Propafenone has minor beta-adrenergic blocking effects with a potency of approximately 1:40 of propranolol. It has saturable clearance, so that plasma concentrations at 900 mg daily are disproportionately greater than at 600 mg/day. Thus, its beta-adrenergic blocking actions will be more pronounced at the highest dosage. Propafenone was not used in CAST.

However, in our experience, propafenone is less proarrhythmic than flecainide or encainide. We use this agent for patients with atrial tachyarrhythmia who are not candidates for endocardial catheter ablation and in patients with sustained ventricular tachyarrhythmias. It should be used cautiously in any patient with a history of congestive heart failure.

## Moricizine

### Antiarrhythmic Efficacy

Ventricular tachycardia and ventricular fibrillation.[72,73]

### Dosing Regimen

Usual daily oral dose is 600 to 900 mg. Most patients require administration of the drug three times daily, but in some twice-a-day dosing is possible.

### Adverse Effects

Proarrhythmia is the most serious side effect. Nausea and dizziness are relatively common side effects but usually occur with doses >750 mg/day.

### Commentary

Limited data suggest that moricizine may be useful in supraventricular tachycardia.[74] It has very limited use in patients with sustained ventricular tachycardia or ventricular fibrillation,[75] and there is a substantial proarrhythmic incidence in these patients. CAST II was discontinued prematurely, and there was an excess mortality during the first 14-day treatment period with moricizine.[76] The drug is useful to suppress highly symptomatic nonsustained ventricular arrhythmias and is relatively safe in patients without structural heart disease. Future studies may demonstrate a role for moricizine in the treatment of patients with atrial tachyarrhythmias.

## Amiodarone

### Antiarrhythmic Efficacy

Atrial tachycardia, atrial flutter, atrial fibrillation, AV node reentry, AV reentry, ventricular tachycardia, ventricular fibrillation.[77-89]

### Dosing Regimen

The usual daily oral dose is 200 to 400 mg. The 200-mg dose is given once daily and 400 mg can be given as a single dose or as 200 mg twice a day. The elimination half-life for amiodarone is approximately 53 days. Because of this, a loading dose is required. There is no standard loading dose regimen. For patients with sustained ventricular tachycardia or ventricular fibrillation, we use a loading dose of approximately 11 g. This can be accomplished in most patients with administration of 800 mg two times per day for 7 days.[90] In patients who cannot tolerate this loading dose, the total amount can be given over several more days. Such an aggressive loading dose is not necessary in most patients treated for supraventricular tachycardia. One study used 600 mg/day for 4 weeks in patients with atrial fibrillation or flutter.[81] An alternative is to use 1200 to 1600 mg per day for approximately 5 days.

A progressively decreasing maintenance dose is prescribed following the total loading dose. For most patients with sustained ventricular tachyarrhythmias, we recommend 400 mg twice daily for 4 weeks, 300 mg twice daily for the next 4 weeks, and then 300 to 400 mg/day. Variations in this drug regimen may be necessary in some patients who develop amiodarone side effects. In patients treated for supraventricular tachycardia, the daily amiodarone dose is 400 to 600 mg for approximately 1 month following the loading dose. Thereafter, it is decreased to 200 to 400 mg/day. In these patients, 200 to 300 mg/day is used whenever possible to reduce the risk of long-term side effects. These low doses often cannot be used in patients with sustained ventricular arrhythmias in whom a recurrence may have more dire consequences.

### Adverse Effects

Amiodarone has a plethora of side effects, many of them serious. Proarrhythmia can occur but is generally less than with many other agents. The most serious side effect is pulmonary toxicity, which has been reported to occur in 1 to 13 percent of patients.[89] We have noted this complication in approximately 3 to 4 percent of patients. There is controversy regarding an increased risk of pulmonary toxicity in patients who have underlying lung disease. Regardless, in these patients it is often difficult to determine whether new abnormalities on a chest roentgenogram or worsening of pulmonary symptoms are caused by the underlying lung disease or amiodarone toxicity. For this reason amiodarone should be used very cautiously in patients with significant pulmonary disease. We recommend a baseline pulmo-

nary function test with carbon monoxide diffusion capacity and a chest roentgenogram every 3 to 4 months for surveillance. Symptoms such as shortness of breath or persistent cough should be investigated immediately. In essence, it is advisable for *both* physician and patient to have a high index of suspicion that any new or worsening pulmonary symptom might be caused by amiodarone toxicity.

Amiodarone has two iodines per molecule. It has been associated with both hyperthyroidism and hypothyroidism, the latter occurring more frequently. If amiodarone therapy is necessary, treatment of the thyroid dysfunction can be accomplished while maintaining amiodarone treatment. Surveillance for thyroid dysfunction is suggested. Thyroid function is assessed at baseline and every 6 months.

Acute hepatitis has been reported but is relatively rare. However, persistent elevation of liver enzymes is common and should be monitored carefully. We obtain baseline liver function tests and repeat them every 3 to 4 months. Patients with persistence of significantly (for example, twice normal) elevated liver enzymes may require discontinuation of amiodarone to prevent chronic liver toxicity.

Corneal microdeposits occur frequently and may produce a halo on viewing bright lights at night. Interference with visual acuity is rare. Patients may also have skin involvement with photosensitivity to the sun and a blue discoloration of the skin, often in sun-exposed areas. We advise patients to use sunscreens that block ultraviolet light and to avoid direct sun exposure if possible. Nausea is a common side effect that is dose-related and usually disappears when the dose is lowered.

In summary, before starting amiodarone treatment, we obtain a pulmonary function test, chest roentgenogram, and thyroid and liver function tests. During follow-up, a chest roentgenogram and liver function tests are evaluated every 3 to 4 months, and thyroid function tests every 6 months.

### Commentary

Like Charles Dickens's *A Tale of Two Cities,* amiodarone often appears to represent the best of times and the worst of times. It is a highly effective drug that is often lifesaving in patients with refractory sustained ventricular tachyarrhythmias. It can also maintain sinus rhythm in many patients with atrial fibrillation refractory to other drugs. Unfortunately, its side-effects profile often limits its use. For this reason, amiodarone is usually relegated to a second- or third-line choice in the United States. We use amiodarone most frequently to prevent recurrent sustained ventricular tachyarrhythmias and in patients with refractory atrial fibrillation. Recent data suggest that "low-dose" (200 mg/day) amiodarone is effective with minimal side effects to prevent atrial fibrillation, and its use in this situation is becoming more widespread. In patients with markedly impaired left ventricular function, we may use amiodarone as a first-line agent.

### Bretylium

#### Antiarrhythmic Efficacy

Ventricular tachycardia and ventricular fibrillation.[91,92]

#### Dosing Regimen

Bretylium can only be administered intravenously. The usual initial dose is 5 mg/kg given over 5 to 10 min. This dose may be repeated in 15 to 30 min if arrhythmia suppression has not been achieved. A maintenance dose of 1 to 4 mg/min may be used if needed.

#### Adverse Effects

The major side effect is hypotension. Postural hypotension may be troublesome and, if bretylium is given for several days, can last days after bretylium has been discontinued. Nausea and vomiting may also occur, especially if the drug is administered rapidly.

#### Commentary

Bretylium is effective to prevent acute recurrences of sustained ventricular arrhythmias in some patients. It is usually given after intravenous lido-

caine, procainamide, or both have been ineffective. In patients who require long-term therapy, oral antiarrhythmic agents should be administered concomitantly and bretylium weaned thereafter.

### Sotalol

#### Antiarrhythmic Efficacy

Atrial tachycardia, AV node reentry, AV reentry, ventricular tachycardia, and ventricular fibrillation.[35,70,93–100]

#### Dosing Regimen

The usual daily oral dose is 160 to 480 mg. Sotalol is usually given twice daily but may be given three times a day in smaller amounts to improve tolerance. Electrophysiologic effects of sotalol to prolong ventricular refractoriness are minimal at dosages 160 mg/day or less.[101,102] At these lower doses, the drug is primarily a beta-adrenergic blocker.

#### Adverse Effects

Serious side effects include ventricular proarrhythmia, especially torsade de pointes, and CHF. Torsade de pointes with sotalol, unlike quinidine, is more dose-related. Thus, caution should be used if dosage is increased during outpatient therapy. Other side effects are usually dose-dependent and related to beta-adrenergic activity. These include fatigue, dizziness, and dyspnea.

#### Commentary

Sotalol is useful for supraventricular and ventricular arrhythmias. Its lack of drug-drug interactions and noncardiac organ toxicity are attractive attributes for long-term use. It should not be administered to patients who cannot tolerate beta-adrenergic blockade. For most patients, daily doses of 320 mg or more are necessary to prevent recurrence of sustained ventricular arrhythmias. The QT interval should be monitored closely during dose titration. Sotalol may have to be discontinued or the dose decreased if marked QT prolongation occurs. There is no absolute QT interval cutoff, but we try to avoid a corrected QT interval more than 520 ms.

## Digoxin

### Antiarrhythmic Efficacy

Prevention of AV node reentry and AV reentry.[103-105] Decreases ventricular response in atrial fibrillation and atrial flutter.[106-108]

### Dosing Regimen

The usual daily oral dose is 0.25 mg. Occasionally higher doses are necessary to control ventricular rate in patients with atrial fibrillation or atrial flutter. An intravenous loading dose of digoxin may be given, 0.5 to 1.0 mg initially with a total 24-h dose <1.5 mg. Oral loading may also be given with similar doses, but the peak onset of action will occur later.

### Adverse Effects

Oral digoxin is extremely well tolerated, with few if any side effects for most patients. Digitalis toxicity can occur, especially in patients with renal disease. Common side effects with digitalis toxicity are anorexia, nausea, vomiting, and—in extreme cases—headache and green and yellow colored vision. Digitalis toxic arrhythmias can be quite serious, including bidirectional ventricular tachycardia and ventricular fibrillation. If any doubt exists as to the presence of digitalis toxicity, digoxin should be withheld, digoxin levels should be immediately obtained, and therapy initiated if needed.

### Commentary

Digitalis blocks the sodium-potassium ATPase pump and is an agonist for cardiac muscarinic receptors.[32] Importantly, direct effects of digoxin on AV nodal function are minimal.[109] Its depression of conduction and prolongation of refractoriness in the AV node is indirect, due to increased vagal tone.[107,108] Because of these indirect actions, therapeutic efficacy

of digoxin often can be negated by changes in autonomic tone.

For example, in patients with atrial fibrillation, it is common for the ventricular response to be controlled at rest but to accelerate inappropriately with light to moderate activity (vagal withdrawal and increased sympathetic tone). Ventricular rate control is much less susceptible to autonomic perturbations with verapamil or diltiazem, agents that directly affect AV nodal function. Thus, we prefer verapamil and diltiazem for rate control in patients with atrial fibrillation or flutter unless CHF is present, when digoxin is the treatment of choice. Digoxin can cause more frequent and prolonged episodes of atrial fibrillation in a small subgroup of patients with vagally mediated atrial fibrillation. In these patients, atrial fibrillation occurs almost exclusively during periods of high vagal tone—for example, during sleep and after eating. Digoxin should not be given to these patients.

We do not use intravenous digoxin to terminate AV or AV node reentry. Adenosine and verapamil are far superior to accomplish this goal.[110] Chronic digoxin therapy is effective in some patients to prevent recurrences of AV node reentry,[103,104] but it is much less effective in patients with AV reentry.[105] Further, in patients with ventricular preexcitation, digitalis can accelerate the preexcited ventricular rate during atrial fibrillation and even result in ventricular fibrillation.[111] We do not recommend the use of digoxin in patients with ventricular preexcitation unless poor anterograde conduction has been demonstrated over the manifest accessory pathway. In patients with concealed accessory pathways with AV reentry, digoxin may be successful. Regardless, in patients with AV and AV node reentry, endocardial catheter ablation should be considered first-line therapy in most instances.

## Verapamil

### Antiarrhythmic Efficacy

Sinus node reentry, inappropriate sinus tachycardia, AV node reentry, AV reentry.[112-116] Selected patients with ventricular tachycardia[116] (Chap. 9).

Decreases ventricular response in atrial fibrillation and atrial flutter.[116]

### Dosing Regimen

The usual daily oral dose is 240 to 480 mg. In most patients, long-acting verapamil given once to twice daily is effective and well tolerated. For acute use, 5 to 10 mg of verapamil is given intravenously over 2 min. Additional verapamil at 3 to 10 mg may be given every 4 to 6 h intravenously as needed.

### Adverse Effects

Extreme bradycardia is relatively rare. Exacerbation of heart failure may occur and the drug should be used with caution in these individuals. Dose-related side effects with chronic oral therapy may include constipation, dizziness, and peripheral edema. Intravenous verapamil is contraindicated in patients with atrial fibrillation and ventricular preexcitation. In these patients, intravenous verapamil can cause an increase in the preexcited ventricular rate and cardiac arrest.[113,117,118]

### Commentary

Intravenous verapamil is an excellent drug to terminate a regular narrow QRS complex tachycardia. We prefer adenosine, which has a very short half-life and decreased chance for complications, as the initial agent in most of these instances, but verapamil is highly effective. It should not be given to patients with a regular wide QRS complex tachycardia unless the mechanism is known to be supraventricular tachycardia. In certain patients with idiopathic ventricular tachycardia, intravenous verapamil may terminate the arrhythmia. Regardless, unless the patient is known to have one of these forms of ventricular tachycardia, intravenous verapamil should not be given. Oral verapamil therapy is useful for prevention of recurrences of AV node and AV reentry. However, we prefer endocardial catheter ablation. Long-acting verapamil is very useful to control ventricular response in patients with atrial tachyarrhythmias, and we

consider it first-line therapy for these individuals. Verapamil may prevent recurrences of some atrial tachycardias.

## Diltiazem

### Antiarrhythmic Efficacy

Sinus node reentry, inappropriate sinus tachycardia, AV node reentry, and AV reentry.[119–121] Decreases ventricular response in patients with atrial fibrillation and atrial flutter.[122]

### Dosing Regimen

Diltiazem is approved for intravenous use in supraventricular tachycardia. The initial dose is 0.25 mg/kg given over 2 min (20 mg average for most patients). If the response is inadequate, a second dose of 0.35 mg/kg may be administered after 15 min. A continuous intravenous infusion may be given afterward to control the ventricular rate of atrial fibrillation or flutter. The initial infusion rate is 10 mg/h, but this should be adjusted to patient response. Infusion can be maintained for 24 h, but few data on safety are documented for longer periods of time. We have used it for several days without problems.

Oral diltiazem may be useful to control ventricular response in atrial fibrillation and flutter, but the data are few compared with verapamil. The daily oral dose is probably 180 to 360 mg, but it should be individualized for each patient. Oral diltiazem may be useful to treat patients with AV and AV node reentry who do not undergo ablation.

### Adverse Effects

Hypotension occurs in approximately 7 percent of patients given intravenous diltiazem but is symptomatic in only 3 percent of patients. Worsening or initiation of CHF is a consideration. However, intravenous diltiazem has been given to patients with substantially decreased ventricular function without causing heart failure. Symptomatic bradyarrhythmias may also occur. Oral diltiazem has side effects similar to verapamil, usually dose-related.

*Commentary*

Intravenous diltiazem is a safe and effective method to control ventricular response in patients with atrial fibrillation and flutter. We do not use it to terminate AV or AV node reentry. We prefer intravenous diltiazem to intravenous verapamil for control of ventricular response during atrial fibrillation or flutter in patients with a history of CHF or those with substantially depressed left ventricular function.

## Adenosine

### Antiarrhythmic Efficacy

Termination of AV node reentry, AV reentry, and some types of atrial tachycardia.[123,124]

### Dosing Regimen

Adenosine is only given intravenously. A rapid bolus of 6 to 12 mg is administered over 1 to 2 s followed by a rapid saline flush. If termination of tachycardia has not occurred, a 12-mg bolus can be given after a 5-min waiting period.

The effects of adenosine are potentiated by dipyridamole. Patients receiving dipyridamole should be given smaller doses of adenosine. Methylxanthines—for example, theophylline—antagonize the effects of adenosine. In these individuals the usual doses of adenosine are likely to be ineffective. Adenosine may exacerbate asthma and should be used cautiously in these patients.

### Adverse Effects

The half-life of adenosine is approximately 10 s. Therefore, adverse effects are very short-lived and usually not serious. Facial flushing is common, as are palpitations, chest pain, and a feeling of shortness of breath. Prolonged bradycardia may occur but usually disappears before any intervention can be given. Theophylline can antagonize the effects of adenosine if necessary.

*Commentary*

Adenosine affects the N region of the AV node.[125] It is highly effective to terminate AV and AV node reentry. It is our drug of choice for any patient with a supraventricular tachycardia with apparent 1:1 AV conduction. Termination of tachycardia does not prove an AV node–dependent mechanism. Adenosine can terminate certain atrial tachycardias. If tachycardia terminates with a QRS complex, it will be difficult to distinguish an AV node–independent from a dependent mechanism. However, if AV block precedes termination of tachycardia, then an AV node–independent mechanism is nearly certain—AV reentry is excluded. Adenosine can also terminate certain forms of ventricular tachycardia, most likely through inhibition of a catecholamine-sensitive cyclic AMP mechanism.

## Beta-Adrenergic Blockers

### Commentary

More than 10 beta-adrenergic blockers have been approved for use, few for cardiac arrhythmias. However, the antiarrhythmic effect of these agents is usually related to beta-adrenergic blockade and not to some specific property of a particular drug. Some agents do have membrane-stabilizing properties that may contribute to efficacy. Beta-adrenergic blockers are first-line treatment for very few cardiac arrhythmias. Exceptions are patients with the idiopathic long QT syndrome and those with adrenergic-dependent tachycardias. However, certain patients with exercise-induced ventricular tachycardia may also have VT without exercise. If these latter patients have structural heart disease, beta-adrenergic blockers are not recommended as monotherapy. In contrast, a trial of beta-adrenergic blockers may be warranted in the absence of structural heart disease.

Beta-adrenergic blockers can depress AV nodal conduction. Thus, they may be useful alone or in combination with digoxin or calcium channel blockers to decrease the ventricular response in patients with atrial fibrillation or flutter. They are effective in a substantial number of patients to prevent AV node reentry but are less useful in patients with AV reentry. Regardless, patients with AV and AV node reentry who require chronic therapy are best treated with endocardial catheter ablation. Not uncommonly, a combination of a beta blocker with a primary antiarrhythmic agent can prevent arrhythmia recurrences that occurred with use of the primary agent alone. One explanation for this success may be blockade of sympathetic tone that can antagonize antiarrhythmic effects of many drugs.

Certain beta-adrenergic blockers are relatively cardioselective. These include acebutolol, atenolol, esmolol, and metoprolol. Some agents can be given intravenously; these include esmolol, labetalol, metoprolol, and propranolol. Labetalol is also an alpha blocker. If rapid beta-adrenergic blockade is necessary, esmolol can be given intravenously as an initial load of 500 μg/kg/min for 1 min followed by 50 μg/kg/min for 4 min. If the response is inadequate, this may be repeated in 5 min with 500 μg/kg/min for 1 min and 100 μg/kg/min for 4 min. The dose should be titrated approximately every 5 min until desired rate effect is present. The usual maintenance dose is 50 to 200 μg/kg/min. We commonly use propranolol beginning with 1 mg/min intravenously to a total dose of 0.15 mg/kg or 12 mg total.

Beta-adrenergic blockers have variable tolerability. We prefer agents that can be given once or at most twice daily and have had excellent success with atenolol and metoprolol.

## Proarrhythmia

Antiarrhythmic drugs are a double-edged sword. These agents, given to control cardiac arrhythmias, can, unfortunately, also cause arrhythmias often more serious than the arrhythmia being treated. Proarrhythmia is a significant new arrhythmia or substantial worsening of a previous arrhythmia in a patient receiving antiarrhythmic drugs. Proarrhythmic effects of drugs can occur in multiple cardiac tissues (Table 19-5).

### Sinus Node and Atrium

Sinus pauses may result from drug suppression of sinus node automaticity, conduction, or both. In our experience, sinus node dysfunction is more common with beta-adrenergic blockers, flecainide, sotalol, and amiodarone. Digoxin very infrequently produces sinus node dysfunction.

There are two types of atrial proarrhythmia. Atrial tachyarrhythmias, especially atrial fibrillation, are often rapid and result in considerable concealed conduction in the AV node. This concealed conduction prevents a very rapid ventricular response. Antiarrhythmic agents may slow the atrial rate enough to allow 2:1 or even 1:1 AV conduction, resulting in a faster ventricular rate. An example might be atrial fibrillation with a ventricular response

*Table 19-5   Proarrhythmia during Antiarrhythmic Drug Therapy*

| Anatomic Site | Effect | Result |
|---|---|---|
| Sinus node | Decrease automaticity/conduction | Sinus pause |
| Atrium | Decrease atrial tachycardia rate | Increase ventricular response |
| | Alter electrophysiologic milieu | Atrial tachyarrhythmia |
| AV node | Depress conduction | AV block |
| His-Purkinje system | Depress conduction | AV block |
| Ventricle | Alter electrophysiologic milieu | VT/VF |

of 120/min that converts to atrial flutter with 2:1 AV conduction and a ventricular rate of 140 to 150/min. Flecainide and propafenone can markedly slow the rate of atrial tachycardias without concurrent AV nodal suppression. Since these two drugs substantially prolong QRS duration, the resulting arrhythmia may have a wide, often bizarre QRS morphology and resemble ventricular tachycardia. Undoubtedly, in some of these cases ventricular proarrhythmia has been diagnosed incorrectly. Adequate AV nodal blocking drugs, usually calcium channel or beta-adrenergic blockers, should be used concomitantly to decrease the chances for an accelerated ventricular rate.

Another form of atrial proarrhythmia occurs when an agent alters the electrophysiologic milieu of atrial tissue, causing a new atrial arrhythmia. Figure 19-3 demonstrates the initiation of atrial fibrillation during a bolus intravenous injection of adenosine. Atrial fibrillation may result in part from hyperpolarization of atrial cells, a decrease in atrial action potential duration, or both.[124] Atrial fibrillation is usually self-terminating and not a significant clinical problem.

However, in some patients with ventricular preexcitation, induction of atrial fibrillation with conduction over the accessory pathway (Fig. 19-4) can yield a rapid preexcited ventricular response.

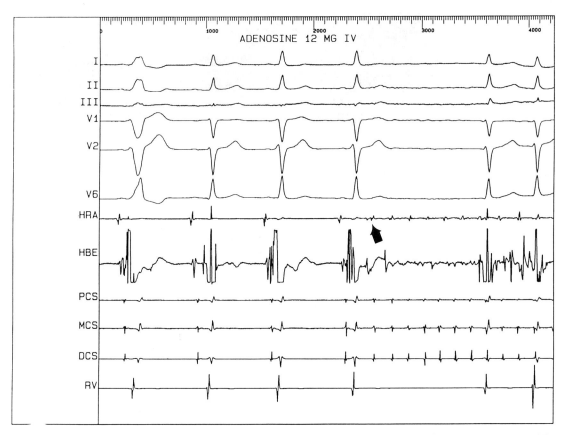

*Figure 19-3*  Initiation of atrial fibrillation with 12 mg IV bolus of adenosine given during sinus rhythm. The first sinus QRS complex demonstrates ventricular preexcitation. The accessory pathway had poor anterograde conduction and, in the presence of adenosine, anterograde block occurred over the accessory pathway. Note the onset of atrial fibrillation (*arrow*).

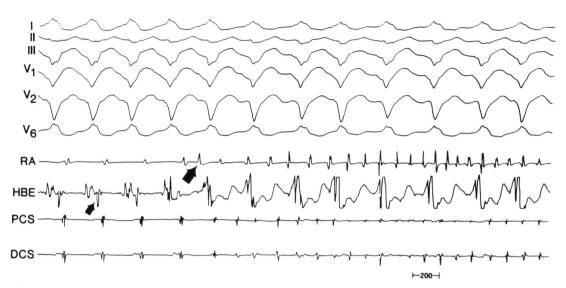

I
II
III
V₁
V₂
V₆
RA
HBE
PCS
DCS

├─200─┤

*Figure 19-4*    Conversion of antidromic reciprocating tachycardia to atrial fibrillation during 12 mg IV bolus of adenosine. All QRS complexes demonstrate conduction over a right free-wall accessory pathway. The first four QRS complexes are generated during antidromic reciprocating tachycardia. Note the concentric retrograde atrial activation sequence with the earliest retrograde atrial activity in the His bundle (HBE) lead (*small arrow*). Atrial fibrillation was initiated during adenosine infusion (*large arrow*), and the rest of the QRS complexes are conducted during atrial fibrillation.

Digoxin can facilitate induction of atrial fibrillation in a subgroup of patients, presumably because of its effects to enhance vagal tone.[126]

### AV Conduction System

Atrioventricular block can occur with drugs that depress conduction in the AV node or His-Purkinje system. An example is shown in Fig. 19-5. This patient with atrial fibrillation had too rapid a ventricular rate with digitoxin. Atenolol was added and the combined effects of these drugs resulted in a very slow ventricular response with substantial symptoms. Undoubtedly, this effect occurred because of block in the AV node, since these agents rarely affect His-Purkinje conduction. Mobitz type II and higher grades of His-Purkinje block can occur with any of the antiarrhythmic drugs that affect His-Purkinje conduction. However, this is a relatively rare complication of drug therapy in our experience. We have treated many patients who have ventricular tachycardia with a variety of drugs that depress His-Purkinje conduction and have rarely noted His-Purkinje block. Regardless, this potential proarrhythmic effect must

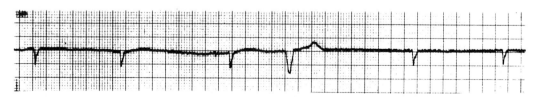

*Figure 19-5*    Marked bradycardia caused by combination therapy with digitoxin (0.1 mg/day) and atenolol (50 mg/day) in a patient with atrial fibrillation. (See text for details.)

always be considered prior to administering these drugs to a patient with preexisting bundle branch block.

### Ventricle

Ventricular proarrhythmia is the most serious and potentially life-threatening side effect of antiarrhythmic drug therapy. It can occur with any antiarrhythmic drug that affects the electrophysiologic properties of ventricular or Purkinje cells (Table 19-3). However, in our experience, lidocaine and mexiletine rarely cause ventricular proarrhythmia. There are various types of ventricular proarrhythmia: drug-associated ventricular fibrillation,[127] incessant ventricular tachycardia, new-onset sustained ventricular tachycardia, torsade de pointes[128] (Fig. 19-6), and marked worsening of previous ventricular arrhythmia

associated with symptoms (Fig. 19-7). Ventricular proarrhythmia can occur in patients being treated for ventricular tachyarrhythmias[127,129,130] or supraventricular tachycardia, most frequently atrial fibrillation.[131–133] The most important predisposing factor is the presence of heart disease, especially a marked depression of ventricular function.[127,129,132,133] The occurrence of ventricular proarrhythmia is rare in patients with normal ventricular function undergoing therapy for supraventricular tachycardia.[133] Proarrhythmia commonly occurs in the initial days of drug therapy,[127,129–131] although there are late proarrhythmic events.[64]

### Initiation of Drug Therapy In Hospital

Drug therapy is initiated in hospital to evaluate the effect of the drug on a patient's arrhythmia or if

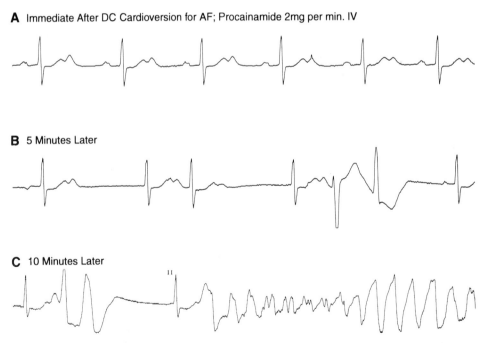

**A** Immediate After DC Cardioversion for AF; Procainamide 2mg per min. IV

**B** 5 Minutes Later

**C** 10 Minutes Later

*Figure 19-6*   Development of torsade de pointes during procainamide therapy. This patient had atrial fibrillation and was given a loading dose of intravenous procainamide followed by a 2-mg/min infusion. Atrial fibrillation persisted and DC cardioversion was administered to restore sinus rhythm. *A.* Sinus rhythm following DC cardioversion was associated with a markedly prolonged QT interval. *B.* At 5 min after DC cardioversion, sinus pauses occurred, followed by ventricular premature complexes. *C.* At 10 min after DC cardioversion, the pauses resulted in greater prolongation of the QT interval and torsade de pointes was initiated (see Chap 8).

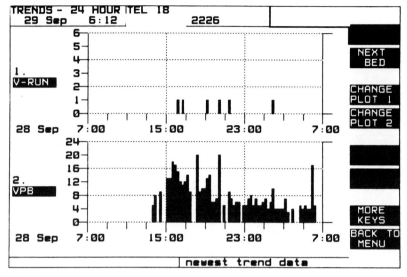

**A**

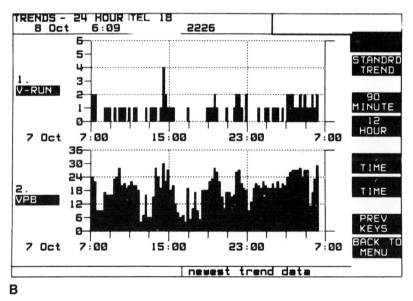

**B**

*Figure 19-7*   Ventricular proarrhythmia during moricizine therapy. *A*. This patient has monomorphic sustained ventricular tachycardia and was continuously monitored by telemetry. Before therapy, he had very few episodes of nonsustained ventricular tachycardia of 3 to 4 beats in duration. Premature ventricular complexes were present. *B*. After the dose of moricizine had been increased to 300 mg every 8 h, the frequency of nonsustained ventricular tachycardia episodes increased, and they were often prolonged, as noted in *C*. The patient was symptomatic with his episodes of nonsustained ventricular tachycardia and the drug was discontinued.

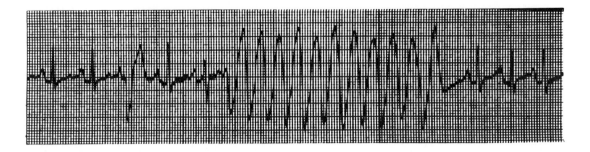

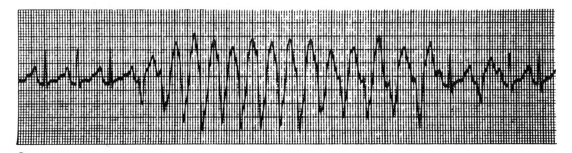

**C**

*Figure 19-7 (Continued)*

there is some concern regarding proarrhythmia. The relative risk of ventricular proarrhythmia depends on the arrhythmia being treated, the presence and degree of structural heart disease, and the drug used. These complex interactions are illustrated with the relative proarrhythmic risk in Fig. 19-8. This figure represents a general approach, but each patient should be considered individually. In this figure, white denotes that it is safe to start drug therapy on an outpatient basis, gray suggests caution in initiating outpatient treatment, and black designates initiation of drug therapy in hospital. Importantly, the relative risk of proarrhythmia depends on multiple factors, which need to be considered together. For example, it is acceptable to start drug therapy on an outpatient basis if the arrhythmia, structural heart disease, and drugs are *all white*. If any of the three is gray, then caution must be exercised. We recommend initiation of therapy in hospital if any of the factors is black. Using this system, a patient with supraventricular

tachycardia with no or minimal structural heart disease can have therapy started as an outpatient with any drug, although caution should be used in some instances. In contrast, regardless of whether structural heart disease is present or which drug is used, patients undergoing therapy for sustained ventricular tachycardia or ventricular fibrillation require hospitalization to start therapy.

## General Commentary

The pharmacologic treatment of patients with cardiac arrhythmias requires substantial knowledge about the arrhythmia and antiarrhythmic drugs. The process begins with a correct diagnosis. A decision is then made whether the patient needs short-term or chronic medical illnesses and drug therapy. In essence, drugs are selected more on the basis of their side-effects

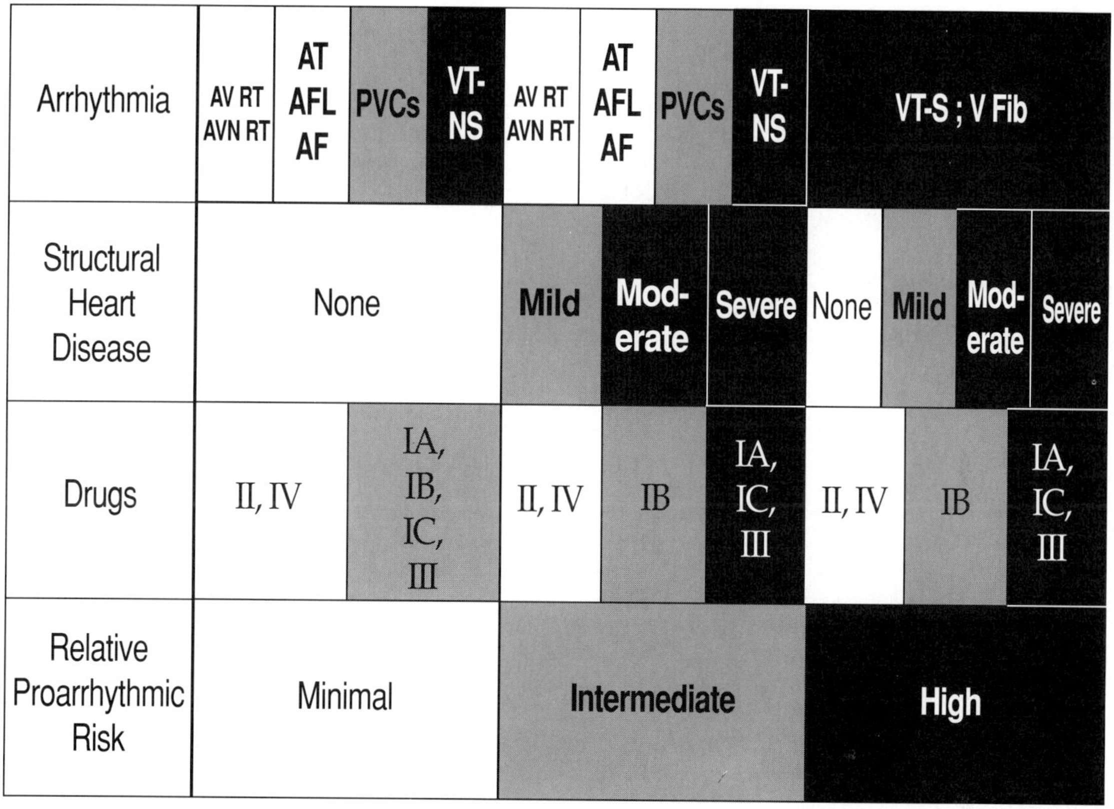

| Arrhythmia | AV RT / AVN RT | AT / AFL / AF | PVCs | VT-NS | AV RT / AVN RT | AT / AFL / AF | PVCs | VT-NS | VT-S ; V Fib | | | |
|---|---|---|---|---|---|---|---|---|---|---|---|---|
| Structural Heart Disease | None | None | None | None | Mild | Moderate | Severe | Severe | None | Mild | Moderate | Severe |
| Drugs | II, IV | II, IV | IA, IB, IC, III | IA, IB, IC, III | II, IV | IB | IA, IC, III | IA, IC, III | II, IV | IB | IA, IC, III | IA, IC, III |
| Relative Proarrhythmic Risk | Minimal | Minimal | Minimal | Minimal | Intermediate | Intermediate | Intermediate | Intermediate | High | High | High | High |

*Figure 19-8*  Relative risk of ventricular proarrhythmia during initiation of drug therapy. (See text for details.) Drugs are listed as shorthand using the Vaughan Williams classification (Table 19-3). Abbreviations: AVRT = atrioventricular reentry; AVNRT = AV node reentry; AT = atrial tachycardia; AFL = atrial flutter; AF = atrial fibrillation; PVCs = premature ventricular complexes; VT-NS = nonsustained ventricular tachycardia; VT-S = sustained ventricular tachycardia; V-FIB = ventricular fibrillation.

therapy and whether nonpharmacologic treatment is preferred. If pharmacologic therapy is chosen, the next step is to select the initial drug. We use an individualized approach to determine which drug is given first. In many patients, several agents are potentially effective for a particular arrhythmia; from there, we try to choose one that is least likely to cause harm to the patient. Thus, factors considered are drug side effects, presence and severity of myocardial, hepatic, and renal dysfunction, and concomitant profile than for efficacy. Last, methods to judge drug

efficacy are employed and may differ for various arrhythmias. For example, serial electrophysiologic-pharmacologic testing is useful to evaluate effectiveness in patients with sustained ventricular tachycardia but is rarely required in evaluating therapy for atrial fibrillation. In conclusion, the seemingly simple process of selecting an antiarrhythmic drug to control a cardiac arrhythmia is actually quite complex if correctly performed. A novice may choose an effective drug, but the seasoned veteran will select the "best" drug(s) for each particular patient.

# *References*

1. Melmon KL et al: *Clinical Pharmacology.* New York, McGraw-Hill, 1992.

2. Gilman AG et al: Goodman and Gilman's *The Pharmacological Basis of Therapeutics.* New York, McGraw-Hill, 1990.

3. Messerli FH: *Cardiovascular Drug Therapy.* Philadelphia, Saunders, 1990.

4. Kessler KM et al: Dynamic variability of binding of antiarrhythmic drugs during the evolution of acute myocardial infarction. *Circulation* 70:472, 1984.

5. Routledge PA et al: Increased alpha-1-acid glycoprotein and lidocaine disposition in myocardial infarction. *Ann Intern Med* 293:701, 1980.

6. Lima JJ et al: Concentration dependence of disopyramide binding to plasma protein and its influence on kinetics and dynamics. *J Pharmacol Exp Ther* 219:741, 1981.

7. Ochs HR et al: Reduction in lidocaine clearance during continuous infusion and by coadministration of propranolol. *N Engl J Med* 303:373, 1980.

8. Feely J et al: Reduction of liver blood flow and propranolol metabolism by cimetidine. *N Engl J Med* 304:692, 1981.

9. Somogyi A, Muirhead M: Pharmacokinetic interactions of cimetidine. *Clin Pharmacokin* 12:321, 1987.

10. Data JL et al: Interaction of quinidine with anticonvulsant drugs. *N Engl J Med* 294:699, 1976.

11. Roden DM, Murray KT: Pharmacokinetics, pharmacodynamics and pharmacogenetics, in Zipes DP, Jalife J (eds): *Cardiac Electrophysiology. From Cell to Bedside,* 2nd ed. Philadelphia, Saunders, (in press).

12. Funck-Brentano C et al: Genetically-determined interaction between propafenone and low dose quinidine: Role of active metabolites in modulating net drug effect. *Br J Clin Pharmacol* 27:435, 1989.

13. Roden DM: Clinical pharmacologic requisites to ensure the adequacy of antiarrhythmic therapy, in Rosen MR, Janse MJ, Wit AL (eds): *Cardiac Electrophysiology: A Textbook.* Mount Kisco, NY, Futura, 1990, pp 1095-1115.

14. Eichelbaum M: Defective oxidation of drugs: Pharmacokinetic and therapeutic implications. *Clin Pharmacokin* 7:1, 1982.

15. Woosley RL et al: Mechanism of the cardiotoxic actions of terfenadine. *JAMA* 269:1532, 1993.

16. Drayer DE, Reidenberg MM: Clinical consequences of polymorphic acetylation of basic drugs. *Clin Pharmacol Ther* 22:251, 1977.

17. Woosley RL et al: Effect of acetylator phenotype on the rate at which procainamide induces antinuclear antibodies and the lupus syndrome. *N Engl J Med* 298:1157, 1978.

18. Windle J et al: Pharmacokinetic and electrophysiologic interactions of amiodarone and procainamide. *Clin Pharmacol Ther* 41:603, 1987.

19. Leahey EB Jr et al: Interactions between quinidine and digoxin. *JAMA* 240:533, 1978.

20. Bennett PB et al: Competition between lidocaine and one of its metabolites, glycylxylidide, for cardiac sodium channels. *Circulation* 78:692, 1988.

21. Roden DM: Are pharmacokinetics helpful for the clinician? *J Cardiovasc Electrophysiol* 2:S178, 1991.

22. Vaughan Williams EM: A classification of antiarrhythmic actions reassessed after a decade of new drugs. *J Clin Pharmacol* 24:129, 1984.

23. Harrison DC: Is there a rational basis for the modified classification of antiarrhythmic drugs? in Morganroth J, Moore EN (eds): *Cardiac Arrhythmias. New Therapeutic Drugs and Devices.* Boston, Nijhoff, 1985, pp 36–47.

24. Grant AO Jr: On the mechanism of action of antiarrhythmic agents. *Am Heart J* 123:1130, 1992.

25. Johnson EA, McKinnon MG: The differential effect of quinidine and pyrilamine on the myocardial action potential at various rates of stimulation. *J Pharmacol Exp Ther* 120:460, 1957.

26. Hille B: Local anesthetics: hydrophillic and hydrophobic pathways for the drug-receptor reaction. *J Gen Physiol* 69:497, 1977.

27. Hondeghem LM, Katzung BG: Time- and voltage-dependent interactions of antiarrhythmic drugs with cardiac sodium channels. *Biochim Biophys Acta* 472:373, 1977.

28. Campbell TJ: Subclassification of Class I antiarrhythmic drugs, in Vaughan Williams EM (ed): *Antirhythmic Drugs Handbook of Exp Pharmacology.* Berlin: Springer-Verlag, 1989, pp 135–155.

29. Hondeghem LM: Antiarrhythmic agents: Modulated receptor applications. *Circulation* 75:514, 1987.

30. Ranger S et al: Kinetics of use-dependent ventricular conduction slowing by antiarrhythmic drugs in humans. *Circulation* 83:1987, 1991.

31. Hondeghem LM, Snyders DJ: Class III antiarrhythmic agents have a lot of potential but a long way to go: Reduced effectiveness and dangers of reverse use dependence. *Circulation* 81:686, 1990.

32. Task Force of the Working Group on Arrhythmias of the European Society of Cardiology: The Sicilian Gambit. A new approach to the classification of antiarrhythmic drugs based on their actions on arrhythmogenic mechanisms. *Circulation* 84:1831, 1991.

33. Arnsdorf MF, Wasserstrom JA: Mechanisms of action of antiarrhythmic drugs: A matrical approach, in Fozzard HA et al (eds): *The Heart and Cardiovascular System.* New York, Raven Press, 1986, pp 1259–1316.

34. Coplen SE et al: Efficacy and safety of quinidine therapy for maintenance of sinus rhythm after cardioversion: A meta-analysis of randomized control trials. *Circulation* 82:1106, 1990.

35. Juul-Moller S et al: Sotalol versus quinidine for the maintenance of sinus rhythm after direct current conversion of atrial fibrillation. *Circulation* 82:1932, 1990.

36. Wellens HJJ, Durrer D: Effect of procaine amide, quinidine, and ajmaline in the Wolff-Parkinson-White syndrome. *Circulation* 50:114, 1974.

37. Sellers TD et al: Effects of procainamide and quinidine sulfate in the Wolff-Parkinson-White syndrome. *Circulation* 55:15, 1977.

38. Wu D et al: Effects of quinidine on atrioventricular nodal reentrant paroxysmal tachycardia. *Circulation* 64:823, 1981.

39. Swerdlow CD et al: Safety and efficacy of intravenous quinidine. *Am J Med* 75:36, 1983.

40. Wu D et al: Effects of procainamide on atrioventricular nodal re-entrant paroxysmal tachycardia. *Circulation* 57:1171, 1978.

41. Miller G et al: The effect of procaine amide in clinical auricular fibrillation and flutter. *Circulation* 6:41, 1952.

42. Greenspan AM et al: Large dose procainamide therapy for ventricular tachyarrhythmia. *Am J Cardiol* 46:453, 1980.

43. Kerr CR et al: Electrophysiologic effects of disopyramide phosphate in patients with Wolff-Parkinson-White syndrome. *Circulation* 65:869, 1982.

44. Wharton JM, Prystowsky EN: Disopyramide, in Messerli FH (ed): *Cardiovascular Drug Therapy.* Philadelphia, Saunders, 1990, pp 1324–1352.

45. Benditt DG et al: Recurrent ventricular tachycardia in man: Evaluation of disopyramide therapy by intracardiac electrical stimulation. *Eur J Cardiol* 9(4):255, 1979.

46. Lerman BB et al: Disopyramide: Evaluation of electrophysiologic effects and clinical efficacy in patients with sustained ventricular tachycardia or ventricular fibrillation. *Am J Cardiol* 51:759, 1983.

47. Teichman SL et al: Disopyramide-pyridostigmine: Report of a beneficial drug interaction. *J Cardiovasc Pharmacol* 7:108, 1985.

48. Podrid PH et al: Congestive heart failure caused by oral disopyramide. *N Engl J Med* 302:614, 1980.

49. Breithardt G et al: Comparison of the antiarrhythmic efficacy of disopyramide and mexiletine against stimulus-induced ventricular tachycardia. *J Cardiovasc Pharmacol* 3:1026, 1981.

50. Waleffe A et al: Combined mexiletine and amiodarone treatment of refractory recurrent ventricular tachycardia. *Am Heart J* 100:788, 1980.

51. Duff JH et al: Mexiletine in the treatment of resistant ventricular arrhythmias: Enhancement of efficacy and reduction of dose-related side effects by combination with quinidine. *Circulation* 67:1124, 1983.

52. Mendes L et al: Role of combination drug therapy with a class IC antiarrhythmic agent and mexiletine for ventricular tachycardia. *J Am Coll Cardiol* 17:1396, 1991.

53. Campbell RWF: Mexiletine. *N Engl J Med* 316:29, 1987.

54. Palileo EV et al: Lack of effectiveness of oral mexiletine in patients with drug-refractory paroxysmal sustained ventricular tachycardia. *Am J Cardiol* 50:1075, 1982.

55. Volosin K et al: Tocainide-associated agranulocytosis. *Am Heart J* 100:1392, 1985.

56. Perlow GM et al: Tocainide-associated interstitial pneumonitis. *Ann Intern Med* 94:489, 1981.

57. Atkinson AJ, Davidson R: Diphenylhydantoin as an antiarrhythmic drug. *Annu Rev Med* 25:99, 1974.

58. Damato AN: Diphenylhydantoin: Pharmacological and clinical use. *Prog Cardiovasc Dis* 12:1, 1969.

59. Neuss H et al: Effects of flecainide on electrophysiological properties of accessory pathways in the Wolff-Parkinson-White syndrome. *Eur Heart J* 4:347, 1983.

60. Hellestrand KJ et al: Cardiac electrophysiologic effects of flecainide acetate for paroxysmal reentrant junctional tachycardias. *Am J Cardiol* 51:770, 1983.

61. Henthorn RW et al: Flecainide acetate prevents recurrence of symptomatic paroxysmal supraventricular tachycardia. *Circulation* 83:119, 1991.

62. Anderson JL et al: Prevention of symptomatic recurrences of paroxysmal atrial fibrillation in patients initially tolerating antiarrhythmic therapy: A multicenter, double-blind, crossover study of flecainide and placebo with transtelephonic monitoring. *Circulation* 80:1157, 1989.

63. Roden DM, Woosley RL: Flecainide. *N Engl J Med* 315:36, 1986.

64. The Cardiac Arrhythmia Suppression Trial (CAST) Investigators: Preliminary report: Effect of encainide and flecainide on mortality in a randomized trial of arrhythmia suppression after myocardial infarction. *N Engl J Med* 321:406, 1989.

65. Herre JM et al: Inefficacy and proarrhythmic effects of flecainide and encainide for sustained ventricular tachycardia and ventricular fibrillation. *Ann Intern Med* 113:671, 1990.

66. Murray KT, Prystowsky EN: Propafenone, in Messerli FH (ed): *Cardiovascular Drug Therapy*. Philadelphia, Saunders, 1990, pp 1353–1365.

67. Waleffe A et al: Electrophysiological effects of propafenone studied with programmed electrical stimulation of the heart in patients with recurrent paroxysmal supraventricular tachycardia. *Eur Heart J* 2:345, 1981.

68. Breithardt G et al: Effect of propafenone in the Wolff-Parkinson-White syndrome: Electrophysiologic findings and long-term follow-up. *Am J Cardiol* 54:29D, 1984.

69. Pritchett ELC et al: Propafenone treatment of symptomatic paroxysmal supraventricular arrhythmias. *Ann Intern Med* 114:539, 1991.

70. Antman EM et al: Therapy of refractory symptomatic atrial fibrillation and atrial flutter: A staged care approach with new antiarrhythmic drugs. *J Am Coll Cardiol* 15:698, 1990.

71. Prystowsky EN et al: Antiarrhythmic and electrophysiologic effects of oral propafenone. *Am J Cardiol* 54:26D, 1984.

72. Clyne CA et al: Moricizine. *N Engl J Med* 327:255, 1992.

73. Fitton A, Buckley MMT: Moricizine: A review of its pharmacological properties and therapeutic efficacy in cardiac arrhythmias. *Drugs* 40(1):138, 1990.

74. Chazov EI et al: Ethmozin. I: Effects of intravenous drug administration on paroxysmal supraventricular tachycardia in the ventricular preexcitation syndrome. *Am Heart J* 108:475, 1984.

75. Mann DA et al: Electrophysiologic effects of ethmozin in patients with ventricular tachycardia. *Am Heart J* 107:674, 1984.

76. The Cardiac Arrhythmia Suppression·Trial II Investigators: Effect of the antiarrhythmic agent moricizine on survival after myocardial infarction. *N Engl J Med* 327:227, 1992.

77. Rosenbaum MB et al: Clinical efficacy of amiodarone as an antiarrhythmic agent. *Am J Cardiol* 38:934, 1976.

78. Wellens HJJ et al: Effect of amiodarone in the Wolff-Parkinson-White syndrome. *Am J Cardiol* 38:189, 1976.

79. Waleffe A et al: Effects of amiodarone studied by programmed electrical stimulation of the heart in patients with paroxysmal re-entrant supraventricular tachycardia. *J Electrocardiol* 11:253, 1978.

80. Horowitz LN et al: Use of amiodarone in the treatment of persistent and paroxysmal atrial fibrillation resistant to quinidine therapy. *J Am Coll Cardiol* 6:1402, 1985.

81. Gosselink ATM et al: Low-dose amiodarone for maintenance of sinus rhythm after cardioversion of atrial fibrillation or flutter. *JAMA* 267:3289, 1992.

82. Heger JJ et al: Amiodarone: Clinical efficacy and electrophysiology during long-term therapy for recurrent ventricular tachycardia or ventricular fibrillation. *N Engl J Med* 305:539, 1981.

83. Heger JJ et al: Clinical efficacy of amiodarone in treatment of recurrent ventricular tachycardia and ventricular fibrillation. *Am Heart J* 106:887, 1983.

84. Fogoros RN et al: Amiodarone: Clinical efficacy and toxicity in 96 patients with recurrent, drug-refractory arrhythmias. *Circulation* 68:88, 1983.

85. McGovern B et al: Long-term clinical outcome of ventricular tachycardia or fibrillation treated with amiodarone. *Am J Cardiol* 53:1558, 1984.

86. Klein LS et al: Prospective evaluation of a discriminant function for prediction of recurrent symptomatic ventricular tachycardia or ventricular fibrillation in coronary artery disease patients receiving amiodarone and having inducible ventricular tachycardia at electrophysiologic study. *Am J Cardiol* 61:1024, 1988.

87. Herre JM et al: Long-term results of amiodarone therapy in patients with recurrent sustained ventricular tachycardia or ventricular fibrillation. *J Am Coll Cardiol* 13:442, 1989.

88. Zipes DP et al: Amiodarone: Electrophysiologic actions, pharmacokinetics and clinical effects. *J Am Coll Cardiol* 3:1059, 1984.

89. Mason JW: Amiodarone. *N Engl J Med* 316:455, 1987.

90. Prystowsky EN et al: Amiodarone: Inter-relationship of dose and time of electrophysiologic and antiarrhythmic effects. *Circulation* 70(II):II-3, 1984.

91. Skale BT, Prystowsky EN: A practitioner's guide to bretylium tosylate. *J Cardiovasc Med* 9(1):79, 1984.

92. Haynes RE et al: Comparison of bretylium tosylate and lidocaine in management of out-of-hospital ventricular fibrillation: A randomized clinical trial. *Am J Cardiol* 48:353, 1981.

93. Rizos I et al: Differential effects of sotalol and metoprolol on induction of paroxysmal supraventricular tachycardia. *Am J Cardiol* 53:1022, 1984.

94. Manz M et al: Sotalol bei supraventrikularer Tachykardie elektrophysiologische Messungen bei Wolff-Parkinson-White Syndrom und AV-knoten-Reentry-tachykardie. *Z Kardiol* 74:500, 1985.

95. Kunze KP et al: Sotalol in patients with Wolff-Parkinson-White syndrome. *Circulation* 75:1050, 1987.

96. Senges J et al: Electrophysiologic testing in assessment of therapy with sotalol for sustained ventricular tachycardia. *Circulation* 69:577, 1984.

97. Steinbeck G et al: Electrophysiologic and antiarrhythmic efficacy of oral sotalol for sustained ventricular tachyarrhythmias: Evaluation by programmed stimulation and ambulatory electrocardiogram. *J Am Coll Cardiol* 8:949, 1986.

98. Dorian P et al: Sotalol and type IA drugs in combination prevent recurrence of sustained ventricular tachycardia. *J Am Coll Cardiol* 22:106, 1993.

99. Mason JW: A comparison of seven antiarrhythmic drugs in patients with ventricular tachyarrhythmias. *N Engl J Med* 329:452, 1993.

100. Singh BN et al: Sotalol: A review of its pharmacodynamic and pharmacokinetic properties, and therapeutic use. *Drugs* 34:311, 1987.

101. Wang T et al: Concentration-dependent pharmacologic properties of sotalol. *Am J Cardiol* 57:1160, 1986.

102. Nattel S et al: Concentration dependence of class III and beta-adrenergic blocking effects of sotalol in anesthetized dogs. *J Am Coll Cardiol* 13:1190, 1989.

103. Wu D et al: The effects of ouabain on induction of

atrioventricular nodal re-entrant paroxysmal supraventricular tachycardia. *Circulation* 52:201, 1975.

104. Wellens HJJ et al: Effect of digitalis in patients with paroxysmal atrioventricular nodal tachycardia. *Circulation* 52:779, 1975.

105. Dhingra RC et al: Electrophysiologic effects of ouabain in patients with preexcitation and circus movement tachycardia. *Am J Cardiol* 47:139, 1981.

106. MacKenzie J: *Diseases of the Heart.* London, Oxford University Press, 1908, pp 270–271.

107. Lewis T: *The Mechanism and Graphic Registration of the Heart Beat.* London, Shaw and Sons, 1925, pp 349–351.

108. Klein HO, Kaplinsky E: Verapamil and digoxin: Their respective effects on atrial fibrillation and their interaction. *Am J Cardiol* 50:894, 1982.

109. Goodman DJ et al: Effect of digoxin on atrioventricular conduction: Studies in patients with and without cardiac autonomic innervation. *Circulation* 51:251, 1975.

110. Greco R et al: Treatment of paroxysmal supraventricular tachycardia in infancy with digitalis, adenosine-5′-triphosphate, and verapamil: A comparative study. *Circulation* 66:504, 1982.

111. Sellers TD Jr et al: Digitalis in the preexcitation syndrome: Analysis during atrial fibrillation. *Circulation* 56:260, 1977.

112. Wellens JHH et al: Effect of verapamil studied by programmed electrical stimulation of the heart in patients with paroxysmal reentrant supraventricular tachycardia. *Br Heart J* 39:1058, 1977.

113. Rinkenberger RL et al: Effects of intravenous and chronic oral verapamil administration in patients with supraventricular tachyarrhythmias. *Circulation* 62:996, 1980.

114. Klein GJ et al: Comparison of the electrophysiological effects of intravenous and oral verapamil in patients with paroxysmal supraventricular tachycardia. *Am J Cardiol* 49:117, 1982.

115. Sung RJ et al: Intravenous verapamil for termination of reentrant supraventricular tachycardias. *Ann Intern Med* 93:682, 1980.

116. Prystowsky EN, Gilmour RF Jr: Role of slow channel blockers in the treatment of arrhythmias: Basic considerations and clinical applications, in Kostis J, Defelice EA (eds): *The Pharmacological Treatment of Cardiovascular Diseases.* New York, Medical Examinators, 1986, pp 213–234.

117. Gulamhusein S et al: Acceleration of the ventricular

response during atrial fibrillation in the Wolff-Parkinson-White syndrome after verapamil. *Circulation* 65:348, 1982.

118. McGovern B et al: Precipitation of cardiac arrest by verapamil in patients with Wolff-Parkinson-White syndrome. *Ann Intern Med* 104:791, 1986.

119. Yeh SJ et al: Effects of oral diltiazem in paroxysmal supraventricular tachycardia. *Am J Cardiol* 52:271, 1983.

120. Betriu A et al: Beneficial effect of intravenous diltiazem in the acute management of paroxysmal supraventricular tachyarrhythmias. *Circulation* 67:88, 1983.

121. Huycke ED et al: Intravenous diltiazem for termination of reentrant supraventricular tachycardia: A placebo-controlled, randomized, double-blind, multicenter study. *J Am Coll Cardiol* 13:538, 1989.

122. Salerno DM et al: Efficacy and safety of intravenous diltiazem for treatment of atrial fibrillation and atrial flutter. *Am J Cardiol* 63:1046, 1989.

123. DiMarco JP et al: Adenosine: Electrophysiologic effects and therapeutic use for terminating paroxysmal supraventricular tachycardia. *Circulation* 68:1254, 1983.

124. Camm AJ, Garratt CJ: Adenosine and supraventricular tachycardia. *N Engl J Med* 325:1621, 1991.

125. Clemo HF, Belardinelli L: Effect of adenosine on atrioventricular conduction: I: Site and characterization of adenosine action in the guinea pig atrioventricular node. *Circulation Res* 59:42, 1986.

126. Coumel P: Neurogenic and humoral influences of the autonomic nervous system in the determination of paroxysmal atrial fibrillation, in Attuel P, Coumel P, Janse MJJ (eds): *The Atrium in Health and Disease.* Mount Kisco, NY, Futura, 1989, pp 213–232.

127. Minardo JD et al: Clinical characteristics of patients with ventricular fibrillation during antiarrhythmic drug therapy. N Engl J Med 319:257, 1988.

128. Jackman WM et al: The long QT syndromes: A critical review, new clinical observations and a unifying hypothesis. *Prog Cardiovasc Dis* 31:15, 1988.

129. Stanton MS et al: Arrhythmogenic effects of antiarrhythmic drugs: A study of 506 patients treated for ventricular tachycardia or fibrillation. *J Am Coll Cardiol* 14:209, 1989.

130. Velebit V et al: Aggravation and provocation of ventricular arrhythmias by antiarrhythmic drugs. *Circulation* 65:886, 1982.

131. Ejvinsson G, Orinius E: Prodromal ventricular premature beats preceded by a diastolic wave. *Acta Med Scand* 208:445, 1980.

132. Flaker GC et al: Antiarrhythmic drug therapy and cardiac mortality in atrial fibrillation. *J Am Coll Cardiol* 20:527, 1992.

133. Prystowsky EN: Inpatient versus outpatient initiation of anti-arrhythmic drug therapy for patients with supraventricular tachycardia (in press).

# Chapter 20

# Operative Therapy of Arrhythmias

## General Principles

Operative therapy may be directed at correcting a primary cardiac abnormality implicated in causing an arrhythmia. For example, coronary revascularization would be a therapy of choice in treating ventricular fibrillation associated with angina pectoris. However, "direct" operative treatment of arrhythmia means preventing arrhythmia by destroying or altering a critical part of a fixed arrhythmia substrate. The traditional model for understanding this concept is the operative ablation of the accessory pathway in the Wolff-Parkinson-White (WPW) syndrome, first performed at Duke University in 1968.[1] The prerequisites for surgery are evident from this model. First, the arrhythmia mechanism must be understood to a sufficient degree to identify myocardial substrate critical to the perpetuation of tachycardia. Second, it must be feasible to ablate this substrate with minimal or at least acceptable impact on cardiac function.

## Indications for Surgery

Indications for surgery depend a great deal on the efficacy and morbidity of a specific operation (Table 20-1) and that of the treatment alternatives. Operative treatment of the WPW syndrome is very efficacious and success rates of over 95 percent with mortality less than 1 percent should be expected in the absence of serious concomitant heart disease.[2] Consequently, operative therapy may be offered as a reasonable alternative to other therapies, if catheter ablation is not successful, especially a lifelong com-

mitment to antiarrhythmic drugs. On the other hand, ventricular tachycardia (VT) is frequently associated with severe, progressive heart disease which contributes to poorer efficacy and higher mortality with operative therapy.[3] In such instances, surgery should generally be offered as a secondary therapy after failure of pharmacologic management. The decision to operate for VT usually requires careful consideration of individual circumstances. Surgery assumes a higher priority in the patient with a smaller, well-circumscribed lesion (usually infarct scar) with well-preserved ventricular function and a lower priority in patients with inoperable concomitant disease and very poor ventricular function. Decisions within the spectrum of these two extremes may be more difficult. Operative ablation of problematic or potentially problematic arrhythmia can also be considered in operating for other cardiac problems.

## The Therapeutic Plan

The overall strategy for operative therapy is the same regardless of the specific arrhythmia or operation planned.[4] This includes

- Complete cardiac assessment
- Preoperative electrophysiologic study
- Formulation of operative plan
- Operative electrophysiologic assessment
- Postoperative electrophysiologic assessment

A general cardiac assessment is necessary to assess factors that could actually cause the arrhythmia, to detect abnormalities that could complicate the surgery if unrecognized, or to delineate concomitant

*Table 20-1   Operative Therapy of Specific Arrhythmias*

| Arrhythmia | Major advantages | Major limitations | Threshold for recommending surgery |
|---|---|---|---|
| Wolff-Parkinson-White syndrome | Effective<br>Low risk | | Low[a] |
| AV node reentry | Effective<br>Low risk | Risk of AV block<br>Operator-dependent | Low to medium[a] |
| Atrial tachycardia | Potentially curative | Arrhythmia may not be inducible<br>Potentially associated with other arrhythmias | Medium to high[a] |
| Atrial flutter | Potentially curative | Limited experience<br>Potentially associated with atrial fibrillation | Medium[a] |
| Atrial fibrillation (corridor operation, maze operation) | May restore normal chronotrophy | Limited experience<br>May not prevent emboli or preserve atrial contractility[b] | Medium to high |
| Ventricular tachycardia | Potentially curative<br>Easier with discrete "lesion" | Limited by associated myocardial disease<br>Mapping may be technically difficult | High |

[a] Assuming failure of endocardial catheter ablation.
[b] Refers specifically to corridor procedure.

abnormalities that could be corrected at the time of surgery. This assessment always includes echocardiography and includes cardiac catheterization for VT patients. The focus of the evaluation is otherwise dependent on clinical suspicion.

The preoperative electrophysiologic assessment must verify the mechanism of clinically observed and other inducible arrhythmias. This study will form the basis for the operative plan and may be relied upon exclusively if the target arrhythmia is not inducible intraoperatively or if an accessory pathway is inadvertently contused and conduction temporarily lost. Knowledge of sinus node function and atrioventricular (AV) node–His bundle function may also affect overall management. Anatomical localization of the tissue in question (for example, accessory pathway or site of "origin" of VT) is a critical part

of the study. Needless to say, operative success depends on accurate information.

The formulation of the operative plan involves discussion between electrophysiologists, surgeons, and, ideally, anesthesiologists to review all the available information. Potential technical or other difficulties can be discussed and points of uncertainty evaluated. Clear communication facilitates optimal results.

The intraoperative electrophysiologic assessment should verify critical preoperative data and, in particular, provide improved resolution of localization. Localization of an accessory pathway with accurate preoperative data may take as little as 10 min, whereas localizing one or more sites of VT may take considerably longer.

Verification of accessory pathway ablation or

noninducibility of VT should be done before closing the chest, the patient's condition permitting. Electrophysiologic testing is repeated postoperatively prior to discharge to assess the efficacy of the procedure. Postoperative testing at its simplest may consist of incremental atrial and ventricular pacing to verify absence of an accessory pathway or may be more complete and involve attempts at VT induction. It is facilitated by temporary atrial and ventricular epicardial wires, implanted intraoperatively, that can be pulled out through the skin prior to discharge.[5]

### Intraoperative Mapping

Mapping involves a systematic analysis of electrical activity at significant anatomical sites.[6,7] Mapping of activation sequence is most widely used to guide surgery. Activation maps during normal and paced rhythms provide a visual representation of electrical activity, much as an angiogram assesses wall motion. The activation map during an arrhythmia usually points to the region that must be ablated and frequently provides clues to the mechanism.

When a mapping electrode is in contact with muscle, a local electrogram is recorded (Fig. 20-1). A rapid deflection (intrinsic deflection) marks the instant that the wave of electrical activity passes the given electrode. If we consider ventricular activation, the onset of the QRS on the surface electrocardiogram (ECG) marks the beginning of ventricular activation and may be considered as time 0 for a given cycle. The designated site at the mapping electrode can then be given a time of activation relative to 0. Summation of these data from multiple electrode sites over the ventricles provides the activation sequence for ventricular depolarization.

Activation sequence is usually represented pictorially as an isochrone map (Fig. 20-2). Electrode sites activated at the same time are joined to provide isochronic lines of equal activation. The functional importance of a given site to a mapped cycle may be obvious in many instances but must frequently be assessed dynamically. If we consider a hypothetical arrhythmia circuit revolving around an anatomical obstacle (perhaps an infarct scar), as illustrated in

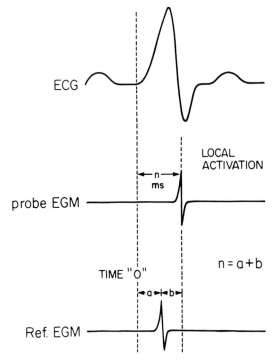

*Figure 20-1* Measurement of activation time at a given electrode site. The onset of ventricular activation, or "time 0" (by convention), is indicated by the onset of depolarization at the earliest ECG lead. At the hypothetical probe site (probe EGM), the rapid deflection of the electrogram represents activation of the muscle at that site that is then timed relative to the onset of depolarization (*n* ms in the example). For ease of measurement, timing is usually made from a fixed site or reference (ref EGM) and subsequently related to the onset of depolarization by adding a correction factor. In the example, the probe time is *b* ms from the reference time and adding *a* ms to *b* provides the activation time of *n* ms. It is technically easier to measure multiple sites from a reference rather than try to relate each one to the onset of ventricular activation from the ECG.

Fig. 20-3, it is obvious that a lesion at site B would be more likely to result in failure of the circuit than at site A. To assess this, site B could be cooled during tachycardia with a cryoprobe ("ice mapping") that causes temporary loss of conduction in the region. Tachycardia will stop if site B is critical to

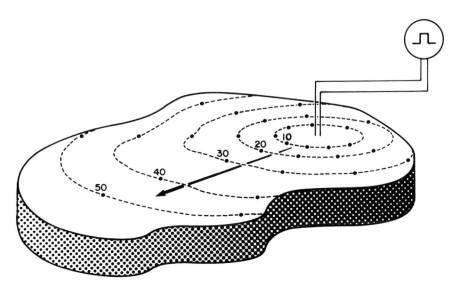

***Figure 20-2***  Activation sequence represented as a simple isochronic map. In this hypothetical myocardium, a paced impulse (⊓) results in progressive myocardial activation. All points measuring the same activation time are joined to represent the wavefront at that point in time in the given plane.

the tachycardia, and the surgeon may then direct efforts to site B. In this example, site B may be the actual generator of the tachycardia (ectopic focus or microreentry) or may just be a part of a larger circuit that narrows at site B.

In its simplest form, mapping can be done with a hand-held probe that is moved sequentially (after each electrogram is recorded) to cover the desired area. This is straightforward and perfectly suitable when the rhythm mapped is stable and uniform, so that many different cycles can be summated to provide a composite representative cycle. Alternatively, more complex mapping systems are available that record the information from many data points simultaneously and provide on-line computer-generated activation maps (Fig. 20-4).[8] This type of system is most useful in ventricular surgery where multiple morphologies of tachycardia are mapped and any given morphology may be observed only transiently. In such a system, only a single cycle is necessary to provide activation sequence provided adequate electrodes are available to cover the area of interest. The area of interest varies with the arrhythmia. For example, the atrioventricular region is important in

the WPW syndrome and the area in and around a chronic infarction is important in a patient with VT related to a previous infarct. Epicardial mapping is adequate for WPW as a rule, but VT may require epicardial, endocardial, and transmural recording.

### Ablative Techniques and Principles

Discrete destruction of a small area or structure crucial to the arrhythmia is the ideal goal when this is feasible, as with accessory pathways in the WPW syndrome. If this is not feasible, the arrhythmogenic zone may be "excluded" electrically, so that the arrhythmia cannot propagate outside the excluded zone.[9] This involves creating a small fibrous barrier around the area harboring the arrhythmia. For example, the left atrium may be electrically excluded if it harbors multiple foci of atrial tachycardia[10] or the right ventricle can be excluded in arrhythmogenic right ventricular dysplasia where multiple sites may cause VT.[11] Scalpel incision with repair or cryosurgery provides the fibrous "fence" that will contain the arrhythmia.

In addition to the scalpel, other tools are

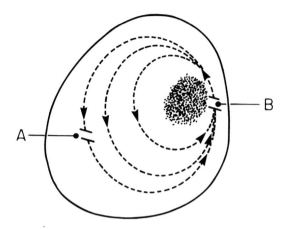

**Figure 20-3** A hypothetical reentrant circuit. The stippled zone represents infarct scar and the lines represent the path of VT. A lesion at the narrow part of the circuit (B) will stop tachycardia, whereas a lesion in the redundant part (A) will not interrupt tachycardia.

available to the surgeon for specific purposes. For example, it may be more logical to "freeze" a papillary muscle harboring VT in order to maintain functional anatomy rather than remove it. Cryosurgery is widely used and versatile and was used early in the development of arrhythmia surgery.[12] The most prevalent systems use expanding nitrous oxide at the tip of a probe to provide freezing. Freezing tissue at a critical temperature results in cellular destruction and ablates conductive tissue and working muscle, allowing healing by fibrosis. The advantages of this technique include the following:

1. Cooling initially causes temporary elimination of conduction and makes it possible to test the functional importance of a site before destroying tissue ("ice mapping").

2. The lesion can be customized by changing the dimensions and shape of the cryoprobe and the time of application.

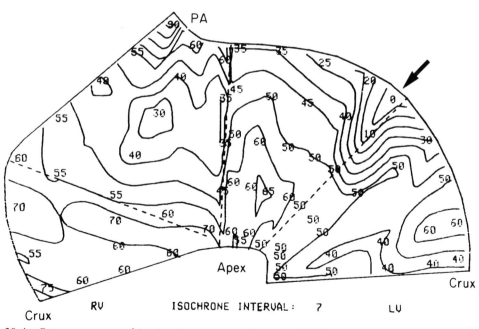

**Figure 20-4** Computer-generated isochronic map in a patient with WPW syndrome. The epicardium is depicted as if the heart were cut along the posterior interventricular groove and flattened. Earliest epicardial activation occurred at the left lateral AV area (*arrow*) in this patient with a left lateral pathway. LV = left ventricle, PA = pulmonary artery, RV = right ventricle.

3. The lesions are discrete and heal by fibrosis, becoming electrically inert and nonarrhythmogenic.

The major disadvantage is the time taken to freeze—several minutes for a small lesion—which can be prohibitive when a relatively large area is to be ablated. More recently, laser photocoagulation has been used as a destructive tool and appears to have many of the advantages of cryosurgery.[13] In addition, relatively large areas can be ablated in a short time.

## Supraventricular Tachycardia

Operative therapy can be considered for virtually any problematic supraventricular tachycardia. In general, the arrhythmia mechanisms are better understood and the feasibility of the procedure is not limited by poor ventricular function.

### The Wolff-Parkinson-White Syndrome

Operative therapy for arrhythmias began with the WPW syndrome, and this remains the classic model for arrhythmia surgery. The target for ablation is the accessory atrioventricular (AV) pathway, a muscular connection bridging the AV groove at any point where there is AV continuity. Accessory pathways are generally classified for operative purposes by location as anterior septal, posterior septal, right free-wall, and left free-wall. The first approximation to pathway localization is provided by the surface ECG, but more definitive localization requires electrophysiologic study (see Chap. 7). The most useful localizing technique is atrial endocardial mapping at the AV ring during AV reciprocating tachycardia (Fig. 20-5). A high index of suspicion should be present for multiple accessory pathways or arrhythmia mechanisms not related to the accessory pathway.

There should be few surprises during intraoperative electrophysiologic testing, the main purpose of which is to provide improved resolution of localization. Indeed, the accessory pathway may become contused intraoperatively and the surgery may have to be done relying solely on the preoperative study. Ventricular epicardial mapping at the AV ring is usually sufficient to define the ventricular insertion of the pathway (Fig. 20-4), while atrial epicardial mapping during AV tachycardia defines the atrial insertion site.

Two approaches are available for the operative procedure, depending on operator preference and training. The endocardial approach[14,15] requires atriotomy, cardiopulmonary bypass, and cardioplegic arrest for left-sided pathways. The epicardial approach[16,17] can be used for all but right anterior septal pathways and does not require atriotomy or bypass (Fig. 20-6). The success rate should be greater than 95 percent for experienced operators regardless of approach, and mortality should be less than 1 percent. A significant potential complication is inadvertent AV block with anterior septal or posterior septal pathways, but this should occur rarely with experience. Mortality and complications usually occur only in the presence of serious heart disease or the requirement for a major adjunctive procedure.

Surgery for WPW syndrome is currently indicated in patients with problematic tachycardia who have failed endocardial catheter ablation. It may also be performed as an adjunctive procedure when other cardiac surgery is performed if surgical expertise permits.

### Atrioventricular Nodal Reentry

The clinical electrophysiology of AV node reentry strongly supports the concept of dual conduction pathways in the AV nodal region as the functional substrate for reentry. The exact anatomical correlates are not known, specifically whether reentry is confined entirely to the AV node or includes atrial perinodal tissue or fibers (Fig. 20-7). Surgery was not attempted for many years, with the view that cure of reentry could not be affected without destroying the AV node. Fortuitous cure of AV node reentry during attempted operative AV nodal ablation suggested

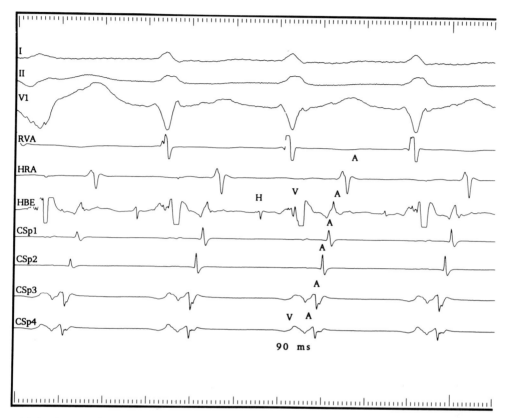

*Figure 20-5*   Atrial endocardial mapping during AV reciprocating tachycardia. Earliest atrial activation during tachycardia occurs at the distal electrode on the coronary sinus catheter ($CS_4$) with a VA interval of 90 ms. The catheter was positioned at the approximate atrial insertion site of the accessory pathway (left lateral). I, II, $V_1$ = surface electrocardiographic leads; $CS_{p1 \text{ to } 4}$ = coronary sinus electrogram from proximal to distal electrode, respectively; HBE = His bundle electrogram; HRA = high right atrium; RVA = right ventricular atrium.

that the reentrant circuit could be interrupted without AV block.[18] Ross and Johnson[19] first demonstrated consistent operative cure of AV node reentry with perinodal dissection.

The preoperative assessment of AV node reentry is straightforward and involves establishing that AV node reentry is indeed the mechanism of observed tachycardia and excluding other tachycardia mechanisms. Activation sequence mapping aimed at delineating the atrial insertion of the retrograde limb of the circuit may not be helpful, since this site is invariably the AV node region and further resolution by conventional catheter techniques is usually diffi-

cult. Ross and Johnson[19] originally described a perinodal operation aimed at disrupting AV node exit sites to the atrium, with the dissection usually focused anteriorly and, less frequently, posteriorly to the AV node. This was based on intraoperative mapping of the retrograde insertion site during tachycardia that was usually observed anterior to the AV node and sometimes posteriorly (Fig. 20-8). Cox[20] described a technique whereby a series of cryolesions surrounded the AV node and prevented reentry, possibly by disrupting the exit site of the circuit. Guiraudon[21] described an anatomically guided procedure (AV node "skeletonization") that

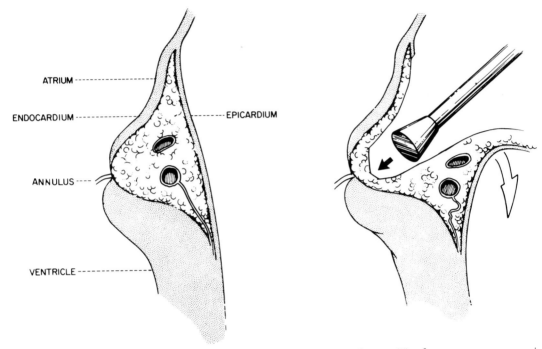

***Figure 20-6*** Epicardial approach for operative ablation of accessory pathways. The figure represents a section through the heart at the level of the annulus. The AV fat pad contains coronary artery and vein and generally harbors the accessory pathway. In this approach, epicardial dissection through the fat pad exposes the annulus. A cryoprobe is then applied to the region of interest, and this is frozen to complete the procedure. *(From Klein et al.[16] Reproduced by permission.)*

achieved a similar result by perinodal dissection. The latter two procedures were not guided by intraoperative mapping, which is technically difficult due to the resolution of standard mapping. However, the development of multiple fine electrodes over the AV node region may one day allow a more discrete, elegant operation.

Centers reporting the results of these procedures suggest a success rate greater than 90 percent should be achievable with mortality less than 1 percent. The major potential complication is inadvertent AV block. This surgery has largely been supplanted by endocardial catheter ablation techniques but may be considered in patients who have failed ablation.

### Atrial Tachycardia

Focal atrial tachycardia due to abnormal automaticity or intraatrial reentry is a much less common mecha-

nism for paroxysmal supraventricular tachycardia than AV node or AV reentry. It is more frequently seen in pediatric patients and after repair of congenital heart lesions such as atrial septal defect or anomalous pulmonary venous return. The major goal of preoperative mapping is localizing the focus or reentrant circuit with atrial endocardial mapping, and the best candidate is one with a consistent atrial morphology documented during repeated clinical episodes. A major obstacle remains the inability to induce some of these arrhythmias (presumably those due to abnormal automaticity) in the laboratory, since accurate mapping is necessary for a successful outcome. The patient with noninducible tachycardia may be taken to the electrophysiology laboratory for mapping during a spontaneous episode of tachycardia. Alternatively, the P wave morphology and/or limited mapping may at least pinpoint the site to either atrium, which could then be "excluded." If an abnormal

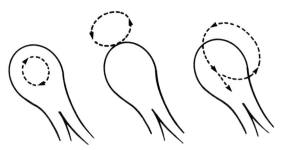

**Figure 20-7**   Anatomic basis for atrioventricular node reentry. The circuit is potentially entirely intranodal (*left panel*), entirely extranodal (*middle panel*), or partially extranodal (*right panel*). The success of perinodal procedures without interrupting AV conduction suggests that the circuit is at least in part perinodal (*right panel*).

region responsible for arrhythmia is identified, it can be ablated by a variety of techniques according to anatomic location or operator preference. These techniques include excision, cryosurgery, or "exclusion."[9,22,23]

Surgery for atrial tachycardia may be considered for medically refractory patients. Major limitations

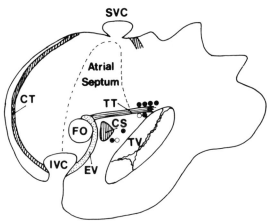

**Figure 20-8**   Site of early retrograde atrial activation during AV node reentrant tachycardia. The right atrium is presented as opened along the anterolateral wall. Sites of early activation in individual patients are represented as solid circles (during tachycardia) or unfilled circles (during ventricular pacing). Activation generally occurs early anterior to the AV node. CT = crista terminalis; EV = eustachian valve; FO = foramen ovale; SVC = superior vena cava; TT = tendon of Tordaro; TV = tricuspid valve, IVC = inferior vena cava. (*From Ross et al.*[19] *Reproduced by permission.*)

include the not infrequent association of multiple atrial sites or atrial fibrillation and inability to induce the clinical arrhythmia consistently for accurate mapping. The increasing success of endocardial catheter ablation for these arrhythmias will limit surgery to patients with ablation failure.

### Atrial Flutter

Abundant clinical and experimental evidence supports the hypothesis that atrial flutter is a macroreentrant atrial arrhythmia.[24] The "common" type of atrial flutter has been best studied and shown to be due to a larger reentrant circuit confined to the right atrium (Fig. 20-9). This arrhythmia can usually be reproducibly initiated in the laboratory and the circuit defined by endocardial mapping. An excitable gap can be demonstrated by entrainment or atrial extrastimuli (Fig. 5-7) and slow conduction or fragmentation can sometimes be demonstrated in the low posteromedial right atrium.

Atrial mapping intraoperatively can define the reentrant circuit with greater resolution. The ablative intervention is directed at the narrowest part of the circuit and cryosurgical ablation of the atrial muscle between the inferior vena cava and tricuspid valve and the region around the coronary sinus orifice has successfully eliminated tachycardia.[24] Surgery for atrial flutter may be considered for medically refractory recurrent atrial flutter. Repeated clinical records should document consistent atrial flutter and not episodic atrial fibrillation that may not be affected by correcting atrial flutter. This surgery should be considered with serious reservations in the presence of diffuse atrial enlargement or disease, since atrial fibrillation is a common accompanying arrhythmia under these circumstances. This surgery too has been relegated to a backup role in patients who have failed endocardial catheter ablation.

### Atrial Fibrillation

Atrial fibrillation is a common and problematic arrhythmia but difficult to study by our standard electrophysiologic techniques. The arrhythmia is probably maintained by multiple reentrant wavelets

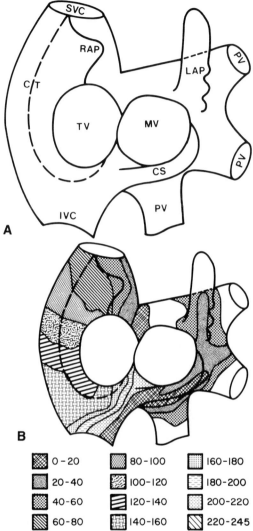

| | | |
|---|---|---|
| ▨ 0 - 20 | ▨ 80-100 | ▨ 160-180 |
| ▨ 20-40 | ▨ 100-120 | ▨ 180-200 |
| ▨ 40-60 | ▨ 120-140 | ▨ 200-220 |
| ▨ 60-80 | ▨ 140-160 | ▨ 220-245 |

*Figure 20-9* Epicardial atrial mapping during the common type of atrial flutter. The heart is depicted as if the ventricles were removed from the AV annulus and the atria are viewed from below. *A*. CS = coronary sinus; CT = crista terminalis; IVC = inferior vena cava; LAP = left atrial appendage; MV = mitral valve; PV = pulmonary vein; RAP = right atrial appendage; SVC = superior vena cava; TV = tricuspid valve. *B*. Shaded areas represent zones of equal activation time (ms) during atrial flutter. Earliest activation is seen in the posteroseptal region and a complete right atrial circuit can be traced. The left atrium is activated passively from both the anteroseptal and posteroseptal regions. *(From Klein et al.[24] Reproduced by permission.)*

changing dynamically and seeking nonrefractory tissue. Our current understanding of the mechanism and pathophysiology does not allow us to identify tissue critical to the perpetuation of the arrhythmia and to perform a discrete, focused ablative procedure. Preoperative electrophysiologic testing may be useful to rule out a primary cause of atrial fibrillation— such as AV reentry degenerating rapidly into fibrillation—or to assess sinus and AV conduction. Otherwise, it is not useful to guide operative therapy. Experimental operative approaches to atrial fibrillation depend on the principle that a large atrial mass is required to sustain it. A large dilated left atrium secondary to mitral valve disease may be electrically excluded (isolated), leaving a relatively normal right atrium to maintain sinus rhythm.[10] The "corridor" operation[25] isolates a corridor of tissue from the sinus node to the AV node from most of the right and left atria and allows normal chronotrophic function regardless of the prevalent rhythms in the isolated atria. Functionally, this operation "fragments" the atria by dissection and cryosurgery into three distinct zones, the left atrium, the right atrial corridor, and the remaining right atrium, each of which is electrically independent (Fig. 20-10).

Although this procedure can achieve normal chronotrophic function if sinus node function is normal, atrial contractility will not be salvaged and embolism may not be prevented. It is technically much simpler to perform His bundle ablation and implant a pacemaker. Therefore, this procedure is only indicated in the younger patient with medically refractory atrial fibrillation who has a strong desire or need to avoid pacemaker implantation. Cox and coworkers[26] have described an atrial procedure that they have called the *maze operation*.[26] This is based on the principle that atrial fibrillation requires a critical contiguous atrial mass to sustain the multiple reentrant circuits. Atrial incisions are designed to channel the sinus impulse through a predefined path, or "maze," which does not permit sufficient contiguous atrial tissue to sustain atrial fibrillation. The procedure offers the potential of maintaining atrial contractility in addition to normal chronotrophic function.

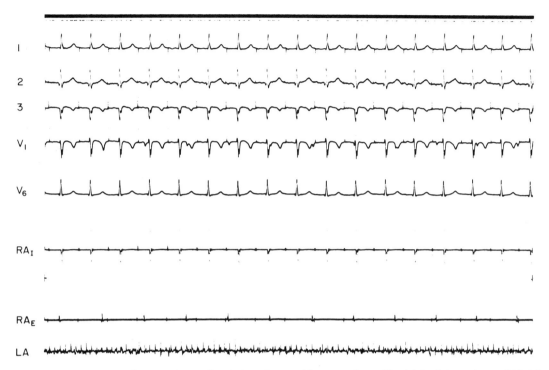

**Figure 20-10**  Dissociated atrial electrical activity after corridor procedure. The high right atrium within the corridor ($RA_1$) is being paced and the ventricles follow. The left atrium (LA) is still fibrillating and the excluded right atrium ($RA_E$) is in a slow atrial rhythm. 2, 3, $V_1$, $V_6$ = surface electrocardiographic leads.

## Ventricular Tachycardia

Recurrent sustained VT is most commonly observed in the setting of previous myocardial infarction but also occurs with any heart disease (cardiomyopathy, valvular, congenital, hypertensive) or, less commonly, in the absence of clinically apparent heart disease. The mechanism of VT in its various settings is certainly not uniform, but the ability to induce it reproducibly by programmed stimulation permits mapping with a view to guiding a discrete operative intervention. A comprehensive cardiac assessment is critical to success. It must first be determined that VT is not secondary to a reversible problem, most commonly acute ischemia, proarrhythmia, or electrolyte disturbance. Cardiac anatomy must be well described to allow concomitant procedures such as coronary bypass grafting, aneurysmectomy, or valve replacement. The anatomic "lesion" (usually infarct scar or aneurysm) must be carefully delineated, as the VT mechanism is invariably in or close to this area. Identification of a lesion is important, since this will focus mapping to the correct region and may provide a basis for a "visually guided" procedure if mapping fails or is otherwise inadequate. The most common lesion is an infarct scar or aneurysm, but others can include a congenital aneurysm, site of previous surgery for congenital heart disease, or more focal cardiomyopathy such as arrhythmogenic right ventricular dysplasia that affects predominantly the right ventricle. In fact, VT without a discrete lesion (normal heart or diffuse disease) should be approached with considerable caution, since the surgery depends entirely on reproducible, detailed intraoperative mapping.

The major goal of preoperative electrophysiologic testing is localization of the so called site or origin of VT. A roving electrode catheter is used to provide a local electrogram from each of several predetermined sites during VT, after which the endocardial activation sequence is determined. The earliest ventricular activation site relative to the onset of the QRS on the surface ECG is considered to be the site of origin and is probably close to the site of exit of activation from the zone of slow conduction necessary to sustain reentry. Consistent, fragmented electrograms in mid to late diastole may be recording a critical zone of slow conduction, although the functional significance of this must be established by demonstrating that the electrograms are necessary during tachycardia. Pace mapping is an ancillary technique based on the principle that pacing at the site of origin of VT will provide QRS morphology identical to that seen in clinical VT. Significant QRS latency between the stimulus artifact and the onset of the paced QRS at this site further suggest stimulation at or near the zone of slow conduction of VT. Mapping during sinus rhythm with late fragmented potentials after the termination of the QRS on the surface ECG helps identify abnormal myocardium but does not necessarily implicate it in the tachycardia mechanism.[27]

Although conceptually simple, endocardial mapping of VT is time-consuming, demanding, and technically difficult. Ventricular tachycardia may not be well tolerated, even after slowing with antiarrhythmic medication. Each of multiple morphologies should be mapped. Not all VT morphologies will be reproducibly induced. Systematically moving a catheter to cover an endocardial "grid" is difficult, and the precision of relating a catheter site to a subsequent anatomic location intraoperatively is not ideal. Nonetheless, preoperative mapping can provide useful localizing information and may be the only data available if VT cannot be induced intraoperatively.

Visually guided surgery without intraoperative mapping may be successful if there is a single discrete lesion or scar that is clearly demarcated from normal muscle.[28] In this circumstance, it is possible to excise or ablate the abnormal arrhythmogenic zone in its entirety. However, mapping is essential for many patients. These include patients with more diffuse disease, patients in whom the scar is large and involves valvular apparatus, patients in whom the scar is not well demarcated from normal muscle, and, finally, patients with VT in the absence of apparent heart disease. In this last group of patients, mapping is clearly necessary to guide the operative procedure, since the arrhythmogenic zone is too diffuse or not visually apparent. Multichannel simultaneous recording with computerized interpretation is the preferred mapping method with VT, mainly because of the extensive surfaces that require mapping. This combined with the frequent occurrence of multiple morphologies and frequent self-termination of VT makes sequential, single-channel recording tedious if not prohibitive at times.

Activation sequence mapping during VT is the most widely used method to guide therapy. A very useful adjunct is "dynamic" mapping, where an intervention is directed at a suspected site during VT to see if this results in termination of VT. For example, consistent termination of VT with cooling to 0°C at a specific site (ice mapping) suggests that the latter site is critical to the maintenance of VT and will be a fruitful site for ablation.[29] Laser ablation has also been used in a similar fashion.[13]

## Operative Techniques

The general goal is excision, ablation, or exclusion of the arrhythmogenic zone or the zone determined to be critical to the maintenance of VT. The earliest attempt at operative treatment of VT utilized ventriculotomy of the right ventricle through muscle determined to be the origin of VT in right ventricular dysplasia.[30] The first operative therapy of VT related to chronic infarct scar was the encircling endocardial ventriculotomy (EEV) described by Guiraudon.[31] This was a circumferential incision around the endocardial border of the scar, attempting to follow the plane between scar and normal muscle (the "border" zone). The intention was to disrupt the border zone or exclude the arrhythmogenic area (Fig. 20-11). Excision of endocardial scar ("peel") in the region

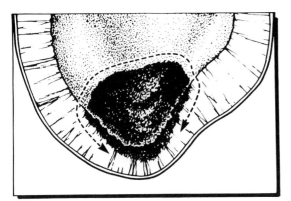

***Figure 20-11*** Encircling endocardial ventriculotomy. The infarct scar is encircled with scalpel incision, carefully following the plane between normal and abnormal muscle, essentially separating the scar from normal muscle. The incision is then sewn over for structural integrity.

of interest or more extensively was subsequently described.[32] Both the EEV and endocardial peel could be guided by mapping or done more extensively without mapping. Variants of these techniques were described using other ablative techniques, including cryosurgery and laser (Fig. 20-12). Cryosurgery is especially useful in ablating sites not amenable to

resection, such as valvular apparatus. A more recently described technique uses introduction of an endocardial balloon with DC shock ablation at electrodes mounted on the balloon at early sites.[33]

It is difficult to compare techniques per se. Arrhythmia surgery is best done with a great deal of individualization, with the surgeon having access to ancillary tools such as cryoprobes or lasers to suit particular circumstances. The intervention may be more discrete and focal if very accurate and unequivocal mapping data are available, or more aggressive in other cases. All VT surgery compromises ventricular function to some degree, and the degree of intervention must be balanced against this. Operative mortality may be 1 percent or less in the patient with excellent ventricular function and a small scar or considerably higher in patients with poor ventricular function.[34,35]

### Indications for Surgery in Ventricular Tachycardia

It is difficult to be dogmatic because decisions to operate are highly individualized and depend on local expertise and experience. However, patients frequently have poor left ventricular function and

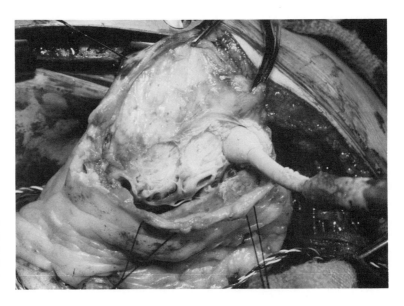

***Figure 20-12*** Encircling cryoablation. In this example of an anterior scar, the aneurysm is removed and the border zone is covered with a series of cryolesions.

progressive disease. The operative mortality increases with the degree of left ventricular dysfunction and extent of coronary artery disease. For these reasons, surgical candidates should be refractory to reasonable drug management. The threshold for surgery should be higher with poorer LV function and diffuse disease. In such cases, the therapeutic decision may swing to a defibrillator antitachycardia device. The threshold for surgery may be lower if a discrete, well-demar-cated lesion is present with good residual LV function. Endocardial catheter ablation has largely supplanted surgery as first-line nonpharmacologic therapy for idiopathic VT in the presence of normal myocardium, which is usually focal and endocardial. Catheter ablation for VT in the presence of cardiomyopathy or chronic infarction needs considerable development but will probably replace surgery for many patients in the future.

# References

1. Cobb FR et al: Successful surgical interruption of the bundle of Kent in a patient with Wolff-Parkinson-White syndrome. *Circulation* 38:1018, 1968.

2. Klein GJ et al: Surgery for tachycardia: indications and electrophysiologic assessment. *Circulation* 75(supp III):186, 1987.

3. Swerdlow C et al: Results of map-guided surgery in 103 patients with VT. *J Am Coll Cardiol* 5:409, 1985.

4. Klein GJ, Guiraudon GM: Surgical therapy of cardiac arrhythmias. *Cardiol Clin* 1:323, 1983.

5. Page PL et al: Value of early postoperative epicardial programmed ventricular stimulation studies after surgery for ventricular tachyarrhythmias. *J Am Coll Cardiol* 2:1046, 1983.

6. Gallagher JJ et al: Technique of intraoperative electrophysiologic mapping. *Am J Cardiol* 49:221, 1982.

7. Gallagher JJ et al: Epicardial mapping in the Wolff-Parkinson-White syndrome. *PACE* 2:523, 1979.

8. Ideker RE et al: A computerized method for the rapid display of ventricular activation during the intraoperative study of arrhythmias. *Circulation* 59:449, 1979.

9. Yee R et al: Refractory paroxysmal sinus tachycardia management by subtotal right atrial exclusion. *J Am Coll Cardiol* 3:400, 1984.

10. Williams JM et al: Left atrial isolation: New technique for the treatment of supraventricular arrhythmias. *J Thor Cardiovasc Surg* 80:373, 1980.

11. Guiraudon GM et al: Total disconnection of the right ventricular freewall: Surgical treatment of right ventricular tachycardia associated with right ventricular dysplasia. *Circulation* 67:463, 1983.

12. Klein GJ et al: Reaction of the myocardium to cryosurgery: Electrophysiology and arrhythmogenic potential. *Circulation* 59:364, 1979.

13. Svenson RH et al: Termination of ventricular tachycardia with epicardial laser photocoagulation: A clinical comparison with patients undergoing successful endocardial photocoagulation alone. *J Am Coll Cardiol* 15:163, 1990.

14. Sealy WC: The Wolff-Parkinson-White syndrome and the beginnings of direct arrhythmia surgery. *Ann Thorac Surg* 8:1, 1984.

15. Cox JL et al: Experience with 118 consecutive patients undergoing operation for the Wolff-Parkinson-White syndrome. *J Thorac Cardiovasc Surg* 90:490, 1985.

16. Klein GJ et al: Surgical correction of the Wolff-Parkinson-White syndrome in the closed heart using cryosurgery. *J Am Coll Cardiol* 3:405, 1984.

17. Guiraudon GM et al: Closed-heart technique for Wolff-Parkinson-White syndrome: Further experience and potential limitations. *Ann Thorac Surg* 42:651, 1986.

18. Pritchett ELC et al: Reentry within the atrioventricular node surgical cure with preservation of atrioventricular conduction. *Circulation* 60:440, 1979.

19. Ross DL et al: Curative surgery for atrioventricular junctional ("AV nodal") reentrant tachycardia. *J Am Coll Cardiol* 6:1392, 1985.

20. Cox JL et al: Cryosurgical treatment of atrioventricular node reentrant tachycardia. *Circulation* 76:1329, 1987.

21. Guiraudon GM et al: Skeletonization of the atrioventricular node for AV node reentrant tachycardia: Experience with 32 patients. *Ann Thorac Surg* 49:565, 1990.

22. Olsson SB et al: Incessant ectopic atrial tachycardia: Successful surgical treatment with regression of dilated cardiomyopathy picture. *Am J Cardiol* 53:1465, 1984.

23. Iwa T et al: Successful surgical treatment of left atrial tachycardia. *Am Heart J* 109:160, 1985.

24. Klein GJ et al: Demonstration of macroreentry and feasibility of operative therapy in the common type of atrial flutter. *Am J Cardiol* 57:587, 1986.

25. Leitch JW et al: Sinus node-atrio-ventricular node isolation: Long term results with the corridor operation for atrial fibrillation. *J Am Coll Cardiol* 17(4):970, 1991.

26. Cox JL et al: The surgical treatment of atrial fibrillation: II. Intraoperative electrophysiologic mapping and description of the electrophysiologic basis of atrial flutter and atrial fibrillation. *J Thorac Cardiovasc Surg* 101:406, 1991.

27. Gallagher JJ et al: Surgical treatment of arrhythmias. *Am J Cardiol* 61:27, 1988.

28. Moran JM et al: Extended endocardial resection for the treatment of ventricular tachycardia and ventricular fibrillation. *Ann Thorac Surg* 34:538, 1982.

29. Galagher JJ et al: Cryoablation of drug-resistant ventricular tachycardia in a patient with a variant of scleroderma. *Circulation* 75:190, 1978.

30. Guiraudon GM et al: Surgical treatment of ventricular tachycardia in 23 patients without coronary artery disease. *Ann Thorac Surg* 32:439, 1981.

31. Guiraudon GM et al: Encircling endocardial ventriculotomy: A new surgical treatment for life-threatening ventricular tachycardias resistant to medical treatment following myocardial infarction. *Ann Thorac Surg* 26:438, 1978.

32. Josephson ME et al: Endocardial excision: A new surgical technique for the treatment of recurrent ventricular tachycardia. *Circulation* 60:1430, 1979.

33. Downar E et al: Intraoperative electrical ablation of ventricular arrhythmias: A "closed heart" procedure. *J Am Coll Cardiol* 10:1048, 1987.

34. Mittleman RS et al: Predictors of surgical mortality and long term results of endocardial resection for drug-refractory ventricular tachycardia. *Am Heart J* 124:1226, 1992.

35. Trappe HJ et al: Role of mapping-guided surgery in patients with recurrent ventricular tachycardia. *Am Heart J* 124:636, 1992.

*Chapter 21*

# Treatment of Tachycardia with Implanted Devices

## Antitachycardia Pacing

### Rationale and Physiologic Basis[1]

Most recurrent tachycardias are reentrant and are theoretically amenable to termination by pacing techniques. The lessons learned in the clinical electrophysiology laboratory have provided the framework subsequently incorporated in a variety of sophisticated implantable devices. The fundamentals of reentry can be understood using a simplified model (Fig. 21-1). The hypothetical reentrant circuit shown surrounds a nonconducting obstacle that defines the pathway anatomically. It has an entrance and an exit, and a zone of slow conduction is incorporated in the circuit. The reentrant circuit is usually started by ectopic activity that finds one limb of the circuit refractory but conducts slowly in the other limb to initiate circus movement.

Once reentry is established (Fig. 21-1), the wave of excitation can be considered to have an advancing "head," followed by a wake of absolute and then relative refractoriness. To terminate tachycardia, stimuli must activate the circuit in advance of the head ("excitable gap"). Activation in the direction of the advancing wave is called *anterograde* or *orthodromic*, while the reverse is *retrograde* or *antidromic*. Depolar-

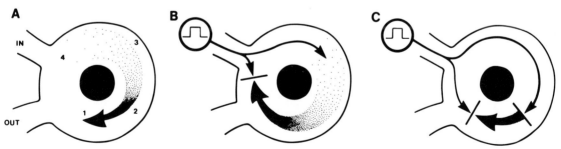

*Figure 21-1*  Effect of pacing on a hypothetical reentrant circuit. The hypothetical circuit represented has a wave of depolarization revolving about an anatomic obstacle and has an entrance and an exit site. In panel A, the "head" of the wave of depolarization (1) is followed by an area of absolute refractoriness (2), relative refractoriness (3), and an excitable gap (4), that is fully excitable. The square wave symbol represents a stimulator generating premature depolarizations. In panel B, the stimulus enters the excitable gap both anterogradely and retrogradely. Retrogradely it collides with the head, which is extinguished. Anterogradely, it "preexcites" the tail and continues to conduct reinitiating circus movement. In panel C, the extrastimulus is more premature. In this instance, reentry is terminated as the extrastimulus collides with both the "head" and the "tail" of the depolarization wave.

ization initiated by stimuli must block both the head and the tail of the circuit to terminate tachycardia, blocking both the orthodromic and antidromic limbs. Preexciting but failing to block the orthodromic limb will only "advance" the next cycle (entrainment).[2] As is evident from Fig. 21-1, termination of a tachycardia by stimulation will be influenced by the following factors:[3]

• The size of the circuit and, more importantly, the size of the excitable gap. The larger the excitable gap, the more easily stimuli penetrate it to influence tachycardia. The gap can also be increased by shortening refractoriness in part of the circuit ("shortening the tail").
• The proximity of the stimulating site to the reentrant circuit. The closer the stimulating site, the better the access to the excitable gap.
• The use of multiple stimulating sites. This may facilitate termination by accessing the circuit at more than one site, perhaps allowing one stimulus to penetrate orthodromically to "block the tail" while another enters antidromically to "block the head."
• The timing of the stimulus. Arriving at the access site to the circuit will be effective only if it is excitable at that moment.
• The use of multiple stimuli at more rapid rates. This increases the probability that one or more stimuli will penetrate the excitable gap. Pacing at more rapid rates also generally shortens refractoriness in working muscle and allows earlier stimuli to penetrate the circuit.
• Access to the circuit. There may be functional or anatomic barriers that limit or impede access of stimuli to the circuit ("protected" circuit). These may or not be overcome by manipulating the number, timing, and location of stimuli. Complex reentrant circuits associated with infarction may be very sensitive to site of pacing for this reason.

## Basic Operation of Antitachycardia Devices[4,5]

The earliest antitachycardia devices relied on patient activation (by a magnet or programmer) of the designated pacing therapy. This strategy had important limitations, a critical one being the dependence on the patient's subjective symptoms to diagnose the arrhythmia accurately and provide therapy. This concept is essentially obsolete. Current devices detect tachycardia, deliver therapy, and reevaluate for tachycardia after each therapy according to programmed criteria. One can consequently divide the function of the unit into two broad categories: arrhythmia recognition or "detection" and pacing therapies.

### Tachycardia Detection

Rate analysis is the cornerstone of arrhythmia detection algorithms.[6] In its most basic form, a device counts signals from a sensing lead and considers a rate greater than a specified rate over a specified time as "tachycardia." These and other detection criteria are programmable in modern devices. Rate criteria work best when the "target" tachycardia has a rate considerably faster than the patient's maximum sinus rate or other "nontarget" arrhythmias. A major problem arises when there is an overlap between the rate of the target arrhythmia and nontarget rhythms (most commonly, sinus tachycardia or atrial fibrillation). A possible approach in such cases is to slow the nontarget rhythm pharmacologically (for example, with beta blockers). Alternatively, the detection algorithm may include additional conditions to be satisfied when high rate is encountered before therapy is delivered.[7] These may include the following:

*Onset criteria.* Most recurrent tachycardias begin abruptly with a sudden rate change, whereas sinus tachycardia classically has a more gradual acceleration. Activation of an onset criterion may "tell" the device to ignore the rapid rate unless it begins abruptly.

*Regularity criteria.* Atrial fibrillation is generally markedly irregular and the algorithm may include a stipulation that the detected tachycardia be regular. However, polymorphic ventricular tachycardia (VT) may also be regular, and this must be considered.

*Analysis of the detected electrocardiogram.*[8] The sensed electrogram will have different characteristics depending on the direction and velocity of impulse propagation. These differences may be sufficiently great that the target arrhythmia can be readily distinguished from others. For example, the electrograms from a sensing lead in the ventricle may be wider and have different polarity during VT then during a supraventricular rhythm. Overlap may occur with aberrantly conducted supraventricular complexes.

*Multiple sensing electrodes.* Multiple sensing electrodes provide information on direction of depolarization, and this may readily distinguish the target rhythm from others. The use of both an atrial and a ventricular sensing electrode makes atrioventricular (AV) dissociation obvious for the diagnosis of VT.

*Mathematical manipulation of the detected signals.* For example, the probability density function of the original automatic defibrillator[9] essentially quantified the time that the electrogram signal was at baseline to distinguish ventricular fibrillation where the baseline is grossly irregular from other rhythms.

*Physiologic sensors.*[7,10] A hemodynamic measure or a surrogate of adequate perfusion could be very useful in an algorithm to identify a poorly tolerated target arrhythmia. Although not incorporated in any approved devices, sensors are an active area of investigation.

The challenge in detection is to identify the target arrhythmia and not treat nontarget arrhythmias whose rate may overlap. Pacing therapies delivered inappropriately may be arrhythmogenic in their own right.[11-13] A careful electrophysiologic assessment is required to program the detection criteria of any manufacturer's device optimally. It is also obvious that programming too many conditions before detection is satisfied involves a risk of the target arrhythmia going undetected.

### Pacing Therapies

After detection of a target tachycardia, a device will deliver pacing stimuli in a pattern that has been determined to be successful during acute testing.[1,14] There are four basic patterns of stimulation, all of which may be useful (Fig. 21-2). *Underdrive pacing* introduces stimuli at a rate slower than tachycardia

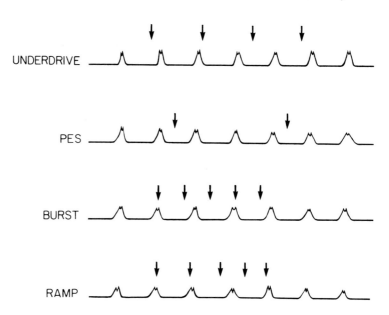

***Figure 21-2*** Basic stimulation patterns. Underdrive pacing involves pacing at a fixed rate less than that of the tachycardia until one of the stimuli fortuitously is optimally timed and terminates the tachycardia. The letters *PES* refer to programmed extrastimuli where one or more extrastimuli are programmed into the cardiac cycle at a coupling interval shown to be effective. The cardiac cycle is then "scanned" at earlier coupling intervals if termination does not occur. *Burst* refers to a series of stimuli at a rate faster than the tachycardia rate with equal intervals between stimuli. *Ramp* refers to a series of stimuli with a progressive decrease (decremental, as shown) or increase (incremental) in the interval between stimuli.

UNDERDRIVE

PES

BURST

RAMP

in a fixed-rate mode until a stimulus arrives at an optimal time fortuitously to terminate tachycardia. This requires a slower tachycardia that can be terminated with a single extrastimulus and is a mode rarely used today. *Single or multiple extrastimuli* can be programmed into the cardiac cycle at intervals determined to be successful at acute testing. If the first sequence is not effective, diastole is "scanned" with one or more stimuli of progressive prematurity. *Burst pacing* introduces a series of stimuli (for example, 10 stimuli at 200/min), while *ramp* (autodecremental) pacing introduces a series of stimuli that are progressively faster within a given ramp (Fig. 21-3). Again, each therapy is followed by a more aggressive one (faster, longer, or earlier) if the previous one is unsuccessful. The use of progressively aggressive therapies is referred to as *staged* or *tiered* therapy, the general philosophy being that initial therapies should

be those that may terminate tachycardia with less risk of acceleration of the target arrhythmia.[15] More complicated combinations and variations of the basic stimulation patterns are also available. Finally, all pacing therapies are optimally "adaptive" in that the therapy is not fixed but dependent on the rate of detected tachycardia. For example, a burst of stimuli might be programmed to begin pacing at a rate that is a percentage of the tachycardia cycle length rather than at a fixed rate. Because of spontaneous variations in tachycardia rate, the adaptive mode is preferred.

Pacing may also be useful for *prevention* of tachycardia. This is most evident when tachycardia is obviously bradycardia-dependent (Figs. 21-4 and 21-5) and with selected arrhythmias such as torsade de pointes due to QT prolongation, which may be completely suppressed by overdrive pacing.[16,17] Pacing at more rapid rates can be antiarrhythmic

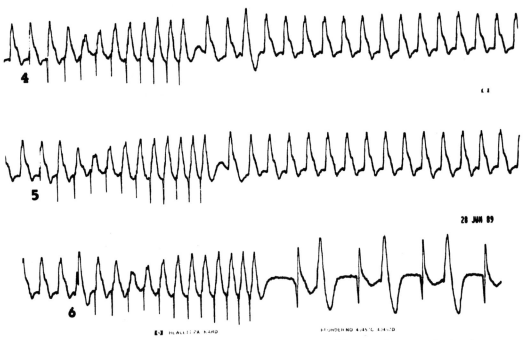

*Figure 21-3*   Clinical example of decremental ramp pacing. The record is a continuous strip showing treatment of a spontaneous tachycardia with an implanted device. The first five therapies (one to three not shown) failed to terminate VT but the sixth one did. With this device, an additional stimulus is added to each ramp to a preset programmed maximum or until tachycardia terminates. Note that each cycle of the ramp is less than the preceding cycle.

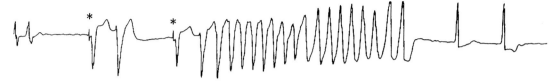

***Figure 21-4***    Ventricular tachycardia related to bradycardia. This patient with an implanted device had frequent nonsustained and sustained VT requiring cardioversion. The VT was clearly related to bradycardia as an increase in pacing rate from 60 to 80 eliminated tachycardia. Pacing spikes are indicated by an asterisk.

by decreasing the dispersion of refractoriness and suppressing ectopic pacemakers. Tachycardia related exclusively to preceding bradycardia is uncommon and one cannot assume that pacing will be effective solely because an episode of tachycardia occurred during slow heart rate. Theoretically, pacing at different sites or multiple sites may alter the dynamics of a reentrant circuit and prevent tachycardia. For example, simultaneous atrial and ventricular pacing may prevent reentrant junctional tachycardia by synchronizing opposite ends of the reentrant circuit. Preventative pacing is an attractive concept whose role may expand in the future.[14]

Finally, pacing can be considered for hemodynamic improvement of a tachycardia even if it cannot be terminated by pacing. The most useful example of this occurs with atrial tachycardias with a rapid ventricular response. Pacing the atrium at rates faster than the tachycardia will increase the degree of AV block, causing a net slowing of the heart rate and allowing the ventricular response to be regulated until more definitive therapy is effective.[5]

## Clinical Application

### Supraventricular Tachycardia[5]

An antitachycardia device can be considered for any patient with recurrent, supraventricular tachycardia (SVT) in which consistent, safe termination can be demonstrated by acute testing and in whom arrhythmia cannot be controlled with a reasonable drug regimen. Tachycardia mechanisms amenable to pacing termination include atrioventricular reentry, atrioventricular node reentry, and atrial reentry including atrial flutter. A device should not be considered in the Wolff-Parkinson-White syndrome, with the potential for a rapid ventricular response during atrial fibrillation. Satisfactory results have been reported for the majority of well-selected patients.[18] Major limitations include the occurrence of atrial fibrillation during therapy, the frequent need for concomitant medications, and the ongoing commitment to attentive care of an implanted device. In spite of the availability of technically sophisticated devices and encouraging reports, these devices have

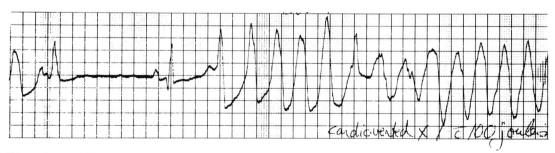

***Figure 21-5***    QT prolongation with torsade de pointes. This patient had idiopathic long QT syndrome presenting in later adulthood and possibly exacerbated by hypokalemia. Atrial pacing at a rate of 90/min prevented VT.

achieved little popularity for SVT due to the limitations cited and the concurrent development of curative therapies such as surgery and catheter ablation. The role of antitachycardia devices is currently limited to unique circumstances where curative procedures are not feasible or where a pacemaker is otherwise indicated for bradycardia.

### Ventricular Tachycardia[13]

Antitachycardia devices can theoretically be considered for any patient with recurrent, drug-refractory VT where consistent and safe termination of tachycardia can be demonstrated by detailed and laborious electrophysiologic testing. Ventricular tachycardia amenable to pace termination is usually monomorphic and relatively slow (less than 200/min). The role of antitachycardia devices is limited because

of the ever-present risk of deterioration of VT (acceleration) to unstable ventricular tachycardia or fibrillation (VF) during therapy even in the most carefully evaluated patient (Fig. 21-6). For this reason, a device limited to pacing therapies has become virtually obsolete for VT.

## Implantable Cardioverter Defibrillator

### Rationale

An implanted device capable of detecting and treating VF is the ultimate therapy in the patient in whom reasonable drug therapy is not effective and curative therapy is not feasible. The first automatic defibrilla-

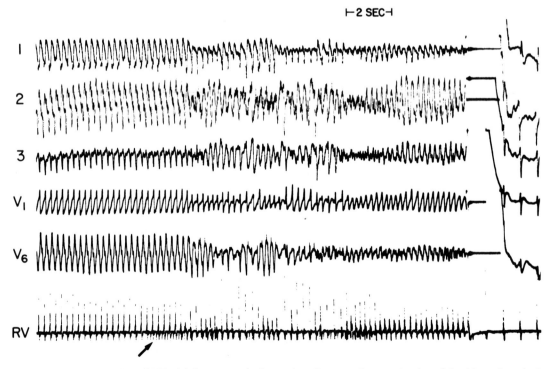

⊢2 SEC⊣

*Figure 21-6*  Acceleration of VT with burst ventricular pacing. Burst pacing was instituted in this patient during electrophysiologic testing (*arrow*) to terminate VT. Arrhythmia quickly accelerated into ventricular fibrillation requiring countershock. Key: 1, 2, 3, $V_1$, $V_6$ = surface ECG leads; RV = right ventricular electrogram.

tor was implanted in patients in 1980, after a decade of development by Michel Mirowski and his colleagues.[9] The next decade witnessed a growing acceptance of the concept and technical evolution that is still continuing at a rapid pace.[19] The implantable cardioverter defibrillator (ICD) is widely considered as a landmark advance in the therapy of patients with life-threatening ventricular arrhythmias. The reasons for the tremendous growth of ICD therapy include

- An increasing appreciation of the limitations of antiarrhythmic drugs, especially in patients with severe, noncorrectable myocardial pathology[20–22]
- A growing awareness of the limitations of electrophysiologic techniques and Holter monitoring in predicting drug efficacy[22,23]
- Increasing reliability and sophistication of ICDs[14,19]

### Basic Operation

The basic ICD has three essential elements (Fig. 21-7). These include sensing electrodes, defibrillation (DF) electrodes, and the device itself. Sensing is ideally accomplished through a close bipolar pair of electrodes capable of providing high-amplitude, narrow electrograms with a rapid intrinsic deflection and minimal far-field effect. Defibrillation electrodes should have a relatively large surface area and be positioned in such a way as to provide current density as uniformly as possible to the heart. These are most commonly in the form of patches sewn directly on the heart. The device itself has a logic system to determine when arrhythmia is present based on the sensed electrograms and the capability to deliver high-energy (up to approximately 35 J) countershock. Newer features added to current devices include bradycardia pacing, antitachycardia pacing, and advanced telemetry.[19]

The standard implant technique requires epicardial positioning of DF electrodes.[19,24] Operative approaches to achieve this include median sternotomy, subxiphoid, subcostal, and left thoracotomy approaches; the choice depends on operator preference and the need to perform concomitant cardiac surgery.

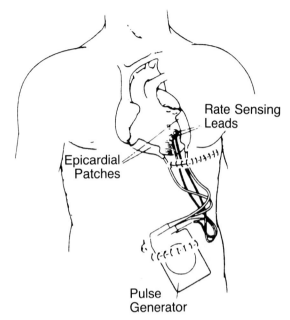

**Figure 21-7** Basic components of an implantable cardioverter defibrillator. The essentials of this system include a pulse generator, rate sensing leads, and defibrillation electrodes. Most pulse generators are implanted in an abdominal site because of their size. The rate-sensing leads shown are monopolar screw-in leads, two of which make a bipolar pair. The defibrillating electrodes shown are two large epicardial patches with one usually positioned anteriorly and one posteriorly. *(From JAMA 252:1363, 1989. Reproduced by permission.)*

Satisfactory positioning of the patches must be verified by ensuring that they can defibrillate the heart consistently (at least two times) at an energy less than (by at least 10 J) the maximum output of the device. The sensing electrodes are positioned to yield an optimum R wave (at least 5 mV) during sinus rhythm. Sensing should also be assessed during ventricular fibrillation to ensure that the signals are of adequate size to be detected by the device. Pacing threshold should also be satisfactory for devices with pacing capabilities. Finally, the generator is implanted and connected to the lead systems. The generator is generally implanted in an abdominal site because of the relatively large size (approximately 200 to 250 g) of current devices. Ventricular fibrillation is again induced prior to leaving the operating room to ensure satisfactory function of the entire system. Testing of the device prior to hospital discharge is also recommended. Nonthoracotomy approaches to lead implantation currently undergoing evaluation will undoubtedly become the method of choice when widely available (see below).

## Clinical Application

### Patient Selection

Patients are considered for ICD implant after recovery from sustained VT or VF when a correctable cause cannot be identified or efficacy of a reasonable prophylactic antiarrhythmic regimen cannot be verified. A NASPE policy conference recently identified four class 1 ("uniform consensus") indications.[24] These are as follows:

1.  Sustained VT or VF where electrophysiologic testing or spontaneous arrhythmias cannot guide therapy
2.  Recurrent VT or VF despite predicted effective antiarrhythmic therapy
3.  Ventricular tachycardia or VF in patients whose drug therapy is limited by intolerance or noncompliance
4.  Persistent inducibility of clinically relevant VT or VF at electrophysiologic study despite best medical therapy

Undiagnosed syncope with uncontrolled inducible VT is considered a class 2 indication (a therapeutic option but without uniform consensus by experts).

The implantation of an ICD is generally not justified when a reversible cause of VT or VF is identified or when VT or VF is incessant or frequently recurrent. In addition, ICD therapy should not be considered when the patient's life span is otherwise severely limited by cardiac or other disease. The latter consideration may sometimes make for difficult decisions on an individual basis. It is highly likely that these indications will evolve as a result of increasing sophistication of devices, and their application will be affected by economic issues and other therapeutic advances. The use of ICDs has been advocated for "prophylactic" therapy in patients thought to be at high risk of cardiac arrest even though they have never had a sustained ventricular tachyarrhythmia. Several large clinical trials[25] are under way to test this concept. The feasibility of prophylactic implantation will depend on highly specific identification of the patient destined to have cardiac arrest, demonstration of improvement in total mortality as well as sudden death mortality, and economic considerations.

### Clinical Results

Abundant documentation of successful automatic recognition and treatment of VT and VF is available,[26–30] establishing, in principle, the utility of the ICD concept (Fig. 21-8). Published series of ICD implants in survivors of cardiac arrest suggest a cumulative 2-year sudden death rate of 0 to 9 percent and a 2-year mortality of 5 to 19 percent.[24] This is considered to be a marked improvement in the expected survival of these patients based on

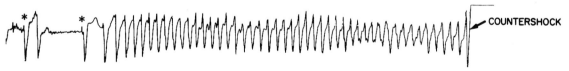

*Figure 21-8*   Automatic defibrillation of spontaneous VF. The figure illustrates spontaneous ventricular fibrillation or polymorphous VT in a patient with an ICD. The device senses and treats this spontaneous arrhythmia automatically with a countershock.

historic controls and is largely responsible for current recommendations and enthusiasm for ICD therapy. However, it has been suggested that 5-year survival in medically treated patients approaches that of ICD patients.[31] This is not surprising, since all survival curves eventually come together. Ultimately, a rigorous prospective, randomized comparison between ICD and best medical therapy is necessary to elucidate the magnitude of benefit of ICD and subgroups gaining the most benefit. At least two such trials are under way. The Canadian Implantable Defibrillator Study (CIDS) compares ICD to empirical amiodarone and a European study[32] compares ICD to best medical therapy.

### Complications[24]

Perioperative mortality for ICD implantation ranges from 1.5 to 5.4 percent. Hardware complications occur in up to 10 percent of cases and include infection, sensing lead problems, migration or fracture of defibrillation leads, and device malfunction (Fig. 21-9). These complications will decrease with device evolution and increasing use of nonthoracot-

omy implantation techniques. A significant source of difficulty after implantation is the "inappropriate" shock delivered for nontarget arrhythmias that reach the rate threshold. The most common nontarget arrhythmias are atrial fibrillation or sinus tachycardia. These can be dealt with by drugs (usually beta blockers) or changes in the detection criteria, as discussed above. Rarely, catheter ablation of the AV node may be considered. The "asymptomatic" shock was a diagnostic problem in older ICDs, as it was difficult to be certain whether this was due to appropriate therapy (detection and therapy of VT or VF may occur rapidly before appreciation of symptoms), device malfunction, or the presence of a nontarget arrhythmia.

### Developmental Goals

The only ICD available for clinical use for most of the 1980s was the AICD line (CPI). In 1992, there are at least six companies manufacturing advanced devices (Table 21-1) approved or in clinical trials. The ICD of the 1990s will expand the scope and sophistication of therapy and bear little resemblance

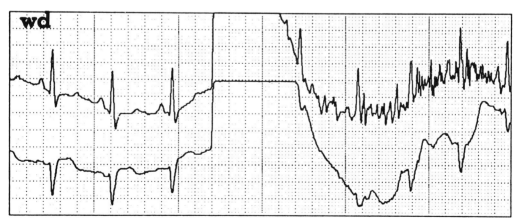

*Figure 21-9*   Inappropriate shock. A Holter record is illustrated during an inappropriate shock in a patient with an ICD. Shocks during sinus rhythm were subsequently traced to a fractured sensing wire, which resulted in false sensing of VF.

*Table 21-1   Advanced Devices Approved or in Clinical Trial*

| | CPI PRX | Medtronic PCD 7217 | Intermedics RES Q | Siemens Siecure | Telectronics Guardian | Ventritex Cadence |
|---|---|---|---|---|---|---|
| Weight (grams) | 220 | 197 | 220 | 210 | 270 | 237 |
| Programmable | yes | yes | yes | yes | yes | yes |
| VVI pacing | yes | yes | yes | yes | yes | yes |
| Antitachy pacing | yes | yes | yes | yes | yes | yes |
| Energy range (J) | 0.1/34 | 0.2/34 | 0.1/40 | 0.5/40 | 0.5/30 | 0.1/38 |
| Pulse waveform | M | M, S | Bp | M | M | M, Bp |
| Tiered therapy | yes | yes | yes | yes | yes | yes |
| Noninvasive EP | yes | yes | yes | yes | yes | yes |
| Event retrieval | yes | yes | yes | yes | yes | yes |
| EGM retrieval | no | no | no | no | yes | yes |
| Committed | no | [a] | yes | yes | no | no |

[a]Committed for VF therapy, not VT therapy. BP = biphasic; EGM = electrogram; M = monophasic; S = sequential.

to the original product. The following will likely serve as key foci for improvement[19]:

*Device size.* Current devices are large and range in weight from 200 to 270 g. This necessitates an abdominal implant site for the generator. Significant size reduction is required to allow for pectoral implantation.

*Nonthoracotomy implantation.* Nonthoracotomy implantation is currently under clinical investigation and will probably obviate the need for epicardial electrodes in the great majority of patients. The electrodes are incorporated in transvenous leads that also incorporate pace-sense electrodes. In addition, a patch or array electrode can be positioned subcutaneously near the cardiac apex to serve as part of the electrode system. Three electrodes are often required to compensate for the smaller defibrillating surface area of transvenous leads. Excellent results have been reported with nonthoracotomy systems.[33] An electrode system utilizing transvenous leads exclusively has been described,[34] raising the possibility of ICD implantation in a fashion similar to standard pacemaker implantation (Fig. 21-10).

*Device longevity.* Early devices had a battery life of 1 to 2 years and current devices have projected battery lives in the range of 4 to 5 years. This will undoubtedly improve and effectively decrease the cost of long-term therapy.

*Efficacy of defibrillation.* Improved electrode design and optimization of the defibrillation pulse will lower the energy requirements for defibrillation. A biphasic pulse[35-37] has been shown to decrease energy requirements for defibrillation with most systems, but this will probably not be the last word in optimal defibrillation pulse. The use of multiple electrodes, as in sequential pulse defibrillation, is especially useful in nonthoracotomy systems where optimal current density must be attained with smaller electrodes.[38-42]

*Event storage and telemetry.* Retrieval of all detected and treated arrhythmias in the form of ECGs and event markers will be available and greatly facilitate analysis of events and optimal device programming (Fig. 21-11). The mysterious "asymptomatic" shock will be a problem of historic interest.

*Improved detection.* The backbone of detection is currently electrogram analysis using detection of a designated rate to "diagnose" the target arrhythmia. The refinements discussed early under antitachycardia pacing will be incorporated, including a physiologic sensor that will provide a surrogate of hemodynamic

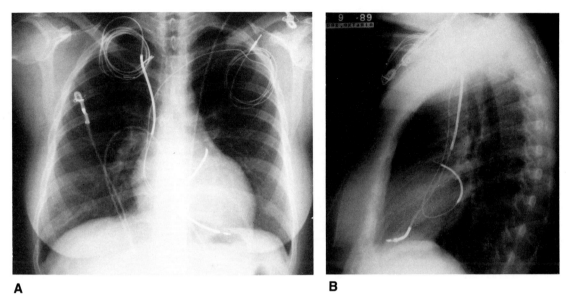

**A**                                             **B**

*Figure 21-10*   Transvenous lead defibrillation system. This lead system incorporates three defibrillating electrodes, all inserted pervenously via the left subclavian vein. Electrode catheters with large defibrillating coils are inserted in the superior vena cava, right ventricular apex, and coronary sinus. A bipolar pacing and sensing pair are also located on the distal portion of the right ventricular lead. In this system, the sequential pulse technique has usually been used, with the right ventricular apex being a common cathode and the superior vena cava and coronary sinus leads serving as anodes.

function. The device will use this hemodynamic information in its selection of therapy.

*Tiered therapy.* Tiered therapy is the norm for all new-generation ICDs. When possible, antitachycardia pacing therapies will be used as initial therapies, with countershock therapies further down the sequence of therapies[43] (Fig. 21-12).

*Bradycardia pacing.* All new-generation devices offer VVI bradycardia pacing. Rate response and dual chamber pacing will be incorporated in future devices.

*Atrial arrhythmia therapy.* Antitachycardia pacing for *supraventricular* arrhythmia, including cardioversion for atrial fibrillation, is a theoretical possibility for future development.

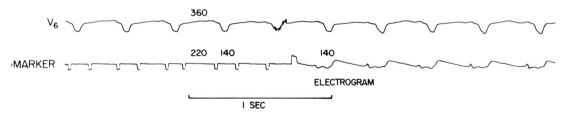

*Figure 21-11*   Troubleshooting using the marker channel and telemetered electrogram. The record is from a patient with an ICD who presented with asymptomatic shocks. Recording of the ECG with display of the marker channel revealed that two events were being sensed for each QRS deflection. Telemetry of the electrogram showed a wide and fractionated electrogram at the sensing lead that was the source of the double sensing. This had to be corrected by repositioning the sensing electrode to an alternate site.

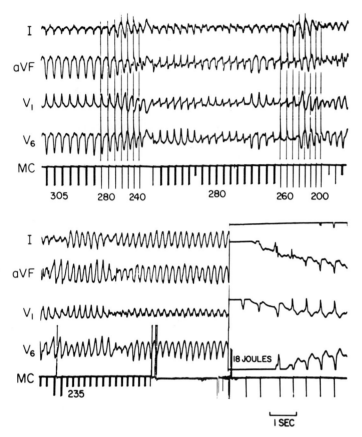

*Figure 21-12* Illustration of tiered therapy. The record is from a patient undergoing evaluation of ICD pacing therapies for termination of induced VT. The first ramp pacing therapy converts monomorphic VT at CL 305 ms to polymorphous tachycardia at CL 280 ms. A second burst further accelerates the arrhythmia to a mean CL of 235 ms. Ventricular fibrillation is then detected, further pacing therapies are aborted, and defibrillation therapy is successfully given. 1, AVF, $V_1$, $V_6$ = surface ECG channels. Key: MC = marker channel. The vertical long solid bars on the marker channel denote VT detection. The vertical short solid bars denote VF detection. (*From Leitch et al.*[40] *Reproduced by permission.*)

## Commentary

A device dedicated exclusively to antitachycardia pacing will have very little role in the future, although antitachycardia pacing can reasonably be added as a feature of bradycardia pacing systems. The ICD will continue to develop and expand its role in the management of serious ventricular arrhythmia. Future devices will be smaller, they will be implanted with nonthoracotomy techniques in the pectoral region, and they will last longer.

## References

1.  Fisher JD et al: Electrical devices for treatment of arrhythmias. *Am J Cardiol* 61:45A, 1988.
2.  Stamato NJ et al: The resetting response of ventricular tachycardia to single and double extrastimuli: Implications for an excitable gap. *Am J Cardiol* 60:596, 1987.
3.  Fisher JD et al: Implantable pacers for tachycardia termination: Stimulation techniques and long-term efficacy. *PACE* 9:1325, 1980.
4.  Kerr CR et al: Use of electrical pacemakers in the treatment of ventricular tachycardia and fibrillation. *Cardiovasc Clin* 1:215, 1985.
5.  Fisher JD: Control of atrial tachycardias using cardiac pacemakers, in Touboul P, Waldo A (eds): *Atrial*

*Arrhythmias: Current Concepts and Management.* St. Louis, Mosby, 1990, p 400.

6. Winkle RA et al: The automatic defibrillator: Local ventricular bipolar sensing to detect ventricular tachycardia and fibrillation. *Am J Cardiol* 52:265, 1983.

7. Sharma AD et al: Right ventricular pressure during ventricular arrhythmias in humans: Potential implications for implantable antitachycardia devices. *JACC* 15:648, 1990.

8. Davies DW et al: Detection of pathological tachycardia by analysis of electrogram morphology. *PACE* 9:200, 1986.

9. Mirowski M et al: Termination of malignant ventricular arrhythmias with an implanted automated defibrillator in human beings. *N Engl J Med* 303:322, 1980.

10. Anderson KM et al: Sensors in pacing. *PACE* 9:954, 1986.

11. Waldecker B: Arrhythmias induced during termination of supraventricular tachycardia. *Am J Cardiol* 55:412, 1985.

12. Roy D et al: Termination of ventricular tachycardia: Role of tachycardia cycle length. *Am J Cardiol* 50:1346, 1982.

13. Fisher JD et al: Comparative effectiveness of pacing techniques for termination of well-tolerated sustained ventricular tachycardia. *PACE* 6:915, 1983.

14. Rosenthal ME et al: Current status of antitachycardia devices. *Circulation* 82:1889, 1990.

15. Naccarelli G et al: Influence of tachycardia cycle length and antiarrhythmic drugs on pacing termination and acceleration of ventricular tachycardia. *Am Heart J* 105:1, 1983.

16. Wilmer CI et al: Atrioventricular pacemaker placement in Romano-Ward syndrome and recurrent torsade de pointes. *Am J Cardiol* 59:171, 1987.

17. Benson, JM et al: Permanent cardiac pacing in patients with the long QT syndrome. *J Am Coll Cardiol* 10:600, 1987.

18. Fisher JD: Clinical results with implanted antitachycardia pacemakers, in Sakseena S, Goldschlager N (eds): *Electrical Therapy for Cardiac Arrhythmias.* Saunders, Philadelphia, 1990, pp 525–535.

19. Troup PJ: Implantable cardioverters and defibrillators, in O'Rouke R (ed): *Current Problems in Cardiology,* vol 14. Chicago, Year Book, 1989, p 675.

20. Veltri E et al: Results of late programmed electrical .stimulation and long-term electrophysiologic effects

21. The Cardiac Arrhythmia Suppression Trial Investigators: Preliminary report: Effect of encainide and flecainide on mortality in a randomized trial of arrhythmia suppression after myocardial infarction. *N Engl J Med* 321:406, 1989.

22. Wilber DJ et al: Out-of-hospital cardiac arrest: Use of electrophysiologic testing in the prediction of long-term outcome. *N Engl J Med* 318:19, 1988.

23. Mitchell LB et al: A randomized clinical trial of the noninvasive and invasive approaches to drug therapy of ventricular tachycardia. *N Engl J Med* 317:1681, 1987.

24. Lehmann MH et al: Implantable cardioverter-defibrillators in cardiovascular practice: Report of the policy conference of the North American Society of Pacing and Electrophysiology. *PACE* 14(6):969, 1991.

25. Bigger JT Jr: Future studies with the implantable cardioverter defibrillation. *PACE* 14:883–889, 1991.

26. Epstein AE et al: Clinical characteristics and outcome of patients with high fibrillation thresholds: A multicenter study. *Circulation* 82:1206, 1992.

27. Tchou PJ et al: Automatic implantable cardioverter defibrillators and survival of patients with left ventricular dysfunction and malignant ventricular arrhythmias. *Ann Intern Med* 109:529, 1988.

28. Furman S, Kim SG: The present status of implantable cardioverter defibrillator therapy. *J Cardiovasc Electrophysiol* 3:602, 1992.

29. Kelly PA et al: The automatic implantable cardioverter-defibrillator: Efficacy complications and survival in patients with malignant ventricular arrhythmias. *J Am Coll Cardiol* 11:1278, 1988.

30. Winkle RA et al: Long-term outcome with the automatic implantable cardioverter-defibrillator. *J Am Coll Cardiol* 13:1353, 1989.

31. Newman D et al: Survival after implantation of the cardioverter defibrillator. *Am J Cardiol* 69:899, 1992.

32. Kuck KH et al: Preliminary results of a randomized trial: AICD vs drugs. *Rev Eur Tech Biomed* 12:110, 1990 (abstract).

33. Saksena S et al: Initial clinical experience with endocardial defibrillation using an implantable cardioverter defibrillator with a triple electrode system. *Arch Intern Med* 149:2333, 1989.

34. Yee R et al: A permanent transvenous lead system for

the implantable pacemaker cardioverter defibrillator: Nonthoracotomy approach to implantation. *Circulation* 85:196, 1992.

35. Jones JL et al: Improved cardiac cell excitation with symmetrical biphasic defibrillator waveforms. *Am J Physiol* 22:H1418, 1987.

36. Tang ASL et al: Ventricular defibrillation using biphasic waveforms of different phasic duration. *PACE* 10:417, 1987.

37. Saksena et al: Prospective comparison of biphasic and monophasic shocks for implantable cardioverter-defibrillators using endocardial leads. *Am J Cardiol* 70:304, 1992.

38. McCowan R et al: Automatic implantable cardioverter-defibrillator implantation without thoracotomy using an endocardial and submuscular patch system. *J Am Coll Cardiol* 17:415, 1991.

39. Bach SM Jr et al: Initial clinical experience: Endotak implantable transvenous defibrillator (abstract). *J Am Coll Cardiol* 13:65A, 1989.

40. Jones DL et al: Sequential pulse defibrillation in humans: Orthogonal sequential pulse defibrillation with epicardial electrodes. *J Am Coll Cardiol* 11:590, 1988.

41. Bardy GH et al: Prospective comparison of sequential pulse and single pulse defibrillation with use of two different clinically available systems. *J Am Coll Cardiol* 14:165, 1989.

42. Jones DL et al: Internal cardiac defibrillation in man: Pronounced improvement with sequential pulse delivery to two different lead orientations. *Circulation* 73:484, 1986.

43. Leitch JW et al: Reduction in defibrillator shocks with an implantable device combining antitachycardia pacing and shock therapies. *J Am Coll Cardiol* 18:145, 1991.

# *Index*

Page numbers in **boldface** indicate tables or illustrations.

ISBN 0-07-050984-0

9 780070 509849

3